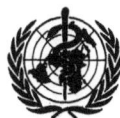

WORLD HEALTH ORGANIZATION

INTERNATIONAL AGENCY FOR RESEARCH ON CANCER

IARC MONOGRAPHS

ON THE

EVALUATION OF THE

CARCINOGENIC RISK

OF CHEMICALS TO HUMANS

Some Food Additives, Feed Additives
and Naturally Occurring Substances

VOLUME 31

This publication represents the views and expert opinions
of an IARC Working Group on the
Evaluation of the Carcinogenic Risk of Chemicals to Humans
which met in Lyon,

19-26 October 1982

July 1983

INTERNATIONAL AGENCY FOR RESEARCH ON CANCER

IARC MONOGRAPHS

In 1971, the International Agency for Research on Cancer (IARC) initiated a programme on the evaluation of the carcinogenic risk of chemicals to humans involving the production of critically evaluated monographs on individual chemicals. In 1980, the programme was expanded to include the evaluation of the carcinogenic risk associated with employment in specific occupations.

The objective of the programme is to elaborate and publish in the form of monographs critical reviews of data on carcinogenicity for chemicals and complex mixtures to which humans are known to be exposed, and on specific occupational exposures, to evaluate these data in terms of human risk with the help of international working groups of experts in chemical carcinogenesis and related fields, and to indicate where additional research efforts are needed.

This project was supported by PHS Grant No. 1 UO1 CA33193-01 awarded by the National Cancer Institute, DHHS.

ISBN 92 832 1231 2 (soft-cover edition)

ISBN 92 832 1531 1 (hard-cover edition)

PRINTED IN FRANCE

CONTENTS

IARC WORKING GROUP ON THE EVALUATION OF THE CARCINOGENIC RISK OF CHEMICALS TO HUMANS: SOME FOOD ADDITIVES, FEED ADDITIVES AND NATURALLY OCCURRING SUBSTANCES

Lyon, 19-26 October 1982

Members[1]

G.T. Bryan, Professor of Human Oncology, Division of Human Oncology, Wisconsin Clinical Cancer Center, University of Wisconsin, 600 Highland Avenue, Madison, WI 53792, USA

C.C. Culvenor, Commonwealth Scientific & Industrial Research Organization, Division of Animal Health, Animal Health Research Laboratory, Private Bag No. 1, Parkville, Victoria 3052, Australia

L. Fishbein, Director, Office of Scientific Intelligence, National Center for Toxicological Research, Jefferson, AR 72079, USA (*Chairman*)

I. Hirono, Professor, Institute of Medical Science, University of Tokyo, 4-6-1, Shirokanedai, Minato-ku, Tokyo 108, Japan

J.C.M. van der Hoeven, Department of Toxicology, Agricultural University, Biotechnion, De Dreijen 12, 6703 BC Wageningen, The Netherlands

O.M. Jensen, Director, Danish Cancer Registry, Finseninstitute, Strandboulevarden 49, 2100 Copenhagen Ø, Denmark (*Rapporteur section 3.3*)

T. Matsushima, Professor & Chairman, Institute of Medical Science, Department of Molecular Oncology, 4-6-1, Shirokanedai, Minato-ku, Tokyo 108, Japan

A.J. McMichael, Commonwealth Scientific & Industrial Research Organization, Division of Human Nutrition, Kintore Avenue, Adelaide, SA 5000, Australia (*Vice-Chairman*)

---

[1]Unable to attend: R. Kroes, Director, Central Institute for Nutrition & Food Research (TNO), Utrechtseweg 48, Zeist, The Netherlands; V.A. Krutovskikh, All-Union Cancer Research Center, Karshirskoye Shosse 6, 115478 Moscow, USSR; Mrs M.-T. van der Venne, Directorate General Employment, Social Affairs and Education, Health & Safety Directorate, Commission of the European Communities, Bâtiment Jean Monnet, Plateau du Kirchberg, BP 1907, Luxembourg, Grand Duchy of Luxembourg

C. Ramel, Wallenberg Laboratory, University of Stockholm, 106 91 Stockholm, Sweden (*Co-rapporteur section 3.2*)

S. Riazuddin, The Nuclear Institute for Agriculture & Biology, PO Box 128, Faisalabad, Pakistan

M. Roberfroid, Professor, Université Catholique de Louvain, Faculté de Médecine, Unité de Biochimie toxicologique et cancerologique, UCL 7369, Avenue Emmanuel Mounier, 73, 1200 Brussels, Belgium (*Co-rapporteur section 3.2*)

A. Somogyi, Professor, Federal Institute of Health, Thielallee 88/92, Postfach 33 0013, 1000 Berlin (West) 33 (*Co-rapporteur section 3.1*)

R. Stahlmann, Institute für Toxikologie und Embryonalpharmakologie (WE 18), Gary-strasse 9, 1000 Berlin (West) 33

R. Truhaut, Centre de Recherches toxicologiques, Faculté des Sciences pharmaceutiques et biologiques de l'Université R. Descartes, 4, avenue de l'Observatoire, 75006 Paris, France

N.M. Woolhouse, University of Ghana Medical School, Department of Biochemistry, PO Box 4236, Accra, Ghana

Representative from the National Cancer Institute

M.I. Kelsey, Division of Cancer Cause and Prevention, National Cancer Institute, Landow Building, Room 3C37, Bethesda, MD 20205, USA

Representative from SRI International

J.G.T. Johansson, Bio-organic Chemistry Department, SRI International, 333 Ravenswood Avenue, Menlo Park, CA 94025, USA (*Co-rapporteur sections 1 and 2*)

Representative from the US Food and Drug Administration

H. Blumenthal, Director, Division of Toxicology HFF-150, Bureau of Foods, Food & Drug Administration, Washington DC 20204, USA

Representative from the US Grocery Manufacturers' Association

R.C. Simpson, Vice-President, Nutrition and Quality, Nabisco Brands Inc., 15 River Road, Wilton, CT 06897, USA

Secretariat

H. Bartsch, Division of Environmental Carcinogenesis (*Co-rapporteur section 3.2*)
J. Cabral, Division of Environmental Carcinogenesis
M. Friesen, Division of Environmental Carcinogenesis
L. Haroun, Division of Environmental Carcinogenesis (*Co-secretary*)
E. Heseltine, Research Training and Liaison (*Editor*)
M. Hollstein[1], Division of Environmental Carcinogenesis
A. Likhachev, Division of Environmental Carcinogenesis
G. Mahon, Division of Epidemiology and Biostatistics
D. Mietton, Division of Environmental Carcinogenesis (*Library assistant*)
R. Montesano, Division of Environmental Carcinogenesis (*Co-rapporteur section 3.1*)
I. O'Neill, Division of Environmental Carcinogenesis (*Co-rapporteur sections 1 and 2*)
M. Parkin, Division of Epidemiology and Biostatistics
C. Partensky, Division of Environmental Carcinogenesis (*Technical officer*)
I. Peterschmitt, Division of Environmental Carcinogenesis, Geneva, Switzerland (*Bibliographic researcher*)
L. Tomatis, Director
J. Wahrendorf, Division of Epidemiology and Biostatistics
J. Wilbourn, Division of Environmental Carcinogenesis (*Co-secretary*)
H. Yamasaki, Division of Environmental Carcinogenesis
D. Zaridze, Division of Epidemiology and Biostatistics

Secretarial assistance

M.-J. Ghess
K. Masters
J. Mitchell
S. Reynaud

---

[1]Present address: Department of Biochemistry, University of California, Berkeley, CA 94720, USA

NOTE TO THE READER

The term 'carcinogenic risk' in the *IARC Monographs* series is taken to mean the probability that exposure to the chemical will lead to cancer in humans.

Inclusion of a chemical in the monographs does not imply that it is a carcinogen, only that the published data have been examined. Equally, the fact that a chemical has not yet been evaluated in a monograph does not mean that it is not carcinogenic.

Anyone who is aware of published data that may alter the evaluation of the carcinogenic risk of a chemical for humans is encouraged to make this information available to the Unit of Retrieval and Coordination of Carcinogenicity Data, International Agency for Research on Cancer, Lyon, France, in order that the chemical may be considered for re-evaluation by a future Working Group.

Although every effort is made to prepare the monographs as accurately as possible, mistakes may occur. Readers are requested to communicate any errors to the Unit of Retrieval and Coordination of Carcinogenicity Data, so that corrections can be reported in future volumes.

IARC MONOGRAPH PROGRAMME ON THE EVALUATION OF THE CARCINOGENIC RISK OF CHEMICALS TO HUMANS[1]

PREAMBLE

1. BACKGROUND

In 1971, the International Agency for Research on Cancer (IARC) initiated a programme on the evaluation of the carcinogenic risk of chemicals to humans with the object of producing monographs on individual chemicals. The criteria established at that time to evaluate carcinogenic risk to humans were adopted by all the working groups whose deliberations resulted in the first 16 volumes of the *IARC Monographs* series. In October 1977, a joint IARC/WHO *ad hoc* Working Group met to re-evaluate these guiding criteria; this preamble reflects the results of their deliberations(1) and those of subsequent IARC *ad hoc* Working Groups which met in April 1978(2)and February 1982(3).

An *ad hoc* Working Group, which met in Lyon in April 1979 to prepare criteria to select chemicals for *IARC Monographs*(4), recommended that the *Monographs* programme be expanded to include consideration of human exposures to complex mixtures which occur, for example, in selected occupations. The Working Group which met in June 1980 therefore considered occupational exposures in the wood, leather and some associated industries; their deliberations resulted in Volume 25 of the *Monographs* series. A further Working Group which met in June 1981 evaluated the carcinogenic risks associated with occupations in the rubber manufacturing industry, and their conclusions were published as Volume 28 of the *Monographs* series.

2. OBJECTIVE AND SCOPE

The objective of the programme is to elaborate and publish in the form of monographs critical reviews of data on carcinogenicity for chemicals, groups of chemicals or industrial processes to which humans are known to be exposed, to evaluate the data in terms of human risk with the help of international working groups of experts in chemical carcinogenesis and related fields, and to indicate where additional research efforts are needed.

---

[1]This project was supported by PHS Grant No. 1 UO1 CA33193-01 awarded by the US National Cancer Institute, DHSS.

The critical analyses of the data are intended to assist national and international authorities in formulating decisions concerning preventive measures. No recommendations are given concerning legislation, since this depends on risk-benefit evaluations, which seem best made by individual governments and/or other international agencies. In this connection, WHO recommendations on food additives(5), drugs(6), pesticides and contaminants(7) and occupational carcinogens(8) are particularly informative.

In February 1982, a special *ad hoc* Working Group met in Lyon to re-evaluate all chemicals, groups of chemicals, industrial processes or occupational exposures evaluated in volumes 1-29 of the *IARC Monographs*(3) and for which some data on carcinogenicity to humans (case reports or epidemiological studies) had been published in the literature. Re-evaluations of the data on humans, the data on experimental animals and the data on short-term tests were made for each agent and an overall evaluation of the carcinogenicity to humans was then made. The Working Group concluded that seven industrial processes or occupational exposures were causally associated with cancer in humans, as were 23 chemicals or groups of chemicals. Sixty-one chemicals, groups of chemicals or industrial processes were considered to be probably carcinogenic to humans. In addition, for 175 chemicals there is *sufficient evidence* of their carcinogenicity in experimental animals.

The *IARC Monographs* are recognized as an authoritative source of information on the carcinogenicity of environmental chemicals. The first users' survey, made in 1976, indicates that the monographs are consulted routinely by various agencies in 24 countries. Up to March 1983, 31 volumes of *Monographs* had been published or were in press; and a cross index of synonyms and trade names in volumes 1 to 26 has been published as Supplement 3 to the *Monographs*(9). Each volume of monographs is printed in 4000 copies for distribution to governments, regulatory agencies and interested scientists. The monographs are also available *via* the WHO Distribution and Sales Service.

3. SELECTION OF CHEMICALS FOR MONOGRAPHS

The chemicals (natural and synthetic, including those which occur as mixtures and in manufacturing processes) are selected for evaluation on the basis of two main criteria: (a) there is evidence of human exposure, and (b) there is some experimental evidence of carcinogenicity and/or there is some evidence or suspicion of a risk to humans. In certain instances, chemical analogues are also considered. The scientific literature is surveyed for published data relevant to the monograph programme. In addition, the IARC *Survey of Chemicals Being Tested for Carcinogenicity*(10) often indicates those chemicals that may be scheduled for future meetings.

Inclusion of a chemical in a volume does not imply that it is carcinogenic, only that the published data have been examined. The evaluations must be consulted to ascertain the conclusions of the Working Group. Equally, the fact that a chemical has not appeared in a monograph does not mean that it is without carcinogenic hazard.

As new data on chemicals for which monographs have already been prepared and new principles for evaluating carcinogenic risk receive acceptance, re-evaluations will be made at subsequent meetings, and revised monographs will be published as necessary.

4. WORKING PROCEDURES

Approximately one year in advance of a meeting of a working group, a list of the substances to be considered is prepared by IARC staff in consultation with other experts. Subsequently, all relevant biological data are collected by IARC; in addition to the published literature, US Public Health Service Publication No. 149(11) has been particularly valuable and has been used in conjunction with other recognized sources of information on chemical carcinogenesis and systems such as CANCERLINE, MEDLINE and TOXLINE. The major collection of data and the preparation of first drafts for the sections on chemical and physical properties, on production, use, occurrence and on analysis are carried out by SRI International, Stanford, CA, USA under a separate contract with the US National Cancer Institute. Most of the data so obtained on production, use and occurrence refer to the United States and Japan; SRI International and IARC supplement this information with that from other sources in Europe. Bibliographical sources for data on mutagenicity and teratogenicity are the Environmental Mutagen Information Center and the Environmental Teratology Information Center, both located at the Oak Ridge National Laboratory, TN, USA.

Six months before the meeting, reprints of articles containing relevant biological data are sent to an expert(s), or are used by the IARC staff, for the preparation of first draft monographs. These drafts are compiled by IARC staff and are sent prior to the meeting to all participants of the Working Group for their comments. The Working Group then meets in Lyon for seven to eight days to discuss and finalize the texts of the monographs and to formulate the evaluations. After the meeting, the master copy of each monograph is verified by consulting the original literature, then edited by a professional editor and prepared for reproduction. The monographs are usually published within six months after the Working Group meeting.

5. DATA FOR EVALUATIONS

With regard to biological data, only reports that have been published or accepted for publication are reviewed by the working groups, although a few ad-hoc exceptions have been made; in certain instances, reports from government agencies that have undergone peer review and are widely available are considered. The monographs do not cite all of the literature on a particular chemical: only those data considered by the Working Group to be relevant to the evaluation of the carcinogenic risk of the chemical to humans are included.

Anyone who is aware of data that have been published or are in press which are relevant to the evaluations of the carcinogenic risk to humans of chemicals for which monographs have appeared is urged to make them available to the Unit of Retrieval and Coordination of Carcinogenicity Data, Division of Environmental Carcinogenesis, International Agency for Research on Cancer, Lyon, France.

6. THE WORKING GROUP

The tasks of the Working Group are five-fold: (a) to ascertain that all data have been collected; (b) to select the data relevant for the evaluation; (c) to ensure that the summaries of the data enable the reader to follow the reasoning of the committee; (d) to judge the significance of the results of experimental and epidemiological studies; and (e) to make an evaluation of the carcinogenic risk of the chemical.

Working Group participants who contributed to the consideration and evaluation of chemicals within a particular volume are listed, with their addresses, at the beginning of each publication. Each member serves as an individual scientist and not as a representative of any organization or government. In addition, observers are often invited from national and international agencies, organizations and industrial associations.

7. GENERAL PRINCIPLES FOR EVALUATING THE CARCINOGENIC RISK OF CHEMICALS

The widely accepted meaning of the term 'chemical carcinogenesis', and that used in these monographs, is the induction by chemicals of neoplasms that are not usually observed, the earlier induction by chemicals of neoplasms that are commonly observed, and/or the induction by chemicals of more neoplasms than are usually found - although fundamentally different mechanisms may be involved in these three situations. Etymologically, the term 'carcinogenesis' means the induction of cancer, that is, of malignant neoplasms; however, the commonly accepted meaning is the induction of various types of neoplasms or of a combination of malignant and benign tumours. In the monographs, the words 'tumour' and 'neoplasm' are used interchangeably. (In scientific literature the terms 'tumourigen', 'oncogen' and 'blastomogen' have all been used synonymously with 'carcinogen', although occasionally 'tumourigen' has been used specifically to denote a substance that induces benign tumours.)

(a) Experimental Evidence

(i) Qualitative aspects

Both the interpretation and evaluation of a particular study as well as the overall assessment of the carcinogenic activity of a chemical involve several qualitatively important considerations, including: (a) the experimental parameters under which the chemical was tested, including route of administration and exposure, species, strain, sex, age, etc.; (b) the consistency with which the chemical has been shown to be carcinogenic, e.g., in how many species and at which target organ(s); (c) the spectrum of neoplastic response, from benign neoplasm to multiple malignant tumours; (d) the stage of tumour formation in which a chemical may be involved: some chemicals act as complete carcinogens and have initiating and promoting activity, while others are promoters only; and (e) the possible role of modifying factors.

There are problems not only of differential survival but of differential toxicity, which may be manifested by unequal growth and weight gain in treated and control animals. These complexities are also considered in the interpretation of data.

Many chemicals induce both benign and malignant tumours. Few instances are recorded in which only benign neoplasms are induced by chemicals that have been studied extensively. Benign tumours may represent a stage in the evolution of a malignant neoplasm or they may be 'end-points' that do not readily undergo transition to malignancy. If a substance is found to induce only benign tumours in experimental animals, it should nevertheless be suspected of being a carcinogen and requires further investigation.

(ii) *Hormonal carcinogenesis*

Hormonal carcinogenesis presents certain distinctive features: the chemicals involved occur both endogenously and exogenously; in many instances, long exposure is required; tumours occur in the target tissue in association with a stimulation of non-neoplastic growth, but in some cases hormones promote the proliferation of tumour cells in a target organ. Hormones that occur in excessive amounts, hormone-mimetic agents and agents that cause hyperactivity or imbalance in the endocrine system may require evaluative methods comparable with those used to identify chemical carcinogens; particular emphasis must be laid on quantitative aspects and duration of exposure. Some chemical carcinogens have significant side effects on the endocrine system, which may also result in hormonal carcinogenesis. Synthetic hormones and anti-hormones can be expected to possess other pharmacological and toxicological actions in addition to those on the endocrine system, and in this respect they must be treated like any other chemical with regard to intrinsic carcinogenic potential.

(iii) *Quantitative aspects*

Dose-response studies are important in the evaluation of carcinogenesis: the confidence with which a carcinogenic effect can be established is strengthened by the observation of an increasing incidence of neoplasms with increasing exposure.

The assessment of carcinogenicity in animals is frequently complicated by recognized differences among the test animals (species, strain, sex, age), route(s) of administration and in dose/duration of exposure; often, target organs at which a cancer occurs and its histological type may vary with these parameters. Nevertheless, indices of carcinogenic potency in particular experimental systems [for instance, the dose-rate required under continuous exposure to halve the probability of the animals remaining tumourless(12)] have been formulated in the hope that, at least among categories of fairly similar agents, such indices may be of some predictive value in other systems, including humans.

Chemical carcinogens differ widely in the dose required to produce a given level of tumour induction, although many of them share common biological properties, which include metabolism to reactive [electrophilic(13-15)] intermediates capable of interacting with DNA. The reason for this variation in dose-response is not understood, but it may be due either to differences within a common metabolic process or to the operation of qualitatively distinct mechanisms.

(iv) *Statistical analysis of animal studies*

Tumours which would have arisen had an animal lived longer may not be observed because of the death of the animal from unrelated causes, and this possibility must be allowed for. Various analytical techniques have been developed which use the assumption of independence of competing risks to allow for the effects of intercurrent mortality on the final numbers of tumour-bearing animals in particular treatment groups.

For externally visible tumours and for neoplasms that cause death, methods such as Kaplan-Meier (i.e., 'lifetable', 'product-limit' or "actuarial') estimates(12), with associated significance tests(16, 17), have been recommended.

For internal neoplasms which are discovered 'incidentally'(16) at autopsy but which did not cause the death of the host, different estimates(18) and significance tests(16,17) may be necessary for the unbiased study of the numbers of tumour-bearing animals.

All of these methods(12,16-18) can be used to analyse the numbers of animals bearing particular tumour types, but they do not distinguish between animals with one or many such tumours. In experiments which end at a particular fixed time, with the simultaneous sacrifice of many animals, analysis of the total numbers of internal neoplasms per animal found at autopsy at the end of the experiment is straightforward. However, there are no adequate statistical methods for analysing the numbers of particular neoplasms that kill an animal. The design and statistical analysis of long-term carcinogenicity experiments were recently reviewed, in Supplement 2 to the *Monograph* series(19).

(b) *Evidence of Carcinogenicity in Humans*

Evidence of carcinogenicity in humans can be derived from three types of study, the first two of which usually provide only suggestive evidence: (i) reports concerning individual cancer patients (case reports), including a history of exposure to the supposed carcinogenic agent; (ii) descriptive epidemiological studies in which the incidence of cancer in human populations is found to vary (spatially or temporally) with exposure to the agent; and (iii) analytical epidemiological studies (e.g., case-control or cohort studies) in which individual exposure to the agent is found to be associated with an increased risk of cancer.

An analytical study that shows a positive association between an agent and a cancer may be interpreted as implying causality to a greater or lesser extent, on the basis of the following criteria: (a) There is no identifiable positive bias. (By 'positive bias' is meant the operation of factors in study design or execution which lead erroneously to a more strongly positive association between an agent and disease than in fact exists. Examples of positive bias include, in case-control studies, better documentation of exposure to the agent for cases than for controls, and, in cohort studies, the use of better means of detecting cancer in individuals exposed to the agent than in individuals not exposed.) (b) The possibility of positive confounding has been considered. (By 'positive confounding' is meant a situation in which the relationship between an agent and a disease is rendered more strongly positive than it truly is as a result of an association between that agent and another agent which either causes or prevents the disease. An example of positive confounding is the association between coffee consumption and lung cancer, which results from their joint association with cigarette smoking.) (c) The association is unlikely to be due to chance alone. (d) The association is strong. (e) There is a dose-response relationship.

In some instances, a single epidemiological study may be strongly indicative of a cause-effect relationship; however, the most convincing evidence of causality comes when several independent studies done under different circumstances result in 'positive' findings.

Analytical epidemiological studies that show no association between an agent and a cancer ('negative' studies) should be interpreted according to criteria analogous to those listed above: (a) there is no identifiable negative bias; (b) the possibility of negative confounding has been considered; and (c) the possible effects of misclassification of exposure or outcome have been weighed. In addition, it must be recognized that in any study there are confidence limits around the estimate of association or relative risk. In a study regarded as 'negative', the upper confidence limit may indicate a relative risk substantially greater than unity; in that case, the study excludes only relative risks that are above the upper limit. This usually means that a 'negative' study must be large to be convincing. Confidence in a 'negative' result is increased when several independent studies carried out under different circumstances are in agreement. Finally, a 'negative' study may be considered to be relevant only to dose levels within or below the range of those observed in the study and is pertinent only if sufficient time has elapsed since first human exposure to the agent. Experience with human cancers of known etiology suggests that the period from first exposure to a chemical carcinogen to development of clinically observed cancer is usually measured in decades and may be in excess of 30 years.

The Working Group whose deliberations resulted in Supplement 4 to the *Monographs*(3) defined the degrees of evidence for carcinogenicity from studies in humans as:

i. *Sufficient evidence* of carcinogenicity, which indicates that there is a causal relationship between the agent and human cancer.

ii. *Limited evidence* of carcinogenicity, which indicates that a causal interpretation is credible, but that alternative explanations, such as chance, bias or confounding, could not adequately be excluded.

iii. *Inadequate evidence*, which applies to both positive and negative evidence, indicates that one of three conditions prevailed: (a) there were few pertinent data; (b) the available studies, while showing evidence of association, did not exclude chance, bias or confounding.

iv. *No evidence* applies when several adequate studies were available which do not show evidence of carcinogenicity.

(c) *Relevance of Experimental Data to the Evaluation of Carcinogenic Risk to Humans*

Information compiled from the first 29 volumes of the *IARC Monographs*(3,20,21) shows that of the chemicals or groups of chemicals now generally accepted to cause or probably to cause cancer in humans (Groups 1 and 2A), all (with the possible exception of arsenic) of those which have been tested appropriately produce cancer in at least one animal species. For several of the chemicals (e.g., aflatoxins, 4-aminobiphenyl, diethylstilboestrol, melphalan, mustard gas and vinyl chloride), evidence of carcinogenicity in experimental animals preceded evidence obtained from epidemiological studies or case reports.

Assessment of evidence of carcinogenicity from studies in experimental animals

Overall evidence of carcinogenicity in experimental animals was classified into four groups:

i. *Sufficient evidence* of carcinogenicity, which indicates that there is an increased incidence of malignant tumours: (a) in multiple species or strains; or (b) in multiple experiments (preferably with different routes of administration or using different dose levels); or (c) to an unusual degree with regard to incidence, site or type of tumour, or age at onset. Additional evidence may be provided by data on dose-response effects, as well as information from short-term tests or on chemical structure.

ii. *Limited evidence* of carcinogenicity, which means that the data suggest a carcinogenic effect but are limited because: (a) the studies involve a single species, strain or experiment; or (b) the experiments are restricted by inadequate dosage levels, inadequate duration of exposure to the agent, inadequate period of follow-up, poor survival, too few animals, or inadequate reporting; or (c) the neoplasms produced often occur spontaneously and, in the past, have been difficult to classify as malignant by histological criteria alone (e.g., lung adenomas and adenocarcinomas and liver tumours in certain strains of mice).

iii. *Inadequate evidence*, which indicates that because of major qualitative or quantitative limitations, the studies cannot be interpreted as showing either the presence or absence of a carcinogenic effect.

iv. *No evidence* applies when several adequate studies show, within the limits of the tests used, that the chemical is not carcinogenic. The number of negative studies is small, since, in general, studies that show no effect are less likely to be published than those suggesting carcinogenicity.

The categories *sufficient evidence* and *limited evidence* refer only to the strength of the experimental evidence that these chemicals are carcinogenic and not to the extent of their carcinogenic activity nor to the mechanism involved. The classification of any chemical may change as new information becomes available.

For many of the chemicals evaluated in the first 31 volumes of the *IARC Monographs* for which there is *sufficient evidence* of carcinogenicity in animals, data relating to carcinogenicity for humans are either insufficient or nonexistent. **In the absence of adequate data on humans, it is reasonable, for practical purposes, to regard chemicals for which there is sufficient evidence of carcinogenicity in animals as if they presented a carcinogenic risk to humans.** The use of the expressions 'for practical purposes' and 'as if they presented a carcinogenic risk' indicates that at the present time a correlation between carcinogenicity in animals and possible human risk cannot be made on a purely scientific basis, but only pragmatically. Such a pragmatical correlation may be useful to regulatory agencies in making decisions related to the primary prevention of cancer.

In the present state of knowledge, it would be difficult to define a predictable relationship between the dose (mg/kg bw/day) of a particular chemical required to produce cancer in test animals and the dose which would produce a similar incidence of cancer in humans. Some data, however, suggest that such a relationship may exist(22,23), at least for certain classes of carcinogenic chemicals, but no acceptable methods are currently available for quantifying the possible errors that may be involved in such an extrapolation procedure.

Assessment of data from short-term tests

In recent years, several short-term tests for the detection of potential carcinogens have been developed. When only inadequate experimental animal data are available, positive results in a variety of validated short-term tests (see section 8(c)(ii)) can be taken as an indication that the compound is a potential carcinogen and that it should be further tested in animals for an assessment of its carcinogenicity. Negative results from short-term tests cannot be considered as evidence to rule out carcinogenicity(3). Whether short-term tests will eventually be as reliable as long-term tests in predicting carcinogenicity in humans will depend on further demonstrations of consistency with long-term experiments and with data from humans.

In view of the limitations of current knowledge about mechanisms of carcinogenesis, certain cautions should be emphasized: (i) at present, these tests should not be used by themselves to conclude whether or not an agent is carcinogenic; (ii) even when positive results are obtained in one or more of these tests, it is not clear that they can be used reliably to predict the relative potencies of compounds as carcinogens in intact animals; (iii) since the currently available tests do not detect all classes of agents that are active in the carcinogenic process (e.g., hormones, promoters), one must be cautious in utilizing these tests as the sole criterion for setting priorities in carcinogenesis research and in selecting compounds for animal bioassays.

The Working Group which met in February 1982 to re-evaluate chemicals and industrial processes associated with cancer in humans(3) sometimes considered the results from short-term tests in making an overall evaluation of the carcinogenic risk of chemicals to humans.

Because of the large number and wide variety of short-term tests that may be relevant for the prediction of potential carcinogens, assessing the overall evidence of activity of a compound in short-term tests is difficult. The data relative to each compound can, however, be classified by grouping results under the type of test used and the biological complexity of the test system. *'DNA damage'* would include evidence for covalent binding to DNA, induction of DNA breakage or repair, induction of prophage in bacteria, and a positive response in tests of comparative survival in DNA repair-proficient and DNA repair-deficient bacteria. *'Mutagenicity'* refers to induction of mutations in cultured cells or in organisms (e.g., heritable alterations in phenotype, including forward or reverse point mutations, recombination, gene conversion, and specific-locus mutation). *'Chromosomal anomalies'* refers to the induction of chromosomal aberrations, including breaks, gaps, rearrangements and micronuclei, sister chromatid exchange and aneuploidy. (This classification does not imply that some chromosomal anomalies are not mutational events.) *'Other'* refers to various additional endpoints, including cell transformation, i.e., morphological transformation and colony formation in agar; dominant lethal tests; morphological abnormalities in sperm; and mitochondrial mutation. Biological systems include: *'Prokaryotes'*, i.e., bacteria, in the presence or absence of a cellular or subcellular metabolic activation system; *'Fungi and plants'*; *'Insects'*, usually *Drosophila melanogaster*; *'Mammalian cells (in vitro)'*, either rodent or human somatic cells or cell lines in culture; *'Mammals (in vivo)'*, studies in which the test compound was administered to intact experimental animals; and *'Humans (in vivo)'*, studies of cells from groups of individuals drawn from a population exposed to the substance in question.

Overall evidence of activity in short-term tests is adjudged to fall into one of four categories, *sufficient*, *limited*, *inadequate* or *no evidence*. The criteria generally used are:

i. *Sufficient evidence*, when there were a total of at least three positive results in at least two of three test systems measuring DNA damage, mutagenicity or chromosomal anomalies. When two of the positive results were for the same biological endpoint, they had to be derived from systems of different biological complexity.

ii. *Limited evidence*, when there were at least two positive results, either for different endpoints or in systems representing two levels of biological complexity.

iii. *Inadequate evidence*, when there were too few data for an adequate evaluation, or when there were contradictory data.

iv. *No evidence*, when there were many negative results from a variety of short-term tests with different endpoints, and at different levels of biological complexity. If certain biological endpoints are not adequately covered this is indicated.

In establishing these categories greater weight may be given to the three primary endpoints - DNA damage, mutagenicity and chromosomal anomalies - and judgements made on the quality as well as on the quantity of the evidence. In a minority of cases, strict interpretation of these criteria may be affected by consideration of a variety of other factors (such as the purity of the test compound, problems of metabolic activation, appropriateness of the test system) such that, in the judgement of the Working Group, a compound may be placed in a lower or higher category.

Assignment of a chemical to one of these categories involves several arbitary decisions, since many of the tests systems are still under validation. Thus, the selection of specific tests remains flexible and should reflect the most advanced state of knowledge in this field.

8. EXPLANATORY NOTES ON THE MONOGRAPH CONTENTS

(a) Chemical and Physical Data (Section 1)

The Chemical Abstracts Services Registry Number, the latest Chemical Abstracts Primary Name (9th Collective Index)(24) and the IUPAC Systematic Name(25) are recorded in section 1. Other synonyms and trade names are given, but no comprehensive list is provided. Further, some of the trade names are those of mixtures in which the compound being evaluated is only one of the ingredients.

The structural and molecular formulae, molecular weight and chemical and physical properties are given. The properties listed refer to the pure substance, unless otherwise specified, and include, in particular, data that might be relevant to carcinogenicity (e.g., lipid solubility) and those that concern identification.

A separate description of the composition of technical products includes available information on impurities and formulated products.

(b) Production, Use, Occurrence and Analysis (Section 2)

The purpose of section 2 is to provide indications of the extent of past and present human exposure to the chemical.

(i) Synthesis

Since cancer is a delayed toxic effect, the dates of first synthesis and of first commercial production of the chemical are provided. In addition, methods of synthesis used in past and present commercial production are described. This information allows a reasonable estimate to be made of the date before which no human exposure could have occurred.

(ii) Production

Since Europe, Japan and the United States are reasonably representative industrialized areas of the world, most data on production, foreign trade and uses are obtained from those countries. It should not, however, be inferred that those nations are the sole or even the major sources or users of any individual chemical.

Production and foreign trade data are obtained from both governmental and trade publications by chemical economists in the three geographical areas. In some cases, separate production data on organic chemicals manufactured in the United States are not available because their publication could disclose confidential information. In such cases, an indication of the minimum quantity produced can be inferred from the number of companies reporting commercial production. Each company is required to report on individual chemicals if the sales value or the weight of the annual production exceeds a specified minimum level. These levels vary for chemicals classified for different uses, e.g., medicinals and plastics; in fact, the minimal annual sales value is between $1000 and $50 000, and the minimal annual weight of production is between 450 and 22 700 kg. Data on production in some European countries are obtained by means of general question-naires sent to companies thought to produce the compounds being evaluated. Informa-tion from the completed questionnaires is compiled by country, and the resulting estimates of production are included in the individual monographs.

(iii) Use

Information on uses is meant to serve as a guide only and is not complete. It is usually obtained from published data but is often complemented by direct contact with manufacturers of the chemical. In the case of drugs, mention of their therapeutic uses does not necessarily represent current practice nor does it imply judgement as to their clinical efficacy.

Statements concerning regulations and standards (e.g., pesticide registrations, maxi-mum levels permitted in foods, occupational standards and allowable limits) in specific countries are mentioned as examples only. They may not reflect the most recent situation, since such legislation is in a constant state of change; nor should it be taken to imply that other countries do not have similar regulations.

(iv) *Occurrence*

Information on the occurrence of a chemical in the environment is obtained from published data, including that derived from the monitoring and surveillance of levels of the chemical in occupational environments, air, water, soil, foods and tissues of animals and humans. When available, data on the generation, persistence and bioaccumulation of a chemical are also included.

(v) *Analysis*

The purpose of the section on analysis is to give the reader an indication, rather than a complete review, of methods cited in the literature. No attempt is made to evaluate critically or to recommend any of the methods.

(c) *Biological Data Relevant to the Evaluation of Carcinogenic Risk to Humans (Section 3)*

In general, the data recorded in section 3 are summarized as given by the author; however, comments made by the Working Group on certain shortcomings of reporting, of statistical analysis or of experimental design are given in square brackets. The nature and extent of impurities/contaminants in the chemicals being tested are given when available.

(i) *Carcinogenicity studies in animals*

The monographs are not intended to cover all reported studies. Some studies are purposely omitted (a) because they are inadequate, as judged from previously described criteria(19,26-29) (e.g., too short a duration, too few animals, poor survival); (b) because they only confirm findings that have already been fully described; or (c) because they are judged irrelevant for the purpose of the evaluation. In certain cases, however, such studies are mentioned briefly, particularly when the information is considered to be a useful supplement to other reports or when it is the only data available. Their inclusion does not, however, imply acceptance of the adequacy of their experimental design or of the analysis and interpretation of their results.

Mention is made of all routes of administration by which the compound has been adequately tested and of all species in which relevant tests have been done(7,28). In most cases, animal strains are given. [General characteristics of mouse strains have been reviewed(30).] Quantitative data are given to indicate the order of magnitude of the effective carcinogenic doses. In general, the doses and schedules are indicated as they appear in the paper; sometimes units have been converted for easier comparison. Experiments in which the compound was administered in conjunction with known carcinogens and experiments on factors that modify the carcinogenic effect are also reported. Experiments on the carcinogenicity of known metabolites and derivatives are also included.

(ii) *Other relevant biological data*

Lethality data are given when available, and other data on toxicity are included when considered relevant. The metabolic data are restricted to studies that show the metabolic fate of the chemical in animals and humans, and comparisons of data from animals and humans are made when possible. Information is also given on absorption, distribution, excretion and placental transfer.

Effects on reproduction and prenatal toxicity. Data on effects on reproduction, teratogenicity and feto- and embryotoxicity from studies in experimental animals and from observations in humans are also included. There appears to be no causal relationship between teratogenicity(31) and carcinogenicity, but chemicals often have both properties. Evidence of prenatal toxicity suggests transplacental transfer, which is a prerequisite for transplacental carcinogenesis.

Indirect tests (mutagenicity and other short-term tests). Data from indirect tests are also included. Since most of these tests have the advantage of taking less time and being less expensive than mammalian carcinogenicity studies, they are generally known as 'short-term' tests. They comprise assay procedures which rely on the induction of biological and biochemical effects in *in vivo* and/or *in vitro* systems. The end-point of the majority of these tests is the production not of neoplasms in animals but of changes at the molecular, cellular or multicellular level as described in section 7(c).

The induction of cancer is thought to proceed by a series of steps, some of which have been distinguished experimentally(32-36). The first step - 'initiation' - is thought to involve damage to DNA resulting in heritable modifications in, or rearrangements of, genetic information. Proliferation of cells whose properties have been permanently altered during initiation (which may involve somatic mutation) is thought to result in the formation of clones of cells whose further progress to malignancy is dependent on a series of events - 'promotion' and 'progression' - the underlying mechanisms of which are largely unknown. Although this is a useful model, it should be kept in mind that the carcinogenic process may not always proceed by such a multi-step mechanism.

The idea that damage to DNA is a critical event in the initiation of carcinogenesis is based on a large body of data which show that many carcinogens are reactive electrophiles *per se*, or can be readily converted to reactive electrophiles by enzymic pathways characteristic of eukaryotic metabolism(37). A variety of DNA-carcinogen adducts, formed by reaction of electrophilic moieties with nucleophilic centres in DNA, have been identified in DNA recovered from reactions performed with carcinogens *in vitro*, or from cultured cells or intact organisms treated with carcinogens(35,38,39). Moreover, the recognition that many classes of carcinogens (including ionizing and ultra-violet radiation and chemicals of a very wide range of structure and reactivity) are mutagenic(40) supports the idea that DNA is a critical target of carcinogenic agents. Assays for mutagenicity and related effects all exploit this characteristic ability of carcinogens to cause DNA damage or chromosomal anomalies either directly or indirectly. It should be noted, however, that some carcinogens may act by mechanisms that do not involve DNA damage (41) and thus would not cause such genetic effects.

In many of the short-term tests, the indicator organism may not possess or may have lost, following culture, the range of enzyme systems known in intact mammals to metabolize chemically unreactive carcinogens to reactive electrophiles. It is often necessary, therefore, to provide an exogenous source of such activity in the form of a tissue extract or cell feeder-layer or whole-cell systems prepared from mammalian sources(19). In-vitro metabolic systems may not accurately reflect the fate of a chemical subjected to the checks and balances afforded by absorption, distribution, metabolism and excretion in mammals(19), and this must be borne in mind when evaluating the results from short-term tests which employ in-vitro metabolic activation.

Tests have been devised which exploit the useful attributes of microbial or cellular genetic systems without compromising the integrity of mammalian pharmacodynamics and metabolism. Such 'host-mediated' assays involve the inoculation of indicator organisms into mammals (usually rodents) which are then dosed with the test chemical. There are limitations to both the numbers and types of organisms which can be introduced and recovered from dosed animals and to the access of indicator organisms to activated metabolites. Lack of sensitivity may therefore be a problem.

A group of short-term tests use 'transformation' of cultured mammalian cells, rather than manifestation of DNA damage or chromosomal anomalies, as an indicator of carcinogenic potential. Some of the assays also employ an exogenous metabolic activation system. Cell transformation is assessed by scoring characteristic changes in cellular and colonial morphology, or changes in growth characteristics (e.g., growth of colonies in soft agar) following treatment with the test compound. In some protocols, the ability of transformed cells to produce tumours is tested by injecting the cells into appropriate animals.

Studies may also be conducted on cells taken from people exposed to putative chemical carcinogens. The cells are examined for mutation and for chromosomal anomalies either directly or after short-term culture *in vitro* or samples of sperm from such individuals may be analysed for morphological abnormalities. Evidence of absorption of putative carcinogens may be adduced from the assay of body fluids and excreta for DNA-damaging activity, using, for example, bacterial mutation assays.

The present state of knowledge does not permit the selection of a specific test(s) as the most appropriate for identifying all classes of potential carcinogens, although certain systems are more sensitive to some classes. Ideally, a compound should be tested in a battery of short term tests. For optimum usefulness, data on purity must be given. For several recent reviews on the use of short-term tests see IARC(19), Montesano *et al.*(42), de Serres and Ashby(43), Sugimura *et al.*(44), Bartsch *et al.*(45) and Hollstein *et al.*(46).

(iii) *Case reports and epidemiological studies*

Observations in humans are summarized in this section. The criteria for including a study in this section are described above (section 7(*b*)).

(*d*) *Summary of Data Reported and Evaluation (Section 4)*

Section 4 summarizes the relevant data from animals and humans and gives the critical views of the Working Group on those data.

(i) *Experimental data*

Data relevant to the evaluation of the carcinogenicity of the chemical in animals are summarized in this section. The animal species mentioned are those in which the carcinogenicity of the substance was clearly demonstrated. Tumour sites are also indicated. If the substance has produced tumours after prenatal exposure or in single-dose experiments, this is indicated. Dose-response data are given when available.

Results from validated mutagenicity and other short-term tests and from tests for prenatal toxicity are reported if the Working Group considered the data to be relevant. The degree of evidence of activity in short-term tests is mentioned in this section.

(ii) *Human data*

Human exposure to the chemical is summarized on the basis of data on production, use and occurrence. Case reports and epidemiological studies that are considered to be pertinent to an assessment of human carcinogenicity are described. Other biological data which are considered to be relevant are also mentioned.

(iii) *Evaluation*

This section comprises the overall evaluation by the Working Group of the carcinogenic risk of the chemical, complex mixture or occupational exposure to humans. All of the data in the monograph, and particularly the summarized experimental and human data, are considered in order to make this evaluation. This section should also be read in conjunction with section 7c of this Preamble.

References

1. IARC (1977) IARC Monograph Programme on the Evaluation of the Carcinogenic Risk of Chemicals to Humans. Preamble. *IARC intern. tech. Rep. No. 77/002*

2. IARC (1978) Chemicals with *sufficient evidence* of carcinogenicity in experimental animals -*IARC Monographs* volumes 1-17. *IARC intern. tech. Rep. No. 78/003*

3. IARC (1982) *IARC Monographs on the Evaluation of the Carcinogenic Risk of Chemicals to Humans*, Supplement 4, *Chemicals and Industrial Processes Associated with Cancer in Humans*, 292 pages

4. IARC (1979) Criteria to select chemicals for *IARC Monographs*. *IARC intern. tech. Rep. No. 79/003*

5. WHO (1961) Fifth Report of the Joint FAO/WHO Expert Committee on Food Additives. Evaluation of carcinogenic hazard of food additives. *WHO tech. Rep. Ser., No. 220*, pp. 5, 18, 19

6. WHO (1969) Report of a WHO Scientific Group. Principles for the testing and evaluation of drugs for carcinogenicity. *WHO tech. Rep. Ser., No. 426*, pp. 19, 21, 22

7. WHO (1974) Report of a WHO Scientific Group. Assessment of the carcinogenicity and mutagenicity of chemicals. *WHO tech. Rep. Ser., No. 546*

8. WHO (1964) Report of a WHO Expert Committee. Prevention of cancer. *WHO tech. Rep. Ser., No. 276*, pp. 29, 30

9. IARC (1972-1983) *IARC Monographs on the Evaluation of the Carcinogenic Risk of Chemicals to Humans*, Volumes 1-31, Lyon, France

    Volume 1 (1972) Some Inorganic Substances, Chlorinated Hydrocarbons, Aromatic Amines, *N*-Nitroso Compounds and Natural Products (19 monographs), 184 pages

    Volume 2 (1973) Some Inorganic and Organometallic Compounds (7 monographs), 181 pages

    Volume 3 (1973) Certain Polycyclic Aromatic Hydrocarbons and Heterocyclic Compounds (17 monographs), 271 pages

    Volume 4 (1974) Some Aromatic Amines, Hydrazine and Related Substances, *N*-Nitroso Compounds and Miscellaneous Alkylating Agents (28 monographs), 286 pages

    Volume 5 (1974) Some Organochlorine Pesticides (12 monographs), 241 pages

    Volume 6 (1974) Sex Hormones (15 monographs), 243 pages

    Volume 7 (1974) Some Anti-thyroid and Related Substances, Nitrofurans and Industrial Chemicals (23 monographs), 326 pages

    Volume 8 (1975) Some Aromatic Azo Compounds (32 monographs), 357 pages

Volume 9 (1975) Some Aziridines, *N*-, *S*- and *O*-Mustards and Selenium (24 monographs), 268 pages

Volume 10 (1976) Some Naturally Occurring Substances (32 monographs), 353 pages

Volume 11 (1976) Cadmium, Nickel, Some Epoxides, Miscellaneous Industrial Chemicals and General Considerations on Volatile Anaesthetics (24 monographs), 306 pages

Volume 12 (1976) Some Carbamates, Thiocarbamates and Carbazides (24 monographs), 282 pages

Volume 13 (1977) Some Miscellaneous Pharmaceutical Substances (17 monographs), 255 pages

Volume 14 (1977) Asbestos (1 monograph), 106 pages

Volume 15 (1977) Some Fumigants, the Herbicides, 2,4-D and 2,4,5-T, Chlorinated Dibenzodioxins and Miscellaneous Industrial Chemicals (18 monographs), 354 pages

Volume 16 (1978) Some Aromatic Amines and Related Nitro Compounds - Hair Dyes, Colouring Agents, and Miscellaneous Industrial Chemicals (32 monographs), 400 pages

Volume 17 (1978) Some *N*-Nitroso Compounds (17 monographs), 365 pages

Volume 18 (1978) Polychlorinated Biphenyls and Polybrominated Biphenyls (2 monographs), 140 pages

Volume 19 (1979) Some Monomers, Plastics and Synthetic Elastomers, and Acrolein (17 monographs), 513 pages

Volume 20 (1979) Some Halogenated Hydrocarbons (25 monographs), 609 pages

Volume 21 (1979) Sex Hormones (II) (22 monographs), 583 pages

Volume 22 (1980) Some Non-Nutritive Sweetening Agents (2 monographs), 208 pages

Volume 23 (1980) Some Metals and Metallic Compounds (4 monographs), 438 pages

Volume 24 (1980) Some Pharmaceutical Drugs (16 monographs), 337 pages

Volume 25 (1981) Wood, Leather and Some Associated Industries (7 monographs), 412 pages

Volume 26 (1981) Some Antineoplastic and Immunosuppressive Agents (18 monographs), 411 pages

Volume 27 (1981) Some Aromatic Amines, Anthraquinones and Nitroso Compounds, and Inorganic Fluorides Used in Drinking-Water and Dental Preparations (18 monographs), 344 pages

Volume 28 (1982) The Rubber Manufacturing Industry (1 monograph), 486 pages

Volume 29 (1982) Some Industrial Chemicals (18 monographs), 416 pages

Volume 30 (1983) Some Miscellaneous Pesticides (18 monographs), 424 pages

Supplement 3 (1982) Cross Index of Synonyms and Trade Names in Volumes 1 to 26, 199 pages

Volume 31 (1983) Some Food Additives, Feed Additives and Naturally Occurring Substances (21 monographs), 314 pages

10. IARC (1973-1981) *Information Bulletin on the Survey of Chemicals Being Tested for Carcinogenicity*, Numbers 1-8, Lyon, France

Number 1 (1973) 52 pages
Number 2 (1973) 77 pages
Number 3 (1974) 67 pages
Number 4 (1974) 97 pages
Number 5 (1975) 88 pages
Number 6 (1976) 360 pages
Number 7 (1978) 460 pages
Number 8 (1979) 604 pages
Number 9 (1981) 294 pages

11. PHS 149 (1951-1980) Public Health Service Publication No. 149, *Survey of Compounds which have been Tested for Carcinogenic Activity*, Washington DC, US Government Printing Office

1951 Hartwell, J.L., 2nd ed., Literature up to 1947 on 1329 compounds, 583 pages

1957 Shubik, P. & Hartwell, J.L., Supplement 1, Literature for the years 1948-1953 on 981 compounds, 388 pages

1969 Shubik, P. & Hartwell, J.L., edited by Peters, J.A., Supplement 2, Literature for the years 1954-1960 on 1048 compounds, 655 pages

1971 National Cancer Institute, Literature for the years 1968-1969 on 882 compounds, 653 pages

1973 National Cancer Institute, Literature for the years 1961-1967 on 1632 compounds, 2343 pages

    1974 National Cancer Institute, Literature for the years 1970-1971 on 750 com-
    pounds, 1667 pages

    1976 National Cancer Institute, Literature for the years 1972-1973 on 966 com-
    pounds, 1638 pages

    1980 National Cancer Institute, Literature for the year 1978 on 664 compounds, 1331
    pages

12. Pike, M.C. & Roe, F.J.C. (1963) An actuarial method of analysis of an experiment in
    two-stage carcinogenesis. *Br. J. Cancer*, *17*, 605-6l0

13. Miller, E.C. & Miller, J.A. (1966) Mechanisms of chemical carcinogenesis: nature of
    proximate carcinogens and interactions with macromolecules. *Pharmacol. Rev.*, *18*,
    805-838

14. Miller, J.A. (1970) Carcinogenesis by chemicals: an overview - G.H.A. Clowes Memorial
    Lecture. *Cancer Res.*, *30*, 559-576

15. Miller, J.A. & Miller, E.C. (1976) *The metabolic activation of chemical carcinogens to
    reactive electrophiles.* In: Yuhas, J.M., Tennant, R.W. & Reagon, J.D., eds, *Biology
    of Radiation Carcinogenesis*, New York, Raven Press

16. Peto, R. (1974) Guidelines on the analysis of tumour rates and death rates in
    experimental animals. *Br. J. Cancer*, *29*, 101-105

17. Peto, R. (1975) Letter to the editor. *Br. J. Cancer*, *31*, 697-699

18. Hoel, D.G. & Walburg, H.E., Jr (1972) Statistical analysis of survival experiments. *J.
    natl Cancer Inst.*, *49*, 361-372

19. IARC (1980) *IARC Monographs on the Evaluation of the Carcinogenic Risk of
    Chemicals to Humans*, Supplement 2, *Long-term and Short-term Screening Assays
    for Carcinogens: A Critical Appraisal*, Lyon

20. IARC Working Group (1980) An evaluation of chemicals and industrial processes
    associated with cancer in humans based on human and animal bata: *IARC Mono-
    graphs* Volumes 1 to 20. *Cancer Res.*, *40*, 1-12

21. IARC (1979) *IARC Monographs on the Evaluation of the Carcinogenic Risk of
    Chemicals to Humans*, Supplement 1, *Chemicals and Industrial Processes Associated
    with Cancer in Humans*, Lyon

22. Rall, D.P. (1977) *Species differences in carcinogenesis testing.* In: Hiatt, H.H., Watson,
    J.D. & Winsten, J.A., eds, *Origins of Human Cancer*, Book C, Cold Spring Harbor,
    NY, Cold Spring Harbor Laboratory, pp. 1383-1390

23. National Academy of Sciences (NAS) (1975) *Contemporary Pest Control Practices and
    Prospects: the Report of the Executive Committee*, Washington DC

24. Chemical Abstracts Services (1978) *Chemical Abstracts Ninth Collective Index (9CI),
    1972-1976*, Vols 76-85, Columbus, OH

25. International Union of Pure & Applied Chemistry (1965) *Nomenclature of Organic Chemistry*, Section C, London, Butterworths

26. WHO (1958) Second Report of the Joint FAO/WHO Expert Committee on Food Additives. Procedures for the testing of intentional food additives to establish their safety and use. *WHO tech. Rep. Ser., No. 144*

27. WHO (1967) Scientific Group. Procedures for investigating intentional and unintentional food additives. *WHO tech. Rep. Ser., No. 348*

28. Berenblum, I., ed. (1969) Carcinogenicity testing. *UICC tech. Rep. Ser., 2*

29. Sontag, J.M., Page, N.P. & Saffiotti, U. (1976) Guidelines for carcinogen bioassay in small rodents. *Natl Cancer Inst. Carcinog. tech. Rep. Ser., No. 1*

30. Committee on Standardized Genetic Nomenclature for Mice (1972) Standardized nomenclature for inbred strains of mice. Fifth listing. *Cancer Res., 32*, 1609-1646

31. Wilson, J.G. & Fraser, F.C. (1977) *Handbook of Teratology*, New York, Plenum Press

32. Berenblum, I. (1975) *Sequential aspects of chemical carcinogenesis: Skin*. In: Becker, F.F., ed., *Cancer. A Comprehensive Treatise*, Vol. 1, New York, Plenum Press, pp. 323-344

33. Foulds, L. (1969) *Neoplastic Development*, Vol. 2, London, Academic Press

34. Farber, E. & Cameron, R. (1980) The sequential analysis of cancer development. *Adv. Cancer Res., 31*, 125-226

35. Weinstein, I.B. (1981) The scientific basis for carcinogen detection and primary cancer prevention. *Cancer, 47*, 1133-1141

36. Slaga, T.J., Sivak, A. & Boutwell, R.K., eds (1978) *Mechanisms of Tumor Promotion and Cocarcinogenesis*, Vol. 2, New York, Raven Press

37. Miller, E.C. & Miller, J.A. (1981) Mechanisms of chemical carcinogenesis. *Cancer, 47*, 1055-1064

38. Brookes, P. & Lawley, P.D. (1964) Evidence for the binding of polynuclear aromatic hydrocarbons to the nucleic acids of mouse skin: relation between carcinogenic power of hydrocarbons and their binding to deoxyribonucleic acid. *Nature, 202*, 781-784

39. Lawley, P.D. (1976) *Carcinogenesis by alkylating agents*. In: Searle, C.E., ed., *Chemical Carcinogens (ACS Monograph 173)*, Washington DC, American Chemical Society, pp. 83-244

40. McCann, J. & Ames, B.N. (1976) Detection of carcinogens as mutagens in the *Salmonella*/microsome test: Assay of 300 chemicals: Discussion. *Proc. natl Acad. Sci. USA, 73*, 950-954

41. Weisburger, J.H. & Williams, G.M. (1980) *Chemical carcinogens*. In: Doull, J., Klaassen, C.D. & Amdur, M.O., eds, *Casarett and Doull's Toxicology: The Basic Science of Poisons*, 2nd ed., New York, MacMillan, pp. 84-138

42. Montesano, R., Bartsch, H. & Tomatis, L., eds (1980) *Molecular and Cellular Aspects of Carcinogen Screening Tests (IARC Scientific Publications No. 27)*, Lyon

43. de Serres, F.J. & Ashby, J., eds (1981) *Evaluation of Short-Term Tests for Carcinogens. Report of the International Collaborative Program,* Amsterdam, Elsevier/North-Holland Biomedical Press

44. Sugimura, T., Sato, S., Nagao, M., Yahagi, T., Matsushima, T., Seino, Y., Takeuchi, M. & Kawachi, T. (1976) *Overlapping of carcinogens and mutagens.* In: Magee, P.N., Takayama, S., Sugimura, T. & Matsushima, T., eds, *Fundamentals in Cancer Prevention,* Tokyo/Baltimore, University of Tokyo/University Park Press, pp. 191-215

45. Bartsch, H., Tomatis, L. & Malaveille, C. (1982) *Qualitative and quantitative comparison between mutagenic and carcinogenic activities of chemicals.* In: Heddle, J.A., ed., *Mutagenicity: New Horizons in Genetic Toxicology,* New York, Academic Press, pp. 35-72

46. Hollstein, M., McCann, J., Angelosanto, F.A. & Nichols, W.W. (1979) Short-term tests for carcinogens and mutagens. *Mutat. Res., 65,* 133-226

GENERAL REMARKS ON THE SUBSTANCES CONSIDERED

This thirty-first volume of *IARC Monographs* covers a number of food additives, naturally occurring substances and veterinary drugs added to animal feeds. Some of the compounds - carrageenan, cholesterol, cinnamyl anthranilate, fusarenon X, ochratoxin A and senkirkine - were considered by previous IARC Working Groups in volumes 10, 11 and 16 of the *Monographs* (IARC, 1976a,b, 1978). Since new data on these compounds had since become available for evaluation, the new information was considered and evaluated in the present monographs.

Three compounds, myristicin, nihydrazone and sulphamethazine, were included in a tentative list of substances to be evaluated, but consideration of these monographs was postponed since no adequate carcinogenicity study was available. Sulphamethazine is presently being tested in mice and rats by administration in the diet (IARC, 1981).

The Working Group noted that for most of the studies on natural products no information on the presence of impurities and/or their levels was available. In those cases in which very high levels were tested in carcinogenicity bioassays, the Group noted that some of the effects observed might be attributable to impurities rather than to the major components of the material fed.

Flavonoids

Interest in the carcinogenicity of flavonoids stems from their presence as glycosides in foods and beverages consumed by humans and domestic animals and the reported carcinogenicity for several species of one which is edible: bracken fern (*Pteridium aquilinum*) (Pamukcu & Bryan, 1979; Bryan & Pamukcu, 1982).

Tea, coffee, cocoa, fruit juices, red wine, beer and even vinegar are important sources of flavonoids. Spices, seasonings and plants used as tea are another important source (Kühnau, 1976).

Although it has been shown that flavonoids are essential requirements for insects, the same has not been shown convincingly for higher animals and humans. However, food flavonoids do have several beneficial effects in mammals. Many of the flavonoids, such as quercetin and myricetin, are strong antioxidants and metal chelators (Heimann & Heinrich, 1959; Kühnau, 1976). Furthermore, flavonoids and related polyphenols have been shown to catalyse or inhibit nitrosation of amino precursors to *N*-nitroso compounds *in vivo* and *in vitro* (Davies *et al.*, 1978; Pignatelli *et al.*, 1982).

There is evidence in experimental animals that some flavonoids have anti-carcinogenic activity (Wattenberg & Leong, 1968, 1970). Flavones are effective inducers of some xenobiotic microsomal enzymes, and for some carcinogenic polycyclic hydrocarbons such induction may favour detoxification (Wattenberg *et al.*, 1968; Wattenberg & Leong, 1968, 1970; Cutroneo *et al.*, 1972; Cutroneo & Bresnick, 1973).

The Working Group examined data on two flavonoids, kaempferol and quercetin, in detail. The 3-rhamnoglucoside of quercetin, rutin, has also been tested for carcinogenicity in experimental animals and for its activity in various short-term tests. These data were included in the monograph on quercetin.

At least 27 aglycones of various flavonoids have been reported to be mutagenic to *Salmonella typhimurium* (Table 1); 40-50 have given negative results. Glycosides of these compounds are mutagenic only after chemical or enzymatic hydrolysis (for a general review on the mutagenicity of flavonoids, see Brown, 1980; Nagao *et al.*, 1981).

Table 1. Plant flavonoids that gave positive results in mutagenicity tests in *Salmonella typhimurium*

Flavonoid	Substitution	References
Flavonols		
4′,7-Di-O-methylquercetin	3,3′,5-OH, 4′,7-OCH$_3$	MacGregor & Jurd (1978)
5,7-Di-O-methylquercetin	3,3′,4′-OH, 5,7-OCH$_3$	MacGregor & Jurd (1978)
Fisetin	3,3′,4′,7-OH	Brown & Dietrich (1979); Sugimura *et al.* (1977); Hardigree & Epler (1978); Nagao *et al.* (1981)
Galangin	3,5,7-OH	Brown & Dietrich (1979); Sugimura *et al.* (1977); MacGregor & Jurd (1978); Nagao *et al.* (1981)
Isorhamnetin	3,4′,5,7-OH, 3′-OCH$_3$	Nagao *et al.* (1981)
Kaempferide	3,5,7-OH, 4′-OCH$_3$	Brown & Dietrich (1979); Nagao *et al.* (1981)
Kaempferol	3,4′,5,7-OH	Brown & Dietrich (1979); Sugimura *et al.* (1977); Hardigree & Epler (1978); MacGregor & Jurd (1978); Nagao *et al.* (1981)
3′-O-Methylquercetin	3,4′,5,7-OH, 3′-OCH$_3$	MacGregor & Jurd (1978)
5-O-Methylquercetin	3,3′,4′,7-OH, 5-OCH$_3$	MacGregor & Jurd (1978)
Morin	2′,3,4′,5,7-OH	Brown & Dietrich (1979); Hardigree & Epler (1978); MacGregor & Jurd (1978); Nagao *et al.* (1981)
Myricetin	3,3′,4′,5,5′,7-OH	Brown & Dietrich (1979); Hardigree & Epler (1978); MacGregor & Jurd (1978)
Myricetin hexaacetate	3,3′,4′,5,5′,7-OCOCH$_3$	Nagao *et al.* (1981)

Quercetin	3,3',4',5,7-OH	Brown & Dietrich (1979); Bjeldanes & Chang (1977); Sugimura et al. (1977); Hardigree & Epler (1978); MacGregor & Jurd (1978); Nagao et al. (1981)
Quercetin pentaacetate	3,3',4',5,7-OCOCH$_3$	Bjeldanes & Chang (1977); Nagao et al. (1981)
Rhamnetin	3,3',4',5-OH, 7-OCH$_3$	Brown & Dietrich (1979); MacGregor & Jurd (1978); Nagao et al. (1981)
Robinetin	3,3',4',5',7-OH	Brown & Dietrich (1979)
Tamarixetin	3,3',5,7-OH, 4'-OCH$_3$	MacGregor & Jurd (1978)

Flavones

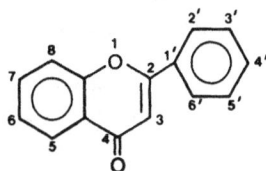

Acacetin	5,7-OH, 4'-OCH$_3$	Nagao et al. (1981)
Apigenin triacetate	4',5,7-OCOCH$_3$	Nagao et al. (1981)
Chrysoeriol	4',5,7-OH, 3'-OCH$_3$	Nagao et al. (1981)
Pedalitin	3',4',5,6-OH, 7-OCH$_3$	Nagao et al. (1981)
Pedalitin tetracetate	3',4',5,6-OCOCH$_3$, 7-OCH$_3$	Nagao et al. (1981)
Wogonin	5,7-OH 8-OCH$_3$	Nagao et al. (1981)

Flavanones

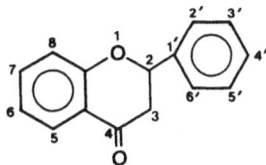

4',7-Dihydroxy flavonone	4',7-OH	Nagao et al. (1981)
Hydrorobinetin	3,3',4',5',7-OH	Nagao et al. (1981)
Taxifolin	3,3',4',5,7-OH	Brown & Dietrich (1979); Nagao et al. (1981)

Isoflavones

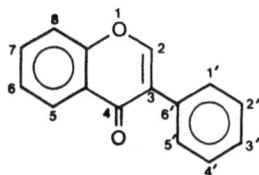

| Tectorigenin | 3',5,7-OH, 6-OCH$_3$ | Nagao et al. (1981) |

Pyrolysis products isolated from foods

The Working Group prepared monographs on two pyrolysis products of tryptophan (Trp-P-1 and Trp-P-2); they were aware also of a recently completed carcinogenicity study on the pyrolysis product, Glu-P-1 (Muramatsu *et al.*, 1983). Charred parts of broiled meat and fish have been shown to possess mutagenic activity, and several heterocyclic amines have been isolated and identified from amino acid pyrolysates (for reviews, see Sugimura *et al.*, 1981, Sugimura, 1982b; Sugimura & Nagao, 1982).

Many other mutagenic pyrolysis products have been isolated and identified, and a number of these have been detected in food. The results of tests for mutagenicity in *Salmonella typhimurium* of pyrolysis products found in food are given in Table 2. The mutagenic activity in the *Salmonella*/microsome assay of some of these pyrolysis products is greater than that of aflatoxin B_1 and of AF-2, which were previously thought to be the compounds the most active in this assay (Sugimura, 1982a,b). Although the mutagenicity of Trp-P-1 and Trp-P-2 has been confirmed in a number of short-term tests (see this volume, pp. 251, 259), only limited data are available on the mutagenic activity of the other pyrolysis products.

The mutagenicity of pyrolysis products can be modified in in-vitro assays by the addition various compounds occurring in food: comutagenic, as well as antimutagenic, activity has been reported. Comutagens are compounds that increase the mutagenicity of a chemical, although they are not mutagenic by themselves. Antimutagens reduce or abolish the mutagenic activity of a mutagen.

The mutagenic activity of pyrolysates of tryptophan is enhanced by harman and norharman (Nagao *et al.*, 1977). These two comutagens are found in tobacco tar (Poindexter & Carpenter, 1962), broiled beef and broiled sardines (Yasuda *et al.*, 1978). The mechanism of the comutagenicity of harman and norharman is not clear; they may exert their comutagenic activity by altering metabolic activation. Since norharman is also comutagenic towards the directly acting mutagen N-acetoxy-2-acetylaminofluorene (Umezawa *et al.*, 1978), other mechanisms cannot be excluded.

Homogenates prepared from certain fresh, uncooked vegetables, such as cabbage, have been reported to reduce the mutagenicity of tryptophan pyrolysates (Kada *et al.*, 1978; Morita *et al.*, 1978). Pigments, like haemin, occurring in mammals also have antimutagenic activity towards Trp-P-1 and Trp-P-2 (Arimoto *et al.*, 1980). Acidic treatment of Trp-P-1 and Trp-P-2 with 2-3 mg/l sodium nitrite resulted in complete loss of their mutagenic activity for *Salmonella typhimurium* (Yoshida & Matsumoto, 1978; Tsuda *et al.*, 1980).

It is difficult to assess the implications of modifying activity *in vitro* for the situation *in vivo*. The fact that a number of compounds occurring in food or in body fluids can reduce the mutagenicity of pyrolysis products may indicate that the effects of these mutagens *in vivo* are less than might be expected from their very high mutagenicity in the *Salmonella*/microsome assay.

Cholesterol

The data from tests in experimental animals on the carcinogenicity of cholesterol metabolites were considered inadequate for an evaluation of the carcinogenicity of cholesterol and were not included in the monograph.

Table 2. Some pyrolysis products isolated from foods and their mutagenicity in *Salmonella typhimurium*[a]

Pyrolysis product (CAS Registry Number)	Structure	Mutagenic activity (rev/μg)[b]		Product from which it was first isolated	Food product from which it has been isolated	Concentration (μg/kg)
		TA98	TA10			
3-Amino-1,4-dimethyl-5H-pyrido[4,3-b]indole (Trp-P-1) [62450-06-0]		39 000[d]	1700[d]	Pyrolysates of tryptophan (Kosuge et al., 1978)	Broiled sun-dried sardine (Yamai-zumi et al., 1980) Broiled beef (Yamaguchi et al., 1980a)	13 53[c]
3-Amino-1-methyl-5H-pyrido[4,3-b]indole (Trp-P-2) [62450-07-1]		104 200[d]	1800[d]	Pyrolysates of tryptophan (Kosuge et al., 1978)	Broiled sun-dried sardine (Yamai-zumi et al., 1980)	13
2-Amino-6-methyldipyrido[1,2-a:3',2'-d]imidazole (Glu-P-1) [67730-11-4]		49 000[e]	3200[e]	Pyrolysates of glutamic acid (Yamamoto et al., 1978)		
2-Aminodipyrido[1,2-a:3',2'-d]imidazole (Glu-P-2) [67730-10-3]		1900[e]	1200[d]	Pyrolysates of glutamic acid (Yamamoto et al., 1978)	Broiled sun-dried cuttle fish (Yamaguchi et al., 1980b)	280
2-Amino-5-phenylpyridine (Phe-P-1) [33421-40-8]		41[f]	23[f]	Pyrolysates of phenylalanine (Tsuji et al., 1978)	Broiled sun-dried sardine (Yamai-zumi et al., 1980)	9
2-Amino-α-carboline (AαC) [26148-68-5]		300[f]	20[f]	Pyrolysates of soya bean globulin (Yoshida et al., 1978)	Grilled beef Grilled chicken Grilled onion (Matsumoto et al., 1981) [Also present in cigarette smoke (Yoshida & Matsumoto, 1980)]	650 180 2 [25-258 ng/cigarette]

Pyrolysis product (CAS Registry Number)	Structure	Mutagenic activity (rev/μg)[b]		Product from which it was first isolated	Food product from which it has been isolated	Concentration (μg/kg)
		TA98	TA100			
2-Amino-3-methyl-α-carboline (MeAαC) [68006-83-7]	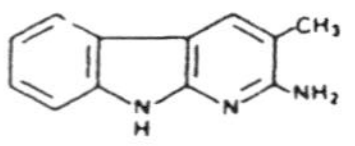	200[f]	120[f]	Pyrolysates of soya bean globulin (Yoshida et al., 1978)	Grilled beef Grilled chicken (Matsumoto et al., 1981) [Also present in cigarette smoke (Yoshida & Matsumoto, 1980)]	64 15 [9-37 ng/cigarette]
2-Amino-3-methylimidazo[4,5-f]quinoline (IQ) [76180-96-6]	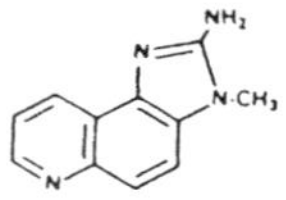	433 000[d]	7000[d]	Broiled sardine (Kasai et al., 1980)	Broiled sun-dried sardine (Sugimura et al., 1981) Broiled beef (Sugimura et al., 1981)	158 1
2-Amino-3,4-dimethylimidazo[4,5-f]quinoline (MeIQ) [77094-11-2]	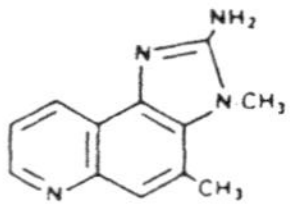	661 000[d]	30 000[d]	Broiled sardine (Kasai et al., 1980)	Broiled sun-dried sardines (Sugimura et al., 1981)	72
2-Amino-3,8-dimethylimidazo[4,5-f]quinoxaline (MeIQx) [77500-04-0]	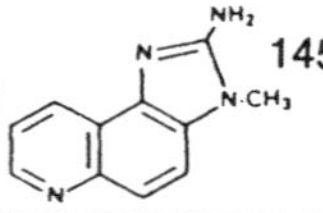	145 000[d]	14 000[d]	Fried beef (Kasai et al., 1981)		

[a]Adapted from Sugimura (1982b)

[b]The mutagenic activities of AF-2 and aflatoxin B, were 6500 (without S9) and 600 (10 μl S9/plate) revertants/μg, respectively, in strain TA98 and 42 000 (without S9) and 28 000 (10 μl S9/plate) revertants/μg, respectively, in strain TA100

[c]per kg raw beef

[d]10 μl S9/plate

[e]30 μl S9/plate

[f]150 μl S9/plate

The Working Group was aware of studies on the mutagenicity of metabolites of cholesterol, including bile acids (Silverman & Andrews, 1977; Kelsey & Pienta, 1981; Ansari et al., 1982), but a discussion of these data was generally considered to be beyond the scope of this monograph. A review on mutagenic products isolated from faeces is available (Venitt, 1982).

Furazolidone and nihydrazone

These compounds were included on the tentative list of substances to be considered. However, carcinogenicity data on these compounds were available only from secondary sources (namely: US Department of Health, Education, & Welfare, 1976a,b; National Academy of Sciences, 1981); according to the principle adopted with regard to use of biological data in evaluating the carcinogenicity of compounds in the *Monographs* programme (see Preamble, p.13), such data could not be used. For this reason, the Working Group discussed deletion of these two monographs from the volume. However, it was decided to retain the monograph on furazolidone because of the widespread use of this compound as a human and veterinary drug and in view of the large amount of information available from mutagenicity and related short-term tests. The data on carcinogenicity in experimental animals for both furazolidone and nihydrazone reported in the *Federal Register* (US Department of Health, Education, & Welfare, 1976a,b) and by the National Academy of Sciences (1981) are summarized below:

Furazolidone was tested in one study in mice and in six studies in rats. In mice, furazolidone increased the incidence of bronchial adenocarcinomas. In female rats, it increased the incidence of multiple benign and malignant mammary tumours; in male rats it increased the incidence of testicular mesotheliomas, basal-cell epitheliomas, squamous-cell carcinomas and dermal fibromas; and in animals of both sexes, it increased the incidence of thyroid adenomas, sebaceous adenomas, pituitary neoplasms and lymphoreticular neoplasms.

Nihydrazone was tested for carcinogenicity in two experiments in rats by administration in the diet. It increased the incidence of benign and malignant mammary tumours in females in both studies.

References

Ansari, G.A.S., Walker, R.D., Smart, V.B. & Smith, L.L. (1982) Further investigations of mutagenic cholesterol preparations. *Food Chem. Toxicol.*, *20*, 35-41

Arimoto, S., Ohara, Y., Namba, T., Negishi, T. & Hayatsu, H. (1980) Inhibition of the mutagenicity of amino acid pyrolysis products by hemin and other biological pyrrole pigments. *Biochem. biophys. Res. Commun.*, *92*, 662-668

Bjeldanes, L.F. & Chang, G.W. (1977) Mutagenic activity of quercetin and related compounds. *Science*, *197*, 577-578

Brown, J.P. (1980) A review of the genetic effects of naturally occurring flavonoids, anthraquinones and related compounds. *Mutat. Res.*, *75*, 243-277

Brown, J.P. & Dietrich, P.S. (1979) Mutagenicity of plant flavonols in the *Salmonella*/mammalian microsome test. Activation of flavonol glycosides by mixed glycosidases from rat cecal bacteria and other sources. *Mutat. Res.*, *66*, 223-240

Bryan, G.T. & Pamukcu, A.M. (1982) *Sources of carcinogens and mutagens in edible plants: Production of urinary bladder and intestinal tumors by bracken fern* (Pteridium aquilinum). In: Stich, H.F., ed., *Carcinogens and Mutagens in the Environment*, Vol. 1, *Food Products*, Boca Raton, FL, CRC Press, Inc., pp. 75-82

Cutroneo, K.R. & Bresnick, E. (1973) Induction of benzpyrene hydroxylase in fetal liver explants by flavones and phenobarbital. *Biochem. Pharmacol.*, *22*, 675-687

Cutroneo, K.R., Seibert, R.A. & Bresnick, E. (1972) Induction of benzpyrene hydroxylase by flavone and its derivatives in fetal rat liver explants. *Biochem. Pharmacol.*, *21*, 937-945

Davies, R., Dennis, M.J., Massey, R.C. & McWeeny, D.J. (1978) *Some effects of phenol- and thiol-nitrosation reactions on* N-*nitrosamine formation*. In: Walker, E.A., Castegnaro, M., Griciute, L. & Lyle, R.E., eds, *Environmental Aspects of* N-*Nitroso Compounds* (*IARC Scientific Publications No. 19*), Lyon, International Agency for Research on Cancer, pp. 183-197

Hardigree, A.A. & Epler, J.L. (1978) Comparative mutagenesis of plant flavonoids in microbial systems. *Mutat. Res.*, *58*, 231-239

Heimann, W. & Heinrich, B. (1959) On the inhibition of the oxidation of ascorbic acid by flavonoids, catalysed by Cu(2) (Ger.). *Fette Seifen Anstrichm.*, *61*, 1024-1029

IARC (1976a) *IARC Monographs on the Evaluation of Carcinogenic Risk of Chemicals to Man*, Vol. 10, *Some Naturally Occurring Substances*, Lyon, pp. 99-111, 181-190, 191-197, 327-331

IARC (1976b) *IARC Monographs on the Evaluation of Carcinogenic Risk of Chemicals to Man*, Vol. 11, *Cadmium, Nickel, Some Epoxides, Miscellaneous Industrial Chemicals and General Considerations on Volatile Anaesthetics*, Lyon, pp. 169-179

IARC (1978) *IARC Monographs on the Evaluation of the Carcinogenic Risk of Chemicals to Man*, Vol. 16, *Some Aromatic Amines and Related Nitro Compounds - Hair Dyes, Colouring Agents and Miscellaneous Industrial Chemicals*, Lyon, pp. 287-299

IARC (1981) *Information Bulletin on the Survey of Chemicals Being Tested for Carcinogenicity*, No. 9, Lyon, p. 156

Kada, T., Morita, K. & Inoue, T. (1978) Anti-mutagenic action of vegetable factor(s) on the mutagenic principle of tryptophan pyrolysate. *Mutat. Res.*, *53*, 351-353

Kasai, H., Yamaizumi, Z., Wakabayashi, K., Nagao, M., Sugimura, T., Yokoyama, S., Miyazawa, T., Spingarn, N.E., Weisburger, J.H. & Nishimura, S. (1980) Potent novel mutagens produced by broiling fish under normal conditions. *Proc. Jpn. Acad.*, *56B*, 278-283

Kasai, H., Yamaizumi, Z., Shiomi, T., Yokoyama, S., Miyazawa, T., Wakabayashi, K., Nagao, M., Sugimura, T. & Nishimura, S. (1981) Structure of a potent mutagen isolated from fried beef. *Chem. Lett.*, 485-488

Kelsey, M.I. & Pienta, R.J. (1981) Transformation of hamster embryo cells by neutral sterols and bile acids. *Toxicol. Lett.*, *9*, 177-182

Kosuge, T., Tsuji, K., Wakabayashi, K., Okamoto, T., Shudo, K., Iitaka, Y., Itai, A., Sugimura, T., Kawachi, T., Nagao, M., Yahagi, T. & Seino, Y. (1978) Isolation and structure studies of mutagenic principles in amino acid pyrolysates. *Chem. pharm. Bull.*, *26*, 611-619

Kühnau, J. (1976) The flavonoids. A class of semi-essential food components: Their role in human nutrition. *World Rev. Nutr. Diet.*, *24*, 117-191

MacGregor, J.T. & Jurd, L. (1978) Mutagenicity of plant flavonoids: Structural requirements for mutagenic activity in *Salmonella typhimurium*. *Mutat. Res.*, *54*, 297-309

Matsumoto, T., Yoshida, D. & Tomita, H. (1981) Determination of mutagens, amino-α-carbolines in grilled food and cigarette smoke condensate. *Cancer Lett.*, *12*, 105-110

Morita, K., Inoue, T. & Kada, T. (1978) Desmutagenic factor of vegetable extracts on mutagenic principles of tryptophan pyrolyzates (Abstract no. 15). *Mutat. Res.*, *54*, 243-244

Muramatsu, M., Saito, D., Araki, A., Matsushima, T. & Hirono, I. (1983) Liver tumor induction by Glu-P-1, pyrolysis product of glutamic acid, in mice. *Gann* (in press)

Nagao, M., Yahagi, T., Kawachi, T., Sugimura, T., Kosuge, T., Tsuji, K., Wakabayashi, K., Mizusaki, S. & Matsumoto, T. (1977) Comutagenic action of norharman and harman. *Proc. Jpn. Acad.*, *53*, 95-98

Nagao, M., Morita, N., Yahagi, T., Shimizu, M., Kuroyanagi, M., Fukuoka, M., Yoshihira, K., Natori, S., Fujino, T. & Sugimura, T. (1981) Mutagenicities of 61 flavonoids and 11 related compounds. *Environ. Mutagenesis*, *3*, 401-419

National Academy of Sciences (1981) *Aromatic Amines: An Assessment of the Biological and Environmental Effects. Report of the Committee on Amines, Board of Toxicology and Environmental Health Hazards, Assembly of Life Sciences*, National Research Council, Washington DC, National Academy Press, pp. 288-319

Pamukcu, A.M. & Bryan, G.T. (1979) *Bracken fern, a natural urinary bladder and intestinal carcinogen*. In: Miller, E.C., Miller, J.A., Hirono, I., Sugimura, T. & Takayama, S., eds, *Naturally Occurring Carcinogens - Mutagens and Modulators of Carcinogenesis*, Tokyo/Baltimore, Japan Scientific Societies Press/University Park Press, pp. 89-99

Pignatelli, B., Béréziat, J.-C., Descotes, G. & Bartsch, H. (1982) Catalysis of nitrosation *in vitro* and *in vivo* in rats by catechin and resorcinol and inhibition by chlorogenic acid. *Carcinogenesis*, *3*, 1045-1049

Poindexter, E.H., Jr & Carpenter, R.D. (1962) The isolation of harmane and norharmane from tobacco and cigarette smoke. *Phytochemistry*, *1*, 215-221

Silverman, S.J. & Andrews, A.W. (1977) Bile acids: Co-mutagenic activity in the *Salmonella*-mammalian-microsome mutagenicity test. *J. natl Cancer Inst.*, *59*, 1557-1559

Sugimura, T. (1982a) *The Ernst W. Bertner memorial award lecture: Tumor initiators and promoters associated with ordinary foods.* In: Arnott, M.S., van Eys, J. & Wang, Y.-M., eds, *Molecular Interrelations of Nutrition and Cancer*, New York, Raven Press, pp. 3-24

Sugimura, T. (1982b) Mutagens, carcinogens, and tumor promoters in our daily food. *Cancer, 49*, 1970-1984

Sugimura, T. & Nagao, M. (1982) *The use of mutagenicity to evaluate carcinogenic hazards in our daily lives.* In: Heddle, J.A., ed., *Mutagenicity: New Horizons in Genetic Toxicology*, New York, Academic Press, pp. 73-88

Sugimura, T., Nagao, M., Matsushima, T., Yahagi, T., Seino, Y., Shirai, A., Sawamura, M., Natori, S., Yoshihira, K., Fukuoka, M. & Kuroyanagi, M. (1977) Mutagenicity of flavone derivatives. *Proc. Jpn. Acad., 53B*, 194-197

Sugimura, T., Nagao, M. & Wakabayashi, K. (1981) *Mutagenic heterocyclic amines in cooked food.* In: Egan, H., Fishbein, L., Castegnaro, M., O'Neill, I.K. & Bartsch, H., eds, *Environmental Carcinogens - Selected Methods of Analysis*, Vol. 4, *Some Aromatic Amines and Azo Dyes in the General and Industrial Environment (IARC Scientific Publications No. 40)*, Lyon, International Agency for Research on Cancer, pp. 251-267

Tsuda, M., Takahashi, Y., Nagao, M., Hirayama, T. & Sugimura, T. (1980) Inactivation of mutagens from pyrolysates of tryptophan and glutamic acid by nitrite and acid solution. *Mutat. Res., 78*, 331-339

Tsuji, K., Yamamoto, T., Zenda, H. & Kosuge, T. (1978) Studies on active principles of tar. VIII. Production of biological active substances in pyrolyses of amino acids. (2) Antifungal constituents in pyrolysis products of phenylalanine. *Takugaku Zasshi, 98*, 910-913

Umezawa, K., Shirai, A., Matsushima, T. & Sugimura, T. (1978) Comutagenic effect of norharman and harman with 2-acetylaminofluorene derivatives. *Proc. natl Acad. Sci. USA, 75*, 928-930

US Department of Health, Education, & Welfare (1976a) Furazolidone (NF-180); Notice of opportunity for hearing on proposal to withdraw approval of certain new animal drug applications. *Fed. Regist., 41*, 19907-19921

US Department of Health, Education, & Welfare (1976b) Furazolidone, nihydrazone, furaltadone, nitrofurazone: Withdrawal of proposals and notice of proposed rule making. *Fed. Regist., 41*, 34884-34921

Venitt, S. (1982) Mutagens in human faeces. Are they relevant to cancer of the large bowel? *Mutat. Res., 98*, 265-286

Wattenberg, L.W. & Leong, J.L. (1968) Inhibition of the carcinogenic action of 7,12-dimethylbenz(a)anthracene by beta-naphthoflavone. *Proc. Soc. exp. Biol. Med., 128*, 940-943

Wattenberg, L.W. & Leong, J.L. (1970) Inhibition of the carcinogenic action of benzo(a)pyrene by flavones. *Cancer Res.*, *30*, 1922-1925

Wattenberg, L.W., Page, M.A. & Leong, J.L. (1968) Induction of increased benzpyrene hydroxylase activity by flavone and related compounds. *Cancer Res.*, *28*, 934-937

Yamaguchi, K., Shudo, K., Okamoto, T., Sugimura, T. & Kosuge, T. (1980a) Presence of 3-amino-1,4-dimethyl-5*H*-pyrido[4,3-*b*]indole in broiled beef. *Gann*, *71*, 745-746

Yamaguchi, K., Shudo, K., Okamoto, T., Sugimura, T. & Kosuge, T. (1980b) Presence of 2-aminodipyrido[1,2-*a*:3′,2′-*d*]imidazole in broiled cuttlefish. *Gann*, *71*, 743-744

Yamaizumi, Z., Shiomi, T., Kasai, H., Nishimura, S., Takahashi, Y., Nagao, M. & Sugimura, T. (1980) Detection of potent mutagens, Trp-P-1 and Trp-P-2, in broiled fish. *Cancer Lett.*, *9*, 75-83

Yamamoto, T., Tsuji, K., Kosuge, T., Okamoto, T., Shudo, K., Takeda, K., Iitaka, Y., Yamaguchi, K., Seino, Y., Yahagi, T., Nagao, M. & Sugimura, T. (1978) Isolation and structure determination of mutagenic substances in L-glutamic acid pyrolysate. *Proc. Jpn. Acad.*, *54B*, 248-250

Yasuda, T., Yamaizumi, Z., Nishimura, S., Nagao, M., Takahashi, T., Fujiki, H., Sugimura, T. & Tsuji, K. (1978) Detection of comutagenic compounds, harman and norharman in pyrolysis product of proteins and food by gas chromatography-mass spectrometry. *Proc. Jpn. Cancer Assoc., 37th Annual Meeting*, p. 21

Yoshida, D. & Matsumoto, T. (1978) Changes in mutagenicity of protein pyrolyzates by reaction with nitrite. *Mutat. Res.*, *58*, 35-40

Yoshida, D. & Matsumoto, T. (1980) Amino-α-carbolines as mutagenic agents in cigarette smoke condensate. *Cancer Lett.*, *10*, 141-149

Yoshida, D., Matsumoto, T., Yoshimura, R. & Matsuzaki, T. (1978) Mutagenicity of amino-α-carbolines in pyrolysis products of soybean globulin. *Biochem. biophys. Res. Commun.*, *83*, 915-920

THE MONOGRAPHS

AF-2 [2-(2-FURYL)-3-(5-NITRO-2-FURYL)ACRYLAMIDE]

1. Chemical and Physical Data

1.1 Synonyms and trade names

Chem. Abstr. Services Reg. No.: 3688-53-7

Chem. Abstr. Name: 2-Furanacetamide, α-[(5-nitro-2-furanyl)methylene]-

IUPAC Systematic Name: α-2-Furyl-5-nitro-2-furanacrylamide

Synonyms: FF; furylfuramide; 2-(2-furyl)-3-(5-nitro-2-furyl)acrylic acid amide; α-(furyl)-β-(5-nitro-2-furyl)acrylic amide; trans-2-(2-furyl)-3-(5-nitro-2-furyl)acrylamide

Trade Names: AF2; Tofuron[1]

1.2 Structural and molecular formulae and molecular weight

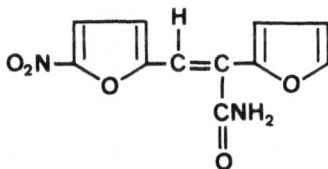

$C_{11}H_8N_2O_5$ Mol. wt: 248.2

---

[1]This product contains 2% AF-2 as the only active compound.

1.3 Chemical and physical properties of the pure substance

    (a) *Description*: Reddish-orange needles

    (b) *Melting-point*: 151-152°C

    (c) *Spectroscopy data*: λ_{max} (ethanol) 303 and 385 nm

    (d) *Solubility*: Slightly soluble in water; soluble in dimethyl formamide, ethanol and methanol

    (e) *Stability*: Sensitive to oxidation and moisture

1.4 Technical products and impurities

No data were available to the Working Group.

2. Production, Use, Occurrence and Analysis

2.1 Production and use

    (a) *Production*

AF-2 was first synthesized in 1958. It can be made by the reaction of 5-nitrofurfural with the potassium salt of 2-furfuryl acetic acid in acetic anhydride and treatment of the resulting compound with sulphur dichloride to form an acid chloride, which is then heated with ammonia (Saikachi & Kanehira, 1962).

Commercial production of AF-2 started in Japan in 1965 or earlier, and annual production by the only Japanese manufacturer is estimated to have reached 25 to 30 thousand kg before the product was withdrawn in 1974. There is no evidence that it is produced commercially in the US or western Europe.

There were no Japanese exports of this chemical during the time that it was produced commercially in Japan.

    (b) *Use*

AF-2 is a synthetic nitrofuran derivative that was approved for use as a food preservative in Japan in 1965; it was withdrawn from the market in 1974 (Tazima, 1979). This compound was used at levels up to 50 mg/kg to protect foods of animal and vegetable origin against attack by a large variety of microorganisms, particularly bacteria. It was added to fish-meat sausage at less than 20 mg/kg, to tôfu (bean curd), to age (fried bean curd) and to animal-meat sausage at less than 5 mg/kg, and to fish cakes at less than 2.5 mg/kg. It has been estimated (de Serres, 1974) that an average individual in Japan consumed about 5 mg of this chemical per year.

2.2 Occurrence

AF-2 is not known to occur as a natural product.

2.3 Analysis

Analytical methods for the determination of AF-2 in food preparations are based on colorimetric methods (Kanno & Okumiya, 1963; Kanno et al., 1966; Nose & Okitsu, 1968). The recovery of 10-80 mg/kg in fish sausage was better than 95%.

Liquid scintillation counting and measurement of radioactivity by thin-layer radiochromatography have been used to determine AF-2 in biological fluids (Tatsumi et al., 1971, 1973a,b, 1975).

3. Biological Data Relevant to the Evaluation of Carcinogenic Risk to Humans

3.1 Carcinogenicity studies in animals

[The Working Group noted that the carcinogenicity of AF-2 for experimental animals was first reported by Ikeda et al. (1974). However, this report is not generally available, and experimental details could not be reported or evaluated.]

(a) Oral administration

Mouse: A group of 10 male ddY mice, six weeks of age, were fed a diet containing 2500 mg/kg AF-2 (purity, 99.66%) for 308 days (total cumulative dose per mouse, 3.9 g), followed by a control diet until termination of the study at 561 days. A group of 10 male mice served as controls; 8 of these were autopsied on day 616 of the study. Nine tumours were reported in 7 treated mice surviving longer than 380 days: 6 were forestomach squamous-cell carcinomas (2 of which had metastases to the liver and 1 to the liver and lung); 1 was a forestomach papilloma; and 2 were pulmonary adenomas. One control mouse had a forestomach papilloma (Sano et al., 1977). [The Working Group noted the small numbers of control and treated animals.]

Groups of 50 male and 50 female CDF_1 mice, weighing 20-25 g, were fed diets containing 800 or 4000 mg/kg AF-2 [purity unspecified] for 18 months, followed by a control diet for 6 months. A group of 50 mice of each sex served as controls. The estimated total cumulative doses of AF-2 per mouse were 6.0 g to high-dose males, 4.0 g to high-dose females, 1.2 g to low-dose males and 1.1 g to low-dose females. The numbers of mice surviving >300 days were 43, 38 and 42 males and 42, 39 and 40 females in the control, low-dose and high-dose groups, respectively. Increases in tumour incidence were observed for the following neoplasms: (a) benign forestomach neoplasms in 0/43 control males, 2/38 low-dose males, 15/42 high-dose males, 0/42 control females, 2/39 low-dose females, and 17/40 high-dose females; malignant forestomach tumours in 14/42 high-dose males and 6/40 females; (b) metastases to liver, lymph nodes, spleen and peritoneal cavity of malignant tumours in 5/14 high-dose males and 3/6 females; and (c) tumours of unspecified type of the oral cavity in 2/42 high-dose males and 2/40 females (Takayama & Kuwabara, 1977a).

Groups of 50 male and 50 female ICR/JCL mice, eight weeks of age, were fed diets containing 800 or 4000 mg/kg AF-2 (purity, 99.66%) for about 440 days. A group of 25 males and 65 females served as controls. The numbers of mice surviving more than three months in the control, low-dose and high-dose groups were 22, 46 and 46 males, and 62, 42 and 50 females, respectively. The following increases in tumour incidence were observed: (a) a dose-related increase in the incidence of benign and malignant forestomach tumours in 0/22 control males, 15/46 low-dose males, 34/46 high-dose males; 0/62 controls females, 13/42 low-dose females and 36/50 high-dose females; (b) a dose-related increase in the incidence of forestomach squamous-cell carcinomas in 0/22 control males, 1/46 low-dose males, 25/46 high-dose males; 0/62 control females, 1/42 low-dose females and 25/50 high-dose females; and (c) a non-significant increase in the incidence of leukaemia in 2/62 control females, 5/42 low-dose females, and 5/50 high-dose females [p = 0.08] (Yokoro et al., 1977).

Rat: A group of 29 weanling female Sprague-Dawley rats, weighing 40-70 g, were fed a diet containing AF-2 (melting-point, 151-152°, with no impurities detected by paper or thin-layer chromatography) at a level of 2000 mg/kg for 46 weeks, followed by a control diet until termination of the study at 66 weeks (estimated total cumulative dose per rat, 10.1 g). The dose was selected on the basis of a range-finding study. A group of 29 weanling female rats served as matched controls. All rats in the treated and control groups were alive at 20 weeks; at the end of the study, 28% of treated and 93% of control rats were still alive. A statistically significant (p < 0.001) increase in the incidence of mammary tumours was seen: 2/29 in controls and 24/29 in treated animals; 17 of the latter were solitary tumours and 7 were multiple. The mean number of mammary tumours per tumour-bearing rat was 2.2 (1.0 in controls). The mammary tumours that occurred in treated rats were 15 adenocarcinomas and 9 fibroadenomas; the two in controls were fibroadenomas (Cohen et al., 1977).

Groups of 50 male and 50 female Wistar rats, weighing 110-120 g, were fed diets containing 800 or 4000 mg/kg AF-2 [purity unspecified] for 18 months, followed by a control diet for 6 months. A group of 50 rats of each sex served as controls. The estimated total cumulative doses of AF-2 per rat were: 13 g for high-dose males and 15 g for females, 6 g for low-dose males and 5 g for females. Body weight gain was reduced in high-dose male and female rats. The numbers of rats surviving >280 days were 47, 42 and 43 males and 48, 48 and 47 females in the control, low-dose and high-dose groups, respectively. Increases in tumour incidence were observed for the following neoplasms: (a) benign and malignant mammary tumours in 0/47 control males, 1/42 low-dose males, 3/43 high-dose males, 3/48 control females, 17/48 low-dose females and 37/47 high-dose females, most of which were adenocarcinomas and were multiple in treated rats; (b) forestomach papillomas in 0/47 control males, 1/42 low-dose males, 10/43 high-dose males, 0/48 control females, 1/48 low-dose females and 12/47 high-dose females. In the high-dose group, a non-significant increase in the incidence of haemangioendothelial sarcomas of the liver was found in 3/43 males and 3/47 females. These tumours did not occur in controls (Takayama & Kuwabara, 1977a,b).

Hamster: A group of 16 male golden hamsters, four weeks of age, were fed a diet containing 2500 mg/kg AF-2 (purity, 99.66%) for up to 565 days (estimated maximum cumulative dose per hamster, 14.1 g). A group of 10 male hamsters served as controls and were observed for 580 days. Body weight gain of treated hamsters was slightly reduced. Increases in tumour incidences were observed for the following neoplasms: (a) forestomach papillomas and squamous-cell carcinomas in 0/7 controls and 11/13 treated animals (7 carcinomas); and (b) a number of other tumours (4 oesophageal papillomas, 6 bile duct adenomas, and 2 lung adenomas) found in treated but not control rats (Sano *et al.*, 1977). [The Working Group noted the small numbers of control and treated animals.]

Groups of 25 male and 25 female golden hamsters, four weeks of age, were fed diets containing 800 or 1600 mg/kg AF-2 (purity, 99.66%) for up to 660 days. Groups of 20 hamsters of each sex served as controls. The estimated total cumulative dose of AF-2 per hamster was: 5.3 g for high-dose males and 4.7 g for females; 2.5 g for low-dose males and 2.4 g for females. Body weight gains of treated hamsters were similar to those of controls. The numbers of hamsters surviving >444 days were 19, 20 and 17 males and 16, 17 and 17 females in the control, low-dose and high-dose groups, respectively. Increases in tumour incidence were observed for the following neoplasms: (a) a dose-related increase in the incidence of benign and malignant forestomach tumours in animals of both sexes: males - 0/19 controls, 13/20 low-dose, 17/17 high-dose; females - 0/16 controls, 10/17 low-dose, 13/17 high-dose [$p < 0.001$]; (b) a statistically significant dose-related increased incidence [$p < 0.05$] of forestomach squamous-cell carcinomas in males: control, 0/19; low-dose, 3/20; high-dose, 8/17 [$p < 0.001$]; and (c) an increase in the incidence of oesophageal tumours in males in the high-dose group: 6 (1 squamous-cell carcinoma)/17; controls, 0/19 [$p = 0.006$] (Kinebuchi *et al.*, 1979).

(b) Subcutaneous administration

Mouse: Groups of 57 male and 51 female ICR/Jcl mice, 21 days of age, received three s.c. injections on days 21, 22 and 23 after birth of 50 μg/g bw AF-2 [purity unspecified] dissolved in propylene glycol. Solvent control groups of 61 males and 56 females were established. When mice were killed 27 weeks after treatment, a statistically significant ($p < 0.001$) increased incidence of lung adenomas (controls, 2/92; treated, 16/55) was observed in mice of both sexes combined (Nomura, 1975).

(c) Perinatal exposure

Mouse: A group of 16 pregnant ICR/Jcl mice, 10 weeks of age, received three s.c. injections on days 13, 15 and 17 of gestation of 50 μg/g bw AF-2 [purity unspecified] dissolved in propylene glycol. A solvent control group of 7 pregnant mice was established. Offspring were separated from mothers four weeks after birth and were killed at week 32 after birth. A statistically significant ($p < 0.02$) increased incidence of lung adenomas (controls, 2/75; treated, 7/41) was observed (Nomura, 1975).

3.2 Other relevant biological data

(a) *Experimental systems*

Toxic effects

The oral LD_{50} of AF-2 is 475 mg/kg bw in female ICR/Jcl mice, 1554 mg/kg bw in Donryu rats (Miyaji, 1971a) and 340 mg/kg bw in Fischer rats (Sodemoto & Enomoto, 1976).

The main acute toxic effect following oral administration of 120-300 mg/kg bw AF-2 to mice was centrilobular necrosis of the liver. This effect was dose-dependent and was reduced by pretreatment with phenobarbital (Horiuchi et al., 1976).

Mice fed diets containing 0.8 or 1.6% AF-2 for 60 days showed lymphoid atrophy and hepatic swelling. All animals fed the highest concentration had died by the end of the fifth week. Some mice given diets containing 0.08 or 0.4% AF-2 for 440 days developed glomerulonephritic lesions (Yokoro et al., 1977). Weanling mice fed diets containing 0.5% AF-2 for six weeks had enlarged livers showing marked cellular degeneration; this effect was increased by high-protein diets (Yanagida et al., 1976).

Male rats fed diets containing 0.4% AF-2 showed atrophy of skeletal muscles within 12 months (Takayama & Kuwabara, 1977a,b). Rats given diets containing 0.2% AF-2 for four weeks showed hypertrophy of the liver with an accumulation of rough endoplasmic reticulum. The hypertrophy was found to be reversible when the chronic treatment was discontinued (Miyaji, 1971a). Feeding of Wistar rats with a diet containing 0.1-0.2% AF-2 reduced the hepatic content of cytochrome P-450 and decreased aminopyrine *N*-demethylase and aniline hydroxylase activities after only one day of treatment (Fukuhara & Takabatake, 1975, 1977). Addition of 0.05 mM also decreased the activities of these enzymes in liver microsomes *in vitro* (Fukuhara & Takabatake, 1977).

When AF-2 was given as a single s.c dose of 0.5 or 1.0 mg/kg bw simultaneously with an antigen, it suppressed the immune response in mice. When administered at a dose of 1.0 mg/kg bw eight or 23 h before or 24 h after the antigen, it augmented antibody response (Sawada & Matsuoka, 1976).

Effects on reproduction and prenatal toxicity

After a single oral dose of 20 mg/kg bw ^{14}C-labelled AF-2 to rats on day 20 of pregnancy, 0.4% of the radioactivity was detected in the foetuses (Tanaka et al., 1976a,b).

No significant teratogenic effect was observed in mice that received single oral doses of up to 313 mg/kg bw AF-2 on day 10 of pregnancy or diets containing up to 0.5% AF-2 on days 7-18 of gestation (Imahori, 1975). In four-generation studies, no effect was observed in mice or rats given diets containing 0.0125% AF-2 (Miyaji, 1971b). Similarly, foetuses of mice receiving dietary levels of up to 0.2% AF-2 showed no effects, although growth retardation was observed in foetuses of dams fed 0.6% AF-2 (Tanaka et al., 1976a,b).

In a group of 16 ICR/Jcl mice given 50 mg/kg bw AF-2 subcutaneously on days 13, 15 and 17 of pregnancy, there was a significant decrease in the number of live births (p < 0.001): only one-third of them lived to the adult stage (Nomura, 1975). In further experiments, 18 pregnant ICR/Jcl mice received daily s.c. injections of 40 mg/kg bw phenobarbital from days 4-8 of gestation and a single s.c. dose of 100 mg/kg bw AF-2 on day 10. Ten mice receiving AF-2 without phenobarbital-pretreatment and 14 phenobar-bital-pretreated mice served as controls. AF-2 induced late foetal deaths only in phenobarbital-pretreated animals; there was a significant increase in the incidence of malformations, including dwarfism and anomalies of the fingers, tail and palate in foetuses of pretreated mothers (Nomura & Kondo, 1976; Nomura et al., 1976).

Absorption, distribution, excretion and metabolism

Following an oral dose of 1.3 mg/kg bw ^{14}C-AF-2 to rats, 83% of the radioactivity was excreted in the faeces and 21% in the urine within 48 hours (Tatsumi et al., 1973a).

AF-2 is metabolized in the rat in the small and large intestine; 70% was degraded during incubation with small-intestinal mucosa for 2 h (Tatsumi et al., 1973a).

Reduction of the nitro group of AF-2 occurs in the small-intestinal mucosae; this reaction has been shown to be catalysed by milk, by rat liver xanthine oxidase and by rat liver microsomes in the presence of an electron donor (Akao et al., 1971; Tatsumi et al., 1973b, 1976, 1978). In the presence of the latter two enzyme systems, AF-2 is converted to 2-(2-furyl)-3-(5-oxo-2-pyrrolin-2-yl)acrylamide. It has been suggested that this product is derived from a 5-amino derivative of AF-2 by ring-cleavage and cyclization (Tatsumi et al., 1976; Swaminathan & Lower, 1978).

The binding of metabolites of AF-2 to proteins in the presence of xanthine oxidase is reduced in the presence of cysteine or glutathione (Tatsumi et al., 1978). The active intermediate(s) may be the N-hydroxylamine derivative, but it has not been identified (Tatsumi et al., 1976). The existence of this pathway is supported by the isolation of 2-(β-carboxypropionyl)-3-(5-methylthio-2-furyl) acrylamide in the urine of rabbits administered 100 mg/kg bw ^{14}C-AF-2 (Ou et al., 1977).

Mutagenicity and other short-term tests

The mutagenicity of nitrofurans, including AF-2, was reviewed by Tazima et al. (1975) and by Klemencic and Wang (1978). Unless otherwise specified, the assays described below were carried out under aerobic conditions.

AF-2 was positive in a *rec* assay in *Bacillus subtilis* (Kada, 1973) and was positive in DNA repair tests in *Salmonella typhimurium* and *Escherichia coli* (Yahagi et al., 1974). It was strongly mutagenic in *S. typhimurium* strains TA98 and TA100 (McCann et al., 1975), but not in strains TA1535, TA1536, TA1537 or TA1538 (Yahagi et al., 1974; McCann et al., 1975). It was, however, mutagenic to TA1535 in a fluctuation test (Green et al., 1977).

Studies of point mutations in *E. coli* strains deficient in excision repair and error-prone repair indicate that the mutagenic mechanism of AF-2 mimics that of ultra-violet light. Excision repair-deficient strains give a greater mutagenic response than wild types; the mutations are induced almost entirely by error-prone and rec A-lex A-dependent misrepair of unexcised lesions (Kondo & Ichikawa-Ryo, 1973; Green et al., 1977; Bryant & McCalla, 1980).

Mutagenicity studies with nitroreductase-deficient strains of *S. typhimurium* (Wang & Lee, 1976) and *E. coli* (Bryant & McCalla, 1980) show that the mutagenicity of AF-2 is due primarily to metabolites formed after reduction by aerobic as well as anaerobic nitroreductase. In-vitro activation of AF-2 by xanthine oxidase has also been demonstrated under aerobic and anaerobic conditions, and the active metabolites were found to bind covalently to DNA (Matsushima *et al.*, 1976; Tatsumi *et al.*, 1977).

The urine of rats fed 0.5% AF-2 in the diet for four days was mutagenic to *S. typhimurium* TA100. No increase in mutagenicity was obtained by treatment of the urine samples with β-glucuronidase (Wang & Lee, 1976).

AF-2 was mutagenic (Shahin & von Borstel, 1976) and caused mitotic recombination (Shahin, 1975) in *Saccharomyces cerevisiae*. It caused a dose-related increase in forward mutations at the ad-3 locus of *Neurospora crassa* (Ong & Shahin, 1974). Characterization of such AF-2-induced mutations revealed that the majority are point mutations, and very few, if any, are multilocus deletions (Ong & de Serres, 1981).

Tazima and Onimaru (1974) reported in an abstract that an increased number of egg colour mutants were induced in the silkworm after treatment of developing oocytes by injection of pupae with AF-2. Similar treatment of spermatozoa in pupae resulted in an increased mutation rate only when tested with a rat liver activation system (Murakami *et al.*, 1976).

Blijleven *et al.* (1977) measured sex-linked recessive lethals in *Drosophila melanogaster* after feeding adult males 0.5-2 mM AF-2. In two out of four experiments, a small but significant increase was recorded. No increase was recorded after feeding larvae 4 mM AF-2 or injecting adult males with 0.4 mM.

AF-2 induced a dose-related increase of chromatid aberrations in cultured human lymphocytes and unscheduled DNA synthesis in cultured human fibroblasts. No effect of AF-2 on unscheduled DNA synthesis was seen in fibroblasts from a xeroderma pigmentosum patient (Tonomura & Sasaki, 1973). This compound induced sister chromatid exchanges in a human lymphoblastoid cell line (Tohda *et al.*, 1980).

Chromatid aberrations were recorded in metaphases of C3H mouse mammary carcinoma cells after treatment with 0.05 and 0.1 mM AF-2 (Umeda *et al.*, 1975). In a Chinese hamster fibroblast cell line, a weak but suggestive increase in the incidence of chromatid aberrations was observed after treatment with 0.04 mM AF-2 (Ishidate & Odashima, 1977). The addition of a 9000 x *g* supernatant of rat liver had no effect (Matsuoka *et al.*, 1979).

AF-2 has also been shown to cause an increase in mutations to 8-azaguanine resistance in C3H mouse mammary carcinoma cells (Umeda *et al.*, 1975) and in V79 hamster cells (Wild, 1975). Nakamura *et al.* (1977), using L5178Y mouse lymphoma cells, found an increase in the incidence of reverse mutations to alanine independence and of forward mutations to methotrexate resistance, but only in the presence of a 9000 x *g* supernatant fraction from rat liver.

The ability of AF-2 to induce 8-azaguanine- and ouabain-resistant mutations was much greater under hypoxic than under aerobic conditions in Chinese hamster V79 cells. The toxicity of AF-2 under hypoxic conditions was also increased in both human fibroblasts and hamster V79 cells; human cells were consistently more sensitive to the compound than hamster cells (McCalla *et al.*, 1978).

Fibroblasts from xeroderma pigmentosum patients, but not from ataxia telangiectasia patients, were clearly more sensitive to AF-2 toxicity than normal human fibroblasts. These findings are consistent with data on bacteria which indicate that AF-2 lesions are repaired by the same pathway as are lesions induced by ultra-violet radiation, but not by the same pathway as those induced by X-rays (McCalla et al., 1978).

AF-2 caused neoplastic transformation of secondary cultures of Syrian hamster embryo fibroblasts (Nishi et al., 1977) and of Syrian hamster embryo cells (Pienta, et al., 1978). The tumorigenicity of transformed cells was confirmed by injecting them into hamsters (Nishi et al., 1977; Pienta et al., 1978).

Transplacental treatment of Syrian hamster embryos in vivo with 20, 50 or 100 mg/kg bw AF-2 injected intraperitoneally gave rise to a significant increase in the incidence of morphological transformations in subsequently cultured embryo cells, some of which produced tumours when tested in hamster cheek pouches. The embryo cells from treated mothers also showed a dose-related increase in the incidence of chromatid aberrations (Inui et al., 1978a). Inui et al. (1976) have also shown that transplacental treatment with AF-2 produces a dose-related increase in the incidence of 8-azaguanine- and 6-thioguanine-resistant mutations, the frequency of which was higher when AF-2 was distributed transplacentally in vivo than when it was applied directly to embryonic cells. The transplacental effect of AF-2 on chromosomal aberrations was enhanced by treatment of the mother with phenobarbital (Nishi et al., 1978). Oral administration of 20 mg/kg bw AF-2 to mothers induced chromosomal aberrations in hamster embryo cells; 8-azaguanine- and 6-thioguanine-resistant mutations were induced with 2 mg/kg bw (Inui et al., 1978b).

AF-2 given intraperitoneally to male rats induced a dose-related increase in the incidence of chromosomal aberrations in bone-marrow cells (Sugiyama et al., 1975). The lowest effective dose was 15 mg/kg bw.

A test on bone-marrow reticulocytes of male rats, with i.p. injection of 60-240 mg/kg bw AF-2, revealed a significant increase in micronuclei at the highest dose when half of the dose was given 30 hours and half 6 hours before sacrifice (Goodman et al., 1977).

No increase in the incidence of dominant lethal mutations was observed in DBA/2J male mice administered 300-450 mg/kg bw AF-2 by gavage (Soares & Sheridan, 1975), nor in a second study in which male mice received 76 and 513 mg/kg bw AF-2 orally (Tutikawa & Kada, 1975).

(b) Humans

No data were available to the Working Group.

3.3 Case reports and epidemiological studies of carcinogenicity in humans

In a descriptive epidemiological study in Japan, Hirayama (1978) examined the correlation in twelve geographic districts between estimated per-caput consumption of AF-2 and dietary fat (reportedly based on a national nutritional survey) in 1968 and the proportional increase in age-adjusted breast cancer mortality rates from 1969 to 1974. There was an apparently strong positive correlation of the breast cancer variable with each of the estimated intakes of animal fat and AF-2, with each analysis controlled [presumably] for the effect of the other factor. [No information was given about the method of estimating per-caput AF-2 intake, nor about possible confounding effects of other factors (dietary or otherwise) upon these correlation analyses. Further, the brief time lapse allowed between exposure and cancer death (1968 to 1969-1974) may not be etiologically appropriate.]

4. Summary of Data Reported and Evaluation

4.1 Experimental data

AF-2 was tested for carcinogenicity in three experiments in mice, in two experiments in rats and in two experiments in hamsters by administration in the diet. It produced benign and malignant forestomach tumours in mice of both sexes, benign and malignant mammary tumours and forestomach papillomas in rats of both sexes and benign and malignant forestomach tumours in hamsters of both sexes and oesophageal tumours in male hamsters. In one experiment in weanling mice by subcutaneous injection, it produced lung tumours. It produced multiple lung tumours in the offspring of mice treated subcutaneously during pregnancy.

AF-2 induced DNA damage in bacteria and in human cells and mutations in bacteria, fungi, insects and mammalian cells *in vivo* and *in vitro*. It caused chromosomal anomalies in mammalian cells, including human cells. AF-2 caused neoplastic transformation in hamster cells. There is *sufficient evidence* that AF-2 is active in short-term tests.

AF-2 induced foetal deaths in mice and was teratogenic to survivors of dams pretreated with phenobarbital.

4.2 Human data

AF-2 has been used in Japan since at least 1965, but it is not used presently. Its use as a food preservative was a source of exposure for the general population.

No data were available to assess the teratogenicity or chromosomal effects of this compound in humans.

The one available epidemiological study in which a regional correlation between AF-2 consumption and breast cancer mortality was analysed was considered inadequate to evaluate the carcinogenicity of AF-2.

4.3 Evaluation

The epidemiological data were inadequate to evaluate the carcinogenicity of AF-2 to humans.

There is *sufficient evidence*[1] for the carcinogenicity of AF-2 in experimental animals.

---

[1]In the absence of adequate data on humans, it is reasonable, for practical purposes, to regard chemicals for which there is sufficient evidence of carcinogenicity in animals as if they presented a carcinogenic risk to humans.

5. References

Akao, M., Kuroda, K. & Miyaki, K. (1971) Metabolic degradations of nitrofurans by rat liver homogenate. *Biochem. Pharmacol.*, *20*, 3091-3096

Blijleven, W.G.H., Kortselius, M.J.H. & Kramers, P.G.N. (1977) Mutagenicity testing of H-193, AF-2 and furazolidone in *Drosophila melanogaster. Mutat. Res.*, *56*, 95-100

Bryant, D.W. & McCalla, D.R. (1980) Nitrofuran induced mutagenesis and error prone repair in *Escherichia coli. Chem.-biol. Interactions*, *31*, 151-166

Cohen, S.M., Ichikawa, M. & Bryan, G.T. (1977) Carcinogenicity of 2-(2-furyl)-3-(5-nitro-2-furyl)acrylamide (AF-2) fed to female Sprague-Dawley rats. *Gann*, *68*, 473-476

Fukuhara, M. & Takabatake, E. (1975) The effect of AF$_2$[2-(2-furyl)-3-(5-nitro-2-furyl)acrylamide] on hepatic microsomal mixed function oxidase system in rats. *Chem. pharm. Bull.*, *23*, 1626-1628

Fukuhara, M. & Takabatake, E. (1977) The effects of nitrofuran derivatives on hepatic microsomal mixed-function oxidase activity in rats. *Toxicol. appl. Pharmacol.*, *42*, 571-581

Goodman, D.R., Hakkinen, P.J., Nemenzo, J.H. & Vore, M. (1977) Mutagenic evaluation of nitrofuran derivatives in *Salmonella typhimurium*, by the micronucleus test, and by *in vivo* cytogenetics. *Mutat. Res.*, *48*, 295-306

Green, M.H.L., Rogers, A.M., Muriel, W.J., Ward, A.C. & McCalla, D.R. (1977) Use of simplified fluctuation test to detect and characterize mutagenesis by nitrofurans. *Mutat. Res.*, *44*, 139-143

Hirayama, T. (1978) Epidemiology of breast cancer with special reference to the role of diet. *Prev. Med.*, *7*, 173-195

Horiuchi, T., Ohtsubo, K.-I. & Saito, M. (1976) Furylfuramide-induced hepatic necrosis in mice and its modification by phenobarbital. *Jpn. J. exp. Med.*, *46*, 111-121

Ikeda, I., Horiuchi, S., Furuyama, T., Uchida, O., Suzuki, K. & Azegami, J. (1974) *Induction of Gastric Tumors in Mice by Feeding of Furylfuramide* (Jpn.). Food Sanitation Council, Ministry of Health and Welfare, Japan, August

Imahori, A. (1975) Effects of furylfuramide on pregnant mice and fetuses. *J. Food Hyg. Soc. Jpn*, *16*, 301-306

Inui, N., Taketomi, M. & Nishi, Y. (1976) Mutagenic effects of AF-2, a food additive, on embryonic cells of the Syrian golden hamster on transplacental application. *Mutat. Res.*, *41*, 351-360

Inui, N., Nishi, Y. & Taketomi, M. (1978a) Chromosome breakage and neoplastic transformation of Syrian golden hamster embryonic cells in tissue culture by transplacental application of 2-(2-furyl)-3-(5-nitro-2-furyl)acrylamide (AF-2). *Mutat. Res.*, *58*, 331-338

Inui, N., Nishi, Y. & Taketomi, M. (1978b) Mutagenic effect of orally given AF-2 on embryonic cells in pregnant Syrian hamsters. *Mutat. Res.*, *57*, 69-75

Ishidate, M., Jr & Odashima, S. (1977) Chromosome tests with 134 compounds on Chinese hamster cells *in vitro* - A screening for chemical carcinogens. *Mutat. Res.*, *48*, 337-354

Kada, T. (1973) *Escherichia coli* mutagenicity of furylfuramide. *Jpn. J. Genet.*, *48*, 301-305

Kanno, S. & Okumiya, T. (1963) Studies on analysis of nitrofuran derivatives. IV. Differential colorimetric determination of nitrofurylacrylamide, α-furyl-β-(5-nitro-2-furyl)-acrylamide, and nitrofurazone. *Shokuhin Eiseigaku Zasshi*, *4*, 198-204 (*Chem. Abstr.*, *60*, 9913c)

Kanno, S., Takuma, M., Watanabe, S. & Murai, A. (1966) Analysis of food additives. X. Determination of 2-(2-furyl)-3-(5-nitro-2-furyl)acrylamide in foods by a new colorimetric method (Jpn.). *Shokuhin Eiseigaku Zasshi*, *7*, 140-144 (*Chem. Abstr.*, *65*, 14329g)

Kinebuchi, M., Kawachi, T., Matsukura, N. & Sugimura, T. (1979) Further studies on the carcinogenicity of a food additive, AF-2, in hamsters. *Food Cosmet. Toxicol.*, *17*, 339-341

Klemencic, J.M. & Wang, C.Y. (1978) *Mutagenicity of nitrofurans*. In: Bryan, G.T., ed., *Carcinogenesis - A Comprehensive Survey*, Vol. 4, *Nitrofurans: Chemistry, Metabolism, Mutagenesis, and Carcinogenesis*, New York, Raven Press, pp. 99-130

Kondo, S. & Ichikawa-Ryo, H. (1973) Testing and classification of mutagenicity of furylfuramide in *Escherichia coli*. *Jpn. J. Genet.*, *48*, 295-300

Matsuoka, A., Hayashi, M. & Ishidate, M., Jr (1979) Chromosomal aberration tests on 29 chemicals combined with S9 mix *in vitro*. *Mutat. Res.*, *66*, 277-290

Matsushima, T., Takeuchi, M., Nagao, M., Yahagi, T. & Sugimura, T. (1976) *Metabolism and binding of nitrofuran, 2-(2-furyl-3-(5-nitro-2-furyl)acrylamide*. In: de Serres, F.J., Fouts, J.R. & Philpot, R.M., eds, *In vitro Metabolic Activation in Mutagenesis Testing*, Amsterdam, Elsevier/North-Holland Biomedical Press, pp. 81-84

McCalla, D.R., Arlett, C.R. & Broughton, B. (1978) The action of AF 2 on cultured hamster and human cells under aerobic and hypoxic conditions. *Chem.-biol. Interactions*, *21*, 89-102

McCann, J., Spingarn, N.E., Kobori, J. & Ames, B.N. (1975) Detection of carcinogens as mutagens: Bacterial tester strains with R factor plasmids. *Proc. natl Acad. Sci. USA*, *72*, 979-983

Miyaji, T. (1971a) Acute and chronic toxicity of furylfuramide in rats and mice. *Tohoku J. exp. Med.*, *103*, 331-369

Miyaji, T. (1971b) Effect of furylfuramide on reproduction and malformation. *Tohoku J. exp. Med.*, *103*, 381-388

Murakami, A., Murota, T., Shimada, Y., & Tazima, Y. (1976) Further studies on the genetic effects of furylfuramide on mature spermatozoa in the silkworm (Abstract no. 13). *Mutat. Res.*, *38*, 342-343

Nakamura, N., Suzuki, N. & Okada, S. (1977) Mutagenicity of furylfuramide, a food preservative, tested by using alanine-requiring mouse L5178Y cells *in vitro* and *in vivo*. *Mutat. Res.*, *46*, 355-364

Nishi, Y., Taketomi, M. & Inui, N. (1977) Neoplastic transformation induced by furylfuramide and nitromethylfuran of embryonic hamster cells in tissue culture. *Int. J. Cancer*, *20*, 607-615

Nishi, Y., Taketomi, M. & Inui, N. (1978) An enhancing effect of phenobarbital and 2-(2-furyl)-3-(5-nitro-2-furyl)acrylamide (AF-2) on Syrian hamster chromsomes by combined transplacental application. *Jpn. J. Genet.*, *53*, 59-62

Nomura, T. (1975) Carcinogenicity of the food additive furylfuramide in foetal and young mice. *Nature*, *258*, 610-611

Nomura, T. & Kondo, S. (1976) The enhancement effect of phenobarbital on toxicity of furylfuramide in mouse embryo. *Mutat. Res.*, *35*, 167-172

Nomura, T., Kimura, S., Isa, Y., Tanaka, H. & Sakamoto, Y. (1976) Teratogenic effects of some antimicrobial agents on mouse embryo (Abstract). *Teratology*, *14*, 250

Nose, N. & Okitsu, T. (1968) Simple method for the separation of furylfuramide in foods (Jpn.). *Shokuhin Eiseigaku Zasshi*, *9*, 374-378 (*Chem. Abstr. 70*, 66850d)

Ong, T.-M. & de Serres, F.J. (1981) Genetic analysis of *ad-3* mutants induced by AF-2 and two other nitrofurans in *Neurospora crassa*. *Environ. Mutagenesis*, *3*, 151-158

Ong, T.-M. & Shahin, M.M. (1974) Mutagenic and recombinogenic activities of the food additive furylfuramide in eukaryotes. *Science*, *184*, 1086-1087

Ou, T., Tatsumi, K. & Yoshimura, H. (1977) Isolation and identification of urinary metabolites of AF-2 [3-(5-nitro-2-furyl)-2-(2-furyl) acrylamide] in rabbits. *Biochem. biophys. Res. Commun.*, *75*, 401-405

Pienta, R.J., Lebherz, W.B., III & Takayama, S. (1978) Malignant transformation of cryopreserved early passage Syrian golden hamster cells by 2-(2-furyl)-3-(5-nitro-2-furyl)-acrylamide. *Cancer Lett.*, *5*, 245-251

Saikachi, H. & Kanehira, O. (1962) Nitrofuranacrylic derivatives. *U.S. Patent 3,031,447* (to Masajiro Ueno) (*Chem. Abstr.*, *57*, 9819a)

Sano, T., Kawachi, T., Matsukura, N., Sasajima, K. & Sugimura, T. (1977) Carcinogenicity of a food additive, AF-2, in hamsters and mice. *Z. Krebsforsch.*, *89*, 61-68

Sawada, H. & Matsuoka, Y. (1976) Effect of a nitrofuran derivative (AF-2) on the immune response of mice. *Gann*, *67*, 693-701

de Serres, F.J. (1974) AF-2 - Food preservative or genetic hazard? *Mutat. Res.*, *26*, 1-2

Shahin, M.M. (1975) Genetic activity of niridazole in yeast. *Mutat. Res., 30,* 191-198

Shahin, M.M. & von Borstel, R.C. (1976) Genetic activity of the antimicrobial food additives AF-2 and H-193 in *Saccharomyces cerevisiae. Mutat. Res., 38,* 215-224

Soares, E.R. & Sheridan, W. (1975) Lack of induction of dominant lethals in mice by orally administered AF-2. *Mutat. Res., 31,* 235-240

Sodemoto, Y. & Enomoto, M. (1976) Acute toxicity of chemical carcinogens. 2. Comparative toxic effect of chemical compounds in rats. *St. Marianna med. J., 4,* 77-90

Sugiyama,T., Goto, K. & Uenaka, H. (1975) Acute cytogenetic effect of 2-(2-furyl)-3-(5-nitro-2-furyl)acrylamide (AF-2, a food preservative) on rat bone marrow cells *in vivo. Mutat. Res., 31,* 241-246

Swaminathan, S. & Lower, G.M., Jr (1978) *Biotransformations and excretion of nitrofurans.* In: Bryan, G.T., ed., *Carcinogenesis - A Comprehensive Survey,* Vol. 4, *Nitrofurans: Chemistry, Metabolism, Mutagenesis and Carcinogenesis,* New York, Raven Press, pp. 59-97

Takayama, S. & Kuwabara, N. (1977a) Carcinogenic activity of 2-(2-furyl)-3-(5-nitro-2-furyl)acrylamide, a food additive, in mice and rats. *Cancer Lett., 3,* 115-120

Takayama, S. & Kuwabara, N. (1977b) The production of skeletal muscle atrophy and mammary tumors in rats by feeding 2-(2-furyl)-3-(5-nitro-2-furyl)acrylamide. *Toxicol. Lett., 1,* 11-16

Tanaka, S., Onoda, K., Kawashima, K., Nakaura, S., Nagao, S., Kuwamura, T. & Omori, Y. (1976a) Studies on the teratogenicity of furylfuramide on the fetuses and offspring of rat in relation to fetal distribution (Abstract). *Teratology, 14,* 257

Tanaka, S., Onoda, K., Kawashima, K., Nakaura, S., Nagao, S., Kuwamura, T. & Omori, Y. (1976b) Studies on the teratogenicity of furylfuramide in fetuses and offspring of rats in relation to fetal distribution. *J. toxicol. Sci., 2,* 149-159

Tatsumi, K., Ou, T., Yoshimura, H. & Tsukamoto, H. (1971) Metabolism of drugs. LXXIII. The metabolic fate of nitrofuran derivatives. (1). Studies on the absorption and excretion. *Chem. pharm. Bull., 19,* 330-334

Tatsumi, K., Ou, T., Yamaguchi, T. & Yoshimura, H. (1973a) Metabolism of drugs. LXXIX. The metabolic fate of nitrofuran derivatives. (2). Degradation by small intestinal mucosa and absorption from gastrointestinal tract. *Chem. pharm. Bull., 21,* 191-201

Tatsumi, K., Yamaguchi, T. & Yoshimura, H. (1973b) Metabolism of drugs. LXXX. The metabolic fate of nitrofuran derivatives. (3). Studies on enzymes in small intestinal mucosa of rat catalysing degradation of nitrofuran derivatives. *Chem. pharm. Bull., 21,* 622-628

Tatsumi, K., Yamaguchi,T. & Yoshimura, H. (1975) Metabolism of drugs. LXXXVI. The metabolic fate of nitrofuran derivatives. (4). The portal absorption of nitrofuran derivatives and the absorption rate as a function of age in rats. *Chem. pharm. Bull., 23,* 1555-1560

Tatsumi, K., Kitamura, S. & Yoshimura, H. (1976) Reduction of nitrofuran derivatives by xanthine oxidase and microsomes. *Arch. Biochem. Biophys.*, *175*, 131-137

Tatsumi, K., Kitamura, S. & Yoshimura, H. (1977) Binding of nitrofuran derivatives to nucleic acids and protein. *Chem. pharm. Bull.*, *25*, 2948-2952

Tatsumi, K., Kitamura, S., Ou, T., Yamada, H. & Yoshimura, H. (1978) Studies on metabolic activation of nitrofurans: formation of active metabolites and their binding to cysteine and glutathione. *J. Pharm. Dyn.*, *1*, 105-113

Tazima, Y. (1979) Consequences of the AF-2 incident in Japan. *Environ. Health Perspect.*, *29*, 183-187

Tazima, Y. & Onimaru, K. (1974) Results of mutagenicity testing for some nitrofuran derivatives in a sensitive test system with silkworm oocytes (Abstract no. 14). *Mutat. Res.*, *26*, 440

Tazima, Y., Kada, T. & Murakami, A. (1975) Mutagenicity of nitrofuran derivatives, including furylfuramide, a food preservative. *Mutat. Res.*, *32*, 55-80

Tohda, H., Horaguchi, K., Takahashi, K., Oikawa, A. & Matsushima, T. (1980) Epstein-Barr virus-transformed human lymphoblastoid cells for study of sister chromatid exchange and their evaluation as a test system. *Cancer Res.*, *40*, 4775-4780

Tonomura, A. & Sasaki, M.S. (1973) Chromosome aberrations and DNA repair synthesis in cultured human cells exposed to nitrofurans. *Jpn. J. Genet.*, *48*, 291-294

Tutikawa, K. & Kada, T. (1975) Studies on the mutagenicity of furylfuramide: results of the host-mediated rec-assay and dominant lethal test in mice (Abstract no. 20). *Mutat. Res.*, *31*, 271

Umeda, M., Tsutsui, T., Kikyo, S. & Saito, M. (1975) Mutagenic activity of furylfuramide on cultured mouse cells. *Jpn. J. exp. Med.*, *45*, 161-170

Wang, C.Y. & Lee, L.H. (1976) Mutagenic activity of carcinogenic and noncarcinogenic nitrofurans and of urine of rats fed these compounds. *Chem.-biol. Interactions*, *15*, 69-75

Wild, D. (1975) Mutagenicity of the food additive AF-2, a nitrofuran, in *Escherichia coli* and Chinese hamster cells in culture. *Mutat. Res.*, *31*, 197-199

Yahagi, T., Nagao, M., Hara, K., Matsushima, T., Sugimura, T. & Bryan,G.T. (1974) Relationships between carcinogenic and mutagenic or DNA-modifying effects of nitrofuran derivatives, including 2-(2-furyl)-3-(5-nitro-2-furyl)acrylamide, a food additive. *Cancer Res.*, *34*, 2266-2273

Yanagida, Y., Yamamoto, K. & Imahori, A. (1976) Furylfuramide (AF-2). Toxicity of furylfuramide (AF-2) on weanling mice - Supplementary effect of casein addition to the diet (Jpn.). *Jpn. J. Nutr.*, *34*, 89-94

Yokoro, K., Kajihara, H., Kodama, Y., Nagao, K., Hamada, K. & Kinomura, A. (1977) Chronic toxicity of 2-(2-furyl)-3-(5-nitro-2-furyl)acrylamide (AF-2) in mice, with special reference to carcinogenicity in the forestomach. *Gann*, *68*, 825-828

AGARITINE (L-GLUTAMIC ACID-5-[2-(4-HYDROXYMETHYL)-PHENYLHYDRAZIDE])

1. Chemical and Physical Data

1.1 Synonyms and trade names

Chem. Abstr. Services Reg. No.: 2757-90-6

Chem. Abstr. Name: L-Glutamic acid, 5-[2-[4-(hydroxymethyl)phenyl]hydrazide]

IUPAC Systematic Name: L-Glutamic acid, 5-[2-(α-hydroxy-*para*-tolyl)hydrazide]

Synonyms: β-*N*-[γ-L(+)glutamyl]4-hydroxymethylphenylhydrazine

1.2 Structural and molecular formulae and molecular weight

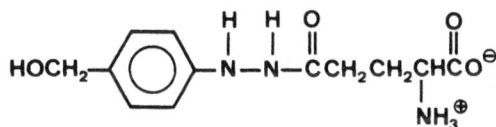

$$HOCH_2 - \bigcirc - \overset{H}{\underset{|}{N}} - \overset{H}{\underset{|}{N}} - \overset{O}{\overset{\|}{C}} CH_2 CH_2 \overset{}{\underset{\underset{NH_3^\oplus}{|}}{C}}HCO^\ominus$$

$C_{12}H_{17}N_3O_4$

Mol. wt: 267.3

1.3 Chemical and physical properties of the pure substance

From Windholz (1976) and Levenberg (1964)

(a) *Description*: Colourless crystals

(b) *Melting-point*: 203-208°C (dec. without melting)

(c) *Optical rotation*: $[\alpha]_D^{25}$ + 6° (c = 1.1 in water)

(d) *Spectroscopy data*: λ_{max} (water) 237.5 nm, A_1^1 = 449; 280 nm, A_1^1 = 52. Infrared and nuclear magnetic resonance spectral data have been reported.

(e) *Solubility*: Very soluble in water; practically insoluble in most anhydrous organic solvents

(f) *Stability*: Stable in solid state; sensitive to oxidation

(g) *Reactivity*: Rapidly oxidized by a variety of oxidants; hydrolysed by hydrochloric acid to L-glutamic acid

1.4 Technical products and impurities

No data were available to the Working Group.

2. Production, Use, Occurrence and Analysis

2.1 Production and use

(a) *Production*

Agaritine occurs naturally in mushrooms. It was first isolated and its structure determined in the early 1960s by Levenberg (1960, 1961, 1964); he isolated it from the cultivated, commonly eaten mushroom *Agaricus bisporus* by extraction with water or methanol and isolation from the extract by one of several methods. The first synthesis of agaritine was reported shortly thereafter (Daniels *et al.*, 1961; Kelly *et al.*, 1962). An improved method for the synthesis of agaritine was reported in 1979, which was used to produce material in amounts sufficient for biological testing (Wallcave *et al.*, 1979).

Agaritine is not produced commercially.

(b) *Use*

The mushroom *Agaricus bisporus*, in which agaritine occurs, is commonly cultivated and eaten (Wallcave *et al.*, 1979). Estimated total US consumption of *Agaricus bisporus* mushrooms was approximately 163 million kg in 1975 and increased to 213 million kg during the 1979-1980 season (US Department of Agriculture, 1980).

2.2 Occurrence

Agaritine has been isolated from the commercial edible mushroom *Agaricus bisporus* in a yield of about 0.4 g/kg fresh weight. It is found predominantly in the fruiting body of young mushrooms, and the concentration diminishes with age (Kelly *et al.*, 1962). Agaritine was also found in boiled press juice preparations, in quantities comparable to those found in *Agaricus bisporus*, in the following ten other species of the genus *Agaricus*: *argentatus*, *campestris*, *comptulis*, *crocodilinus*, *edulis*, *hortensis*, *microme-gathus*, *pattersonii*, *perrarus*, and *xanthodermus* (Levenberg, 1964).

2.3 Analysis

Methods have been reported for the analysis of agaritine in *Agaricus bisporus* by ion-exchange column chromatography, high-performance thin-layer chromatography, paper chromatography and electrophoresis (Levenberg, 1964; Chiarlo *et al.*, 1979; Oka *et al.*, 1981).

3. Biological Data Relevant to the Evaluation of Carcinogenic Risk to Humans

3.1 Carcinogenicity studies in animals

(a) Oral administration

Mouse: Groups of 50 outbred albino Swiss mice of each sex, six weeks old, were administered agaritine (purity, 98%) at a concentration of 625 mg/l in the drinking-water daily for life; a group of 50 male mice was administered 312 mg/l. Groups of 100 mice of each sex, five weeks old, served as controls. All survivors were killed at 120 weeks of age. A significant difference in the survival rate was observed between the groups: at 50 weeks of age 24/50 high-dose males, 39/50 low-dose males, 80/100 male controls, 48/50 high-dose females and 88/100 female controls were still alive. No compound-related increase in the incidence of tumours was observed (Toth *et al.*, 1981a).

(b) Carcinogenicity of derivatives of agaritine

Mouse: Groups of 50 male and 50 female albino Swiss mice, six weeks of age, received *N'*-acetyl-4-(hydroxymethyl)phenylhydrazine (purity > 97%) [a stable synthetic derivative of 4-(hydroxymethyl)phenylhydrazine, a fungal break-down product of agaritine, which contains the $HOCH_2(C_6H_4)$-NH-NH-CO- substructure of agaritine] at a concentration of 625 mg/l in the drinking-water continuously for life. Groups of 100 mice of each sex served as controls. The survival of experimental and control animals was not significantly different. The incidences of lung tumours and the average age at death in control and treated animals were as follows: males - 22/100 (22%) (70 weeks) and 24/50 (48%) (79 weeks) (p < 0.001); females - 15/100 (15%) (90 weeks) and 17/50 (34%) (90 weeks) (p < 0.007). Eight of the treated males had adenocarcinomas, and 16 had only adenomas; of the females, seven had adenocarcinomas and ten had only adenomas. Blood-vessel tumours occurred in 5/100 (5%) male and 8/100 (8%) female controls *versus* 15/50 (30%) (p < 0.001) and 16/50 (32%) (p < 0.001) treated males and females, respectively. The tumour types were specified only for the treated groups: seven males had angiomas and eight had angiosarcomas, whereas nine females had angiomas and seven had angiosarcomas (Toth *et al.*, 1978).

4-(Hydroxymethyl)benzenediazonium ion has been detected in an aqueous extract of *Agaricus bisporus*, and in-vitro tests indicate that it is also generated by an enzyme system found in *A. bisporus* which acts *in situ* and on synthetic agaritine. Groups of 50 male and 50 female Swiss mice, six weeks old, were given single weekly s.c. injections of 50 mg/kg bw 4-(hydroxymethyl)benzenediazonium tetrafluoroborate [purity unspecified] in sodium chloride for 26 weeks; an equal number of mice injected with equimolar amounts of sodium tetrafluoroborate in saline served as controls. All treated mice had died within 75 weeks; the last control died at 115 weeks. Sarcomas at the site of injection were observed in 11/50 treated females (10 fibrosarcomas) and 9/50 treated males (5 fibrosarcomas). Of the sodium tetrafluoroborate-injected controls, three females developed fibrosarcomas, two males each developed a fibrosarcoma and one a fibroma at the injection site. In addition, three treated males and nine treated females developed squamous-cell carcinomas or papillomas of the skin at the injection site. No skin tumour occurred in controls (Toth *et al.*, 1981b).

3.2 Other relevant biological data

Toxic effects

It was reported in an abstract that agaritine was given as single injections of 25, 50, 100, 200 or 400 mg/kg bw to Swiss mice. With high doses, excitation, uncoordinated running, convulsions, and paralyzed lower backs were observed. Histopathological findings included vacuolated cells in the liver and kidney tubules, oedema and desquamation of bladder epithelium and hyperaemia and haemorrhages of the lung (Toth *et al.*, 1975).

Effects on reproduction and prenatal toxicity

No data were available to the Working Group.

Absorption, distribution, excretion and metabolism

No data on agaritine itself were available.

Sporophores of *A. bisporus* contain γ-glutamyl transferase, which cleaves agaratine to L-glutamate and 4-(hydroxymethyl)phenylhydrazine (Levenberg, 1961; Gigliotti & Levenberg, 1964). This hydrolysis may also be catalysed by enzymes found in mammalian gut (Klosterman, 1974).

Two enzymic pathways in *A. bisporus* generate the 4-(hydroxymethyl)benzenediazonium ion from agaritine: (i) conversion of agaritine to 4-(hydroxymethyl)phenylhydrazine and further oxidation to the respective diazonium ion (Levenberg, 1961; Gigliotti, 1963; Gigliotti & Levenberg, 1964). (ii) conversion of agaritine to 4-(hydroxymethyl)benzenediazonium ion, without formation of the hydrazine intermediate (Ross *et al.*, 1982). These enzyme systems appear to be responsible for the occurrence of the 4-(hydroxymethyl)benzenediazonium ion at a level of 0.6 ppm in the mushroom (Ross *et al.*, 1982).

Mutagenicity and other short-term tests

A 'weak' mutagenic effect of agaritine was reported in a spot test in *Salmonella typhimurium* TA100 but not TA98. Addition of an Aroclor-induced rat liver 9000 x *g* supernatant fraction had no effect (De Flora, 1981).

(b) Humans

No data were available to the Working Group.

3.3 Case reports and epidemiological studies of carcinogenicity in humans

No data were available to the Working Group.

4. Summary of Data Reported and Evaluation

4.1 Experimental data[1]

Agaritine was tested for carcinogenicity in mice by administration in the drinking-water; no increase in the incidence of tumours was observed. *N'*-Acetyl-4-(hydroxymethyl)phenylhydrazine (a stable derivative of the hydrolysis product of agaritine) was tested in one experiment in mice by administration in the drinking-water, producing increased incidences of lung tumours and of blood-vessel tumours. 4-(Hydroxymethyl)benzenediazonium ion tetrafluoroborate (another stabilized hydrolysis product of agaritine) was tested in mice by subcutaneous injection, increasing the incidence of fibrosarcomas and of skin papillomas and carcinomas at the injection site.

---

[1]Subsequent to the meeting, the Secretariat became aware of a study in which 4-(hydroxymethyl)benzenediazonium tetrafluoroborate was administered to Swiss mice as a single intragastric instillation of 400 mg/kg bw, producing glandular stomach tumours (Toth *et al.*, 1982).

Agaritine was weakly mutagenic in *Salmonella typhimurium*. The data were *inadequate* to evaluate the activity of agaritine in short-term tests.

No data were available to evaluate the teratogenicity of agaritine to experimental animals.

4.2 Human data

Agaritine is a natural substance found in several mushrooms of the *Agaricus* species, which are eaten both raw and cooked in many parts of the world.

No data were available to evaluate the teratogenicity or chromosomal effects of this compound in humans.

No case report or epidemiological study of the carcinogenicity of agaritine was available to the Working Group.

4.3 Evaluation

The results of one experiment in mice do not provide evidence of carcinogenicity of agaritine to experimental animals. There is *limited evidence*[1] of the carcinogenicity of derivatives of two fungal metabolites of agaritine in experimental animals. In the absence of epidemiological data, no evaluation of the carcinogenicity of agaritine to humans could be made.

5. References

Chiarlo, B., Cajelli, E. & Acerbo, C. (1979) The presence of agaritine in a mushroom (*Agaricus bisporus*) commonly cultivated in Italy. *Fitoterapia, 50,* 111-113

Daniels, E.G., Kelly, R.B. & Hinman, J.W. (1961) Agaritine: An improved isolation procedure and confirmation of structure by synthesis. *J. Am. chem. Soc., 83,* 3333-3334

De Flora, S. (1981) Study of 106 organic and inorganic compounds in the *Salmonella*/microsome test. *Carcinogenesis, 2,* 283-298

Gigliotti, H.J. (1963) The γ-glutamyltransferase and arylhydrazine oxidase activities of *Agaricus bisporus*. Thesis Dissertation, Ann Arbor, MI, University of Michigan

---

[1]See preamble, p. 18.

Gigliotti, H.J. & Levenberg, B. (1964) Studies on the γ-glutamyltransferase of *Agaricus bisporus. J. biol. Chem.*, *239*, 2274-2284

Kelly, R.B., Daniels, E.G. & Hinman, J.W. (1962) Agaritine: Isolation, degradation, and synthesis. *J. org. Chem.*, *27*, 3229-3231

Klosterman, H.J. (1974) Vitamin B_6 antagonists of natural origin. *J. agric. Food Chem.*, *22*, 13-16

Levenberg, B. (1960) Isolation and enzymatic reactions of agaritine, a new amino acid derivative from *Agaricaceae* (Abstract no. 15). *Fed. Proc.*, *19*, 6

Levenberg, B. (1961) Structure and enzymatic cleavage of agaritine, a phenylhydrazide of L-glutamic acid isolated from *Agaricaceae. J. Am. chem. Soc.*, *83*, 503-504

Levenberg, B. (1964) Isolation and structure of agaritine, a γ-glutamyl-substituted arylhydrazine derivative from *Agaricaceae. J. biol. Chem.*, *239*, 2267-2273

Oka, Y., Tsuji, H., Ogawa, T. & Sasaoka, K. (1981) Quantitative determination of the free amino acids and their derivatives in the common edible mushroom, *Agaricus bisporus. J. Nutr. Sci. Vitaminol.*, *27*, 253-262

Ross, A.E., Nagel, D.L. & Toth, B. (1982) Evidence for the occurrence and formation of diazonium ions in the *Agaricus bisporus* mushroom and its extracts. *J. agric. Food Chem.*, *30*, 521-525

Toth, B., Nagel, D., Shimizu, H., Sornson, H., Issenberg, P. & Erickson, J. (1975) Tumorigenicity of *n*-propyl-, *n*-amyl- and *n*-allyl-hydrazines. Toxicity of agaritine (Abstract no. 243). *Proc. Am. Assoc. Cancer Res.*, *16*, 61

Toth, B., Nagel. D., Patil, K., Erickson, J. & Antonson, K. (1978) Tumor induction with the N'-acetyl derivative of 4-hydroxymethylphenylhydrazine, a metabolite of agaritine of *Agaricus bisporus. Cancer Res.*, *38*, 177-180

Toth, B., Raha, C.R., Wallcave, L. & Nagel, D. (1981a) Attempted tumor induction with agaritine in mice. *Anticancer Res.*, *1*, 255-258

Toth, B., Patil, K. & Jae, H.-S. (1981b) Carcinogenesis of 4-(hydroxymethyl)benzenediazonium ion (tetrafluroborate) of *Agaricus bisporus. Cancer Res.*, *41*, 2444-2449

Toth, B., Nagel, D. & Ross, A. (1982) Gastric tumorigenesis by a single dose of 4-(hydroxymethyl)benzenediazonium ion of *Agaricus bisporus. Br. J. Cancer*, *46*, 417-422

US Department of Agriculture (1980) *Mushrooms*, Washington DC, Economics, Statistics & Cooperatives Service, pp. 1-4

Wallcave, L., Nagel, D.L., Raha, C.R., Jae, H.-S., Bronczyk, S., Kupper, R. & Toth, B. (1979) An improved synthesis of agaritine. *J. org. Chem.*, *44*, 3752-3755

Windholz, M., ed. (1976) *The Merck Index*, 9th ed., Rahway, NJ, Merck & Co., Inc., p. 26

2-AMINO-5-NITROTHIAZOLE

1. Chemical and Physical Data

1.1 Synonyms and trade names

Chem. Abstr. Services Reg. No.: 121-66-4

Chem. Abstr. Name: 2-Thiazolamine, 5-nitro-

IUPAC Systematic Name: 2-Amino-5-nitrothiazole

Synonyms: Aminonitrothiazole; aminonitrothiazolum; NCI CO3065; 5-nitro-2-aminothiazole; 5-nitro-2-thiazolylamine

Trade Names: Amnizol soluble; Enheptin; Enheptin Premix; Enheptin T; Entramin; Nitramin; Nitramine; Nitramin Ido

1.2 Structural and molecular formulae and molecular weight

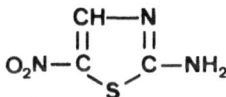

$C_3H_3N_3O_2S$ Mol. wt: 145.2

1.3 Chemical and physical properties of the pure substance

From Windholz (1976) and Wade (1977), unless otherwise specified

(a) *Description*: Greenish-yellow to orange-yellow powder with a slightly bitter taste

(b) *Melting-point*: 202°C (dec.)

(c) *Spectroscopy data*: λ_{max} 386 nm; mass spectral data have been reported (NIH/EPA Chemical Information System, 1982).

(d) *Solubility*: Sparingly soluble in water; soluble in diethyl ether (4 g/l), 95% ethanol (8 g/l) and dilute mineral acid almost insoluble in chloroform

1.4 Technical products and impurities

No data were available to the Working Group.

2. Production, Use, Occurrence and Analysis

2.1 Production and use

(a) *Production*

2-Amino-5-nitrothiazole can be prepared by nitration of acetamidothiazole followed by deacetylation (Hubbard, 1951; Steahly, 1951a,b). It can also be made from *N,N*-dimethyl-2-nitroetheneamine by bromination and treatment with thiourea [see IARC, 1974] and then with water (Cheng & Chamberlin, 1981).

2-Amino-5-nitrothiazole was first produced commercially in the US in 1950 (US Tariff Commission, 1951). Because there is only one US commercial producer, separate production data for 2-amino-5-nitrothiazole are not reported (see Preamble, p. 21). However, the company reported that its 1977 production was in the range of 4.5-45.4 thousand kg (NIH/EPA Chemical Information System, 1981). Separate data on US imports and exports of 2-amino-5-nitrothiazole are not published.

The only Japanese producer of 2-amino-5-nitrothiazole is estimated to have produced about 10 thousand kg in 1981, down from an estimated 30 thousand kg in 1978. Japanese exports of 2-amino-5-nitrothiazole in 1981 are believed to have been negligible.

2-Amino-5-nitrothiazole is believed to be produced by one company in the United Kingdom.

(b) *Use*

2-Amino-5-nitrothiazole has been used as an antiprotozoal agent in veterinary medicine for the prevention and treatment of blackhead (histomoniasis) in turkeys and chickens, and the treatment of canker (trichomoniasis) in pigeons (Wade, 1977). Whether it is still used for these purposes at the present time is not known.

2-Amino-5-nitrothiazole has been used in the synthesis of another antiprotozoal agent, nithiazide, which is the subject of a monograph in this volume (see p. 179). It was also used to make the antischistosomal drug niridazole [1-(5-nitro-2-thiazolyl)-2-imidazolidinone], which was formerly produced by one company in Switzerland (IARC, 1977). It can be used in the synthesis of the antiprotozoal agent atrican [N-(5-nitro-2-thiazolyl)-2-thiophenecarboxamide], which is produced by one company in France.

Although it was reported (Fisher, 1969) that disperse azo dyes can be prepared from 2-amino-5-nitrothiazole, this chemical is not listed in the *Colour Index* as an intermediate in the production of any dyes of known structure. Since the US producer of 2-amino-5-nitrothiazole is also a manufacturer of textile dyes, it seems likely that the chemical is used on site for the manufacture of one or more dyes of proprietary composition.

On 14 November 1980, the US Food and Drug Administration announced withdrawal of its approval of use of a premix containing 2-amino-5-nitrothiazole in turkey feed (which had been originally approved in 1950) as an aid in prevention of blackhead. The manufacturer of the premix had requested that the approval be withdrawn because the product was no longer being marketed (US Food & Drug Administration, 1980).

2.2 Occurrence

2-Amino-5-nitrothiazole is not known to occur as a natural product. No data were available to the Working Group on its persistence in the edible tissues of food-producing animals.

2.3 Analysis

No information on analytical methods for 2-amino-5-nitrothiazole was available to the Working Group.

3. Biological Data Relevant to the Evaluation of Carcinogenic Risk to Humans

3.1 Carcinogenicity studies in animals

Oral administration

Mouse: Groups of 50 male and 50 female B6C3F1 hybrid mice, 53 days of age, were fed diets containing 50 or 100 mg/kg 2-amino-5-nitrothiazole (purity, 99.0 $\pm$ 0.5%) for 104 weeks. The dietary concentrations were selected on the basis of a range-finding study. A group of 50 mice of each sex served as matched controls. No significant dose-related trend in mortality was seen for animals of either sex: by the end of the study, 76, 74 and 66% of males and 70, 76 and 82% of females were still alive in the control, low-dose and high-dose groups, respectively. No significant increase in the incidence of tumours in treated mice of either sex was observed when compared with controls (National Cancer Institute, 1978).

Rat: A group of 35 weanling female Sprague-Dawley rats were fed a diet containing 2-amino-5-nitrothiazole (melting point, 196-197°C, with no impurities detected by paper chromatography) at a level of 1140 mg/kg for one week, then 750 mg/kg until the ninth week, then 1000 mg/kg until the 46th week, followed by a control diet until the end of the study at the 66th week (total cumulative dose per rat, 4.6 g). A group of 39 weanling female rats served as controls. Long-acting penicillin was administered intramuscularly to all rats to control infection. Rats fed 2-amino-5-nitrothiazole exhibited initial growth retardation, which required reduction of the dose, and continued to weigh about 15% less than control rats throughout the study. All rats in the treated and control groups were alive at 10 weeks, and no significant survival difference was seen at 66 weeks. Seven solitary mammary fibroadenomas and one mammary adenocarcinoma were observed in 8/35 treated rats and 2 fibroadenomas in 39 controls ($p < 0.03$); 6/35 treated animals developed renal pelvis hyperplasia, 2/35 renal pelvis transitional-cell carcinomas and 2/35 pulmonary alveolar-cell carcinomas (Cohen *et al.*, 1975). [The Working Group noted the short duration of this experiment.]

Groups of 50 male and 50 female Fischer 344 rats, 50 days of age, were fed diets containing 300 or 600 mg/kg 2-amino-5-nitrothiazole (purity, $99 \pm 0.5\%$) for 110 weeks, followed by one week of control diet. The doses were selected on the basis of a range-finding study. A group of 50 rats of each sex served as matched controls. In male rats, there was a dose-related trend in mortality: by the end of the study, 60, 52 and 42% of males and 66, 66 and 70% of females were still alive in the control, low-dose and high-dose groups, respectively. Statistically significant increases in tumour incidence were observed for the following neoplasms: (1) dose-related trends ($p = 0.044$) in the incidences of malignant lymphomas, lymphocytic leukaemias and undifferentiated leukaemias in males: controls, 11/50; low-dose, 15/50; high-dose, 19/49; (b) a dose-related trend ($p = 0.014$) in the incidence of granulocytic leukaemia in males: controls, 2/50; low-dose, 4/50; high-dose, 9/49 ($p = 0.023$); (c) a dose-related trend (females: $p = 0.016$ and males: $p = 0.048$) in the incidence of chromophobe adenomas of the pituitary gland in 19/45 female controls, 29/47 low-dose females ($p = 0.048$), 29/44 high-dose females ($p = 0.021$), 3/46 male controls, 3/45 low-dose males and 8/43 high-dose males; and (d) a higher incidence of endometrial stromal polyps of the uterus in low-dose females, 9/49 ($p = 0.023$) than in matched controls, 2/50 (National Cancer Institute, 1978). [The Working Group noted that the average incidence of pituitary gland tumours in historical control groups was 40% in females and 20.3% in males (Tarone *et al.*, 1981) and the average incidence of endometrial stromal polyps in female Fischer rats was 12.7-14.9% (Goodman *et al.*, 1979; Tarone *et al.*, 1981).]

3.2 Other relevant biological data

(a) *Experimental systems*

Toxic effects

The i.p. LD_{50} of 2-amino-5-nitrothiazole in BALB/c mice is 420 mg/kg bw (Rockwell, 1978).

Effects on reproduction and prenatal toxicity

No data were available to the Working Group.

Absorption, distribution, excretion and metabolism

No data were available to the Working Group.

Mutagenicity and other short-term tests

2-Amino-5-nitrothiazole was mutagenic in *Salmonella typhimurium* TA100 at concentrations greater than 100 µg/plate, but not in TA1535, TA1537, TA1538 or TA98; activity was not affected by exogenous metabolic activation (Dunkel & Simmon, 1980).

It was reported in an abstract that 2-amino-5-nitrothiazole was mutagenic in a fluctuation test in a *Klebsiella pneumoniae* strain, requiring uracil and proline for growth (Voogd, 1976).

(*b*) Humans

No data were available to the Working Group.

3.3 Case reports and epidemiological studies of carcinogenicity in humans

No data were available to the Working Group.

4. Summary of Data Reported and Evaluation

4.1 Experimental data

2-Amino-5-nitrothiazole was tested for carcinogenicity in one experiment in mice and in two experiments in two strains of rats by administration in the diet. In one experiment in female rats, 2-amino-5-nitrothiazole increased the incidence of benign mammary tumours. In the other experiment in rats it increased the incidences of malignant lymphomas, lymphocytic and undifferentiated leukaemias, and granulocytic leukaemias in male rats. The results of studies in mice were not indicative of a carcinogenic effect.

2-Amino-4-nitrothiazole was mutagenic in bacteria. The data were *inadequate* to evaluate the activity of this compound in short-term tests.

No data were available to evaluate the teratogenicity of this compound to experimental animals.

4.2 Human data

2-Amino-5-nitrothiazole, a synthetic veterinary antiprotozoal agent, has been produced and used since 1950. It is also used as an intermediate in the manufacture of disperse azo dyes. Manufacturers of the compound itself, handlers of feed and people involved in the synthesis of the dyes concerned are exposed to 2-amino-5-nitrothiazole.

No data were available to assess the teratogenicity or chromosomal effects of this compound in humans.

No case report or epidemiological study of the carcinogenicity of 2-amino-5-nitrothiazole was available to the Working Group.

4.3 Evaluation

There is *limited evidence*[1] for the carcinogenicity of 2-amino-5-nitrothiazole in experimental animals. In the absence of epidemiological data, no evaluation of the carcinogenicity of 2-amino-5-nitrothiazole to humans could be made.

5. References

Cheng, D.-C.O. & Chamberlin, K.S. (1981) Process for the preparation of 2-amino-5-nitrothiazole. *US Patent 4,269,985*

Cohen, S.M., Ertürk, E., Von Esch, A.M., Crovetti, A.J. & Bryan, G.T. (1975) Carcinogenicity of 5-nitrofurans and related compounds with amino-heterocyclic substituents. *J. natl Cancer Inst., 54,* 841-850

Dunkel, V.C. & Simmon, V.F. (1980) *Mutagenic activity of chemicals previously tested for carcinogenicity in the National Cancer Institute bioassay program.* In: Montesano, R., Bartsch, H. & Tomatis, L., eds, *Molecular and Cellular Aspects of Carcinogen Screening Tests (IARC Scientific Publications No. 27),* Lyon, pp. 283-302

Fisher, J.G. (1969) *Thiazole dyes.* In: Kirk, R.E. & Othmer, D.F., eds, *Encyclopedia of Chemical Technology,* 2nd ed., Vol. 20, New York, John Wiley & Sons, pp. 193, 194, 197

Goodman, D.G., Ward, J.M., Squire, R.A., Chu, K.C. & Linhart, M.S. (1979) Neoplastic and nonneoplastic lesions in aging F344 rats. *Toxicol. appl. Pharmacol., 48,* 237-248

Hubbard, H.L. (1951) Neutralization of the mineral acid salts of aminonitrothiazole. *US Patent 2,573,641* (to Monsanto Chemical Co.) [*Chem. Abstr., 46,* 3573g]

IARC (1974) *IARC Monographs on the Evaluation of Carcinogenic Risk of Chemicals to Man,* Vol. 7, *Some Anti-thyroid and Related Substances, Nitrofurans and Industrial Chemicals,* Lyon, pp. 95-109

IARC (1977) *IARC Monographs on the Evaluation of Carcinogenic Risk of Chemicals to Man,* Vol. 13, *Some Miscellaneous Pharmaceutical Substances,* Lyon, pp. 123-130

---

[1]See preamble, p. 18.

National Cancer Institute (1978) *Bioassay of 2-Amino-5-nitrothiazole for Possible Carcinogenicity (Tech. Rep. Ser. No. 53; DHEW Publ. No. (NIH) 78-1359)*, Washington DC, US Department of Health, Education, & Welfare

NIH/EPA Chemical Information System (1981) *TSCA Plant and Production Data Base*, Washington DC, CIS Project, Information Sciences Corporation

NIH/EPA Chemical Information System (1982) *Mass Spectral Search System*, Washington DC, CIS Project, Information Sciences Corporation

Rockwell, S. (1978) Cytotoxic and radiosensitizing effects of hypoxic cell sensitizers on EMT6 mouse mammary tumour cells *in vivo* and *in vitro. Br. J. Cancer, 37*, Suppl. III, 212-215

Steahly, G.W. (1951a) Hydrolysis of acetamidonitrothiazole. *US Patent 2,573,656* (to Monsanto Chemical Co.) [*Chem. Abstr., 46*, 3573h]

Steahly, G.W. (1951b) Neutralization of the mineral acid salts of aminonitrothiazole. *US Patent 2,573,657* (to Monsanto Chemical Co.) [*Chem. Abstr., 46*, 3573h]

Tarone, R.E., Chu, K.C. & Ward, J.M. (1981) Variability in the ratio of some common naturally occurring tumors in Fischer 344 rats and (C57BL/6N x C3H/HeN)F_1 (B6C3F$_1$) mice. *J. natl Cancer Inst., 66*, 1175-1181

US Food & Drug Administration (1980) American Cyanamid Co., Enheptin premix; withdrawal of approval of NADA. *Fed. Regist., 45*, 75327, 75328

US Tariff Commission (1951) *Synthetic Organic Chemicals, US Production and Sales, 1950 (Report No. 173)*, Second Series, Washington DC, US Government Printing Office, p. 58

Voogd, C.E. (1976) The mutagenic action of some nitrothiazoles and nitrothiophenes (Abstract no. 30). *Mutat. Res., 38*, 117

Wade, A., ed. (1977) *Martindale, The Extra Pharmacopoeia*, 27th ed., London, The Pharmaceutical Press, p. 1718

Windholz, M., ed. (1976) *The Merck Index*, 9th ed., Rahway, NJ, Merck & Co., Inc., p. 63

CARRAGEENAN

This substance was considered by a previous working group, in October 1975 (IARC, 1976). Since that time, new data have become available, and these have been incorporated into the monograph and taken into account in the present evaluation.

1. Chemical and Physical Data

1.1 Synonyms and trade names

Chem. Abstr. Services Reg. No.: 9000-07-1

Chem. Abstr. Name: Carrageenan

IUPAC Systematic Name: Carrageenan

Synonyms: Carrageen; *kappa*, *lambda* and *iota*-carrageenan; carrageenan gum; carrageenin; carragheanin; carragheen; carragheenan; chondrus extract; gum carrageenan; gum chon 2; gum chond; Irish gum; Irish moss extract*; sulphate ester of a polysaccharide of galactose

Trade Names: Aubygel GS, LGA, MR5O, TRS, X52, X100 & X120; Aubygum DM; Burtonite V-40-E; Carastay; Carastay C, E, K, M, S, & X; Colloid 775; Coreine; Eucheuma spinosum gum; Flanogen ELA, RS1; RS2, 531 & 553; Galozone; Gelcarin; Gelcarin HMR, LA, SI; Gelogen 2, 4, 8, P10, 28, 406 & 440; Gelozone; Genu; Genugel; Genugel CJ, CMJ-2, CMJ-343, CWG, CWG-122, KWG, LC-1, LC-4,MGW, PWG, UE & WG; Genugol RLV; Genulacta; Genulacta CL-126, CP-100, K-100, L-100, MDS, P-100 & PL-93; Genuvisco J; Lygomme CDS, DP, GB3, LA60, 34, 35 & 267/3; Pellugel; Pellugel ID;Pencogel; Satiagel GS350, HV, HVX, K40 & K80; Satiagum 3; Satiagum standard; Seakem Carrageenin; Seakem 3 & LCM; Seaspen PF; Viscarin; Viscarin 402 & TP-4

---

*The terms 'Irish moss', 'chondrus', 'killeen', 'pearl moss', 'pig-wrack',and 'self rock moss' are also sometimes used to describe carrageenan, although they are actually names for the seaweeds that are extracted to produce carrageenan.

1.2 Structural and molecular formulae and molecular weight

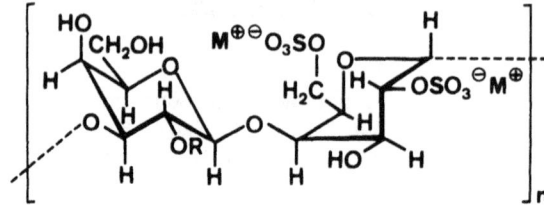

lambda-Carrageenan $R = SO_3^- \ M^+$ or H^+
    Chem. Abstr. Services Reg. No.: 9064-57-7
    Av. mol. wt: No data were available to the Working Group.

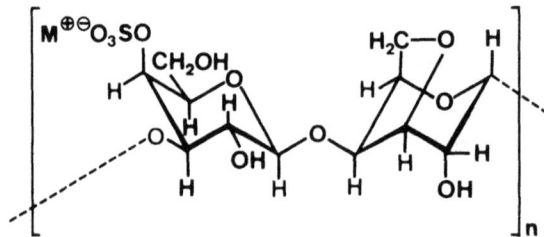

kappa-Carrageenan $R = H$
    Chem. Abstr. Services Reg. No.: 11114-20-8
    Av. mol. wt: 2×10^7 (Tong *et al.*, 1980)

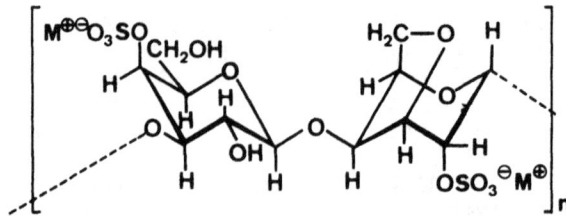

iota-Carrageenan $R = SO_3^- M^+$
    Chem. Abstr. Services Reg. No.: 9062-07-1
    Av. mol. wt: $1.5\text{-}2 \times 10^6$ (Tong *et al.*, 1980)

M = ammonium, calcium, magnesium, potassium or sodium

1.3 Chemical and physical properties

Native carrageenan

Native carrageenan is a hydrocolloid isolated from various red algae (seaweed) and consisting mainly of varying amounts (depending on the processing methods) of the ammonium, calcium, magnesium, potassium or sodium salts of sulphate esters of galactose and 3,6-anhydrogalactose copolymers (the two hexose units are alternately linked *alpha*-1,3 and *beta*-1,4 in the polymer). The sulphate ester content of carrageenan ranges from 18-40%. The principal copolymers are designated *kappa*-, *iota*- and *lambda*- and differ both in structure and in their ability to form gels upon the addition of potassium ions to dilute solutions of carrageenan (National Research Council, 1981).

The carrageenan extracted from the seaweeds *Chondrus crispus* and *Gigartina stellata* contains mainly *kappa*-carrageenan, which is gelled by potassium ion, and *lambda*-carrageenan, which does not form a gel (Tong *et al.*, 1980; Windholz, 1976). The third type of carrageenan, *iota*-carrageenan, which forms a gel, is the principal component of extracts of the seaweed *Eucheuma spinosum* (Guiseley, 1968).

Commercial product

A product called 'degraded carrageenan' has been produced from extracts of *Eucheuma spinosum* seaweed by treatment with dilute hydrochloric acid (WHO, 1974). It has an average molecular weight of 20 000-30 000 and dissolves readily (Anderson & Soman, 1966; Anderson, 1967). No evidence was found that this depolymerized material, which reportedly was sold as an antipeptic agent in Europe (Wade, 1977), is currently being produced commercially.

From National Research Council (1981) and Windholz (1976)

(a) *Description*: Yellowish or tan to white, coarse to fine powder; practically odourless, with a mucilaginous taste

(b) *Spectroscopy data*: Infra-red spectra for have been reported for *iota*, *kappa* and *lambda* carrageenan.

(c) *Identity and purity test*: A series of gelation tests and infra-red spectra can be used to identify the *iota*, *kappa* and *lambda* fractions of carrageenan.

(d) *Solubility*: Soluble in hot water and anhydrous hydrazine; sparingly soluble in formamide and methyl sulphoxide; swells but does not dissolve in dimethyl formamide; generally insoluble in oils and organic solvents (e) *Stability*: Solutions are most stable at pH 9; depolymerized by acids

(f) *Reactivity*: Treatment of aqueous solutions with potassium ion precipitates *kappa* carrageenan. Precipitates or agglomerates certain proteins from solution

1.4 Technical products and impurities

In the US, to meet the requirements of the Food Chemicals Codex, carrageenan and its derived calcium, potassium and sodium salts must pass certain identification tests involving gelling properties and infra-red spectral measurements and meet the following requirements: maxima of 3 mg/kg arsenic, 1.0% acid-insoluble ash, 35.0% total ash, 0.004% heavy metals, 10 mg/kg (0.001%) lead, 12% loss on drying and 18-40% sulphate (dry-weight basis); the viscosity of a 1.5% solution at 75°C should be 5 cps min. The alcohols used for alcohol precipitation of carrageenan are restricted to methanol, ethanol and isopropanol. Carrageenan recovered by drum-roll drying may contain mono- and diglycerides or up to 5% polysorbate 80 used as roll-stripping agents (National Research Council, 1981). Degraded carrageenan need not meet these requirements.

2. Production, Use, Occurrence and Analysis

Two comprehensive reviews on carrageenan have been published (Towle, 1973; CECA SA, undated).

2.1 Production and use

(a) Production

The use of dried carrageenan-containing seaweeds to produce puddings from milk reportedly goes back at least two centuries, and the Irish are reported to have used a seaweed in foods and medicines for about six hundred years. Carrageenan was first extracted only in 1837; the structure was not investigated until the 1840s and was not clarified until the mid-1950s. Commercial production of carrageenan started in 1937; it remained an almost exclusively US industry until the 1950s when it began to be carried out on a large scale in European countries (CECA SA, undated; Guiseley, 1968; Cottrell & Baird, 1980).

Carrageenan is recovered commercially from *Chondrus* seaweed in the US and from *Chondrus* and *Gigartina* seaweed in Europe (Informatics, Inc., 1972). Processing steps used to recover carrageenan vary considerably and are closely-guarded trade secrets. Cottrell and Baird (1980) state that patent literature indicates that the process generally includes the following steps: The seaweed is washed to remove soluble salts and debris before being extracted with slightly alkaline hot water. The extract is concentrated to about 3% carrageenan before alcohol is added to precipitate it; alternatively, the extract can be drum dried to produce a less pure product.

World production of carrageenan in 1971 was approximately 4.5 million kg, with US production accounting for 2.3 million kg of the total (Towle, 1973). World production in 1973 has been estimated at 6 million kg (CECA SA, undated). Whistler and Zysk (1978) estimated that US production of carrageenan in 1978 was 4.2 million kg. US imports of carrageenan in 1979 amounted to 478 thousand kg (US Department of Commerce, 1980). Separate data on US exports of carrageenan are not available.

Carrageenan is believed to be produced by two companies in Denmark and one company in France.

It was first imported into Japan in around 1955, and imports in 1981 are estimated to have been 750 thousand kg. Carrageenan has been produced commercially by several Japanese companies since 1955; the two companies making it in 1981 had a total production of about 450 thousand kg.

(b) Use

Carrageenan and its derived calcium, potassium and sodium salts are used in foods, cosmetics, pharmaceuticals and other products in which their ability to stabilize mixtures, emulsify ingredients and thicken or gel solutions are utilized. Total US consumption in 1978 is estimated to have been 4-5 million kg (Whistler & Zysk, 1978).

The major use of carrageenan is in food products, particularly dairy products. In addition to the functions listed above, it imparts the desired body and texture to food products. It is reportedly used at levels of 0.01-1.0% in such dairy products as pasteurized, evaporated and chocolate milk, infant milk formulas, pudding and pie fillings, and ice cream. It is added at levels of 0.05-1% in the following non-dairy food products: water dessert gels, dietetic jellies, syrups, fruit drink powders and frozen concentrates, imitation coffee creams, sauces, soups, bread doughs and cake batters, icings and glazes, soft drinks and hard drinks (Informatics, Inc., 1972). In 1974, the World Health Organization set the acceptable daily intake of carrageenan at up to 75 mg/kg bw and recommended that low molecular weight or degraded carrageenan not be used in food (FAO/WHO, 1974).

Carrageenan and its derived sodium salt have been used as ingredients in the following cosmetics: bath oil tablets, foundations, make-up preparations, dentifrices (believed to be the major cosmetics use), deodorants, other personal cleaning products, cleansing creams, face, body and hand preparations, moisturizing creams, night preparations, paste masks, skin fresheners, wrinkle smoothing preparations, and other skin preparations (US Food & Drug Administration, 1978).

Carrageenan is used as an emulsifier in mineral oil emulsions used as laxatives, in liquid petrolatum, and in cod liver oil (Swinyard, 1975; Wade, 1977; Boyd, 1982). A modified carrageenan has also been reported to be used as a dispersing agent in reconstitutable powders, such as some antibiotics (Idson & Bachynsky, 1978).

Carrageenan with a minimum molecular weight of 10^5 is also used as a thickener in pesticide formulations (US Environmental Protection Agency, 1980), and it has had very limited use as an oilwell drilling fluid component to reduce filtrate loss (Huebotter & Gray, 1965). Production or importation of a cross-linked polymer of carrageenan, glyoxal and formaldehyde by one US company has been reported (US Environmental Protection Agency, 1979), but no information was available on its use. Although carrageenan has been reported to be used in making suspensions for a variety of industrial uses and for making gels for the release of air-treating compounds (Towle, 1973), no evidence was found that it is presently used in these applications.

Most of the estimated 1.2 million kg of carrageenan used in Japan in 1981 was used, usually in combination with locust bean gum, in the food industry.

The numerous uses of carrageenan and its derived ammonium, calcium, potassium and sodium salts as food additives (e.g., in baking products, cheeses, fruit jellies, macaroni products), as components of paper and paperboard in contact with foods, and as inert ingredients in pesticide formulations, are subject to numerous regulations in the US. In general, the food additive regulations require that it be used only in the amount necessary to function as an emulsifier, stabilizer or thickener in foods (US Food & Drug Administration, 1980).

2.2 Occurrence

Carrageenan has been reported to occur in the following species of Gigartinaceae and Solieraceae orders of the Rhodophyceae class of red seaweed: *Aeodes orbitose*, *Chondrus canaliculatus*, *Chondrus crispus*, *Chondrus ocellatus*, *Eucheuma cottonii*, *Eucheuma edule*, *Eucheuma muricatum* (*E. spinosum*, *E. denticulatum*), *Gigartina acicularis*, *Gigartina asperifolia*, *Gigartina canaliculata*, *Gigartina decipiens*, *Gigartina pistillata*, *Gigartina radula*, *Gigartina stellata* (*G. mamillose*), *Gloiopeltis coliformis*, *Gloiopeltis furcata*, *Gloiopeltis tenax*, *Gymnogongrus norvegicus*, *Gymnogongrus patens*, *Iridaea laminarioides*, *Iridaea capensis* (*Iridophycus capensis*), and *Iridaea flaccida* (*Iridophycus flaccidum* (Informatics, Inc., 1972).

2.3 Analysis

Although numerous methods have been described to characterize the components of carrageenan, methods for detecting the presence of carrageenan in various matrices are relatively limited in number. Methods have been reported for the isolation of carrageenan from dairy products, which are based on detection either by precipitation with a series of reagents or by determining the infra-red spectra. A quantitative method for determinating carrageenan in milk products has also been described in which digestion with papain, clarification, and precipitation with cetyl pyridinium chloride are used to produce a complex, the carrageenan content of which is determined by treatment with phenol and sulphuric acid (Informatics, Inc., 1972). Methods involving infra-red spectrometry for isolating carrageenan and identifying the various types of this compound have been reported, and several other special methods have been reviewed (Craigie & Leigh, 1978), including infra-red analysis of films, colorimetric measurement of 3,6-anhydrogalactose, hexose analysis, sulphate analysis, and viscosity measurements.

3. Biological Data Relevant to the Evaluation of Carcinogenic Risk to Humans

A review on carrageenan is available (Salminen & Hallikainen, 1983).

3.1 Carcinogenicity studies in animals

Carrageenan varies in structure and composition, depending on its source, and has been studied in both native and degraded forms.

A. Native (undegraded) carrageenan

(a) Oral administration

Rat: Groups of 30 male and 30 female MRC outbred rats, seven weeks old, were given 0.5, 2.5 or 5% carrageenan (Gelcarin HMR, largely composed of *kappa* components, high molecular weight) in the diet for life. A group of 100 male and 100 female rats served as controls. Survival of the treated animals was not different from that of controls. No significant increase in tumour incidence was seen (Rustia *et al.*, 1980).

Hamster: Groups of 30 male and 30 female Syrian golden hamsters, seven weeks old, were given 0.5, 2.5 or 5% carrageenan (Gelcarin HMR, largely composed of *kappa* components, high molecular weight) in the diet for life. A group of 100 males and 100 females served as controls. Survival was similar in treated and control groups. No significant increase in tumour incidence was seen (Rustia *et al.*, 1980).

(b) Subcutaneous administration

[An experiment in which carrageenan was administered subcutaneously to female rats (Cater, 1961) was considered inconclusive by the Working Group.]

(c) Co-carcinogenicity experiments

Rat: The effect of undegraded (native) carrageenan (Viscarin 402) upon colon carcinogenesis was studied in female Fischer 344 rats. Weanling rats, five weeks old, were divided into the following treatment groups: 15 rats received control diet; 15 rats received control diet with 15% carrageenan; 30 rats received 15% carrageenan plus 10 weekly s.c. injections of 8 mg/kg bw azoxymethane (AOM); 30 rats received three twice weekly intrarectal instillations of 2 mg *N*-nitrosomethylurea (NMU). Two groups of 30 rats received AOM or NMU alone. Administration of AOM and NMU was started at seven weeks of age, and animals were killed 40 weeks after the first injection of AOM or 30 weeks after the first injection of NMU. Carrageenan enhanced the incidence of colonic tumours in AOM- and NMU-treated rats ($p < 0.01$): AOM + carrageenan, 26/26 (100%) *versus* 17/30 (57%) in rats given AOM alone; NMU + carrageenan, 29/29 (100%) *versus* 20/29 (69%) in rats given NMU alone; control diet, 0/15 (0%); and carrageenan diet, 1/15 (7%) (Watanabe *et al.*, 1978).

B. Degraded carrageenan

Oral administration

Rat: A series of experiments with degraded carrageenan (from *Eucheuma spinosum*; degraded by acid hydrolysis, average molecular weight 20 000-40 000) were conducted in male (250 g) and female (175 g) Sprague-Dawley rats (Wakabayashi *et al.*, 1978; Wakabayashi, 1981). In one experiment, four groups of 30 males and 30 females were fed a diet containing 0 (control), 1, 5 or 10% degraded carrageenan. Animals in each group were sacrificed at 6, 12, 18 and 24 months. Colorectal squamous metaplasia was found in 59/60 and 53/60 rats fed 10% and 5%, respectively. Colorectal tumours were found in 19/60 rats fed 10% (12 squamous-cell carcinomas, 8 adenocarcinomas and 3 adenomas) and in 12/60 rats fed 5% (3 squamous-cell carcinomas, 1 adenocarcinoma and 8 adenomas). No colorectal tumour nor squamous metaplasia was observed in the low-dose group or in controls. In the second experiment, degraded carrageenan was given in the drinking-water (5%) to 20 male and 20 female rats for 15 months. Colorectal squamous metaplasia was found in all rats after 15 months, and 11/40 treated rats developed colorectal tumours (4 squamous-cell carcinomas, 4 adenocarcinomas, 3 adenomas and I myosarcoma); no such tumour was observed in the 15 male and 15 female controls. In the third experiment, 0 (control), 1 or 5 g/kg bw degraded carrageenan was administered by intragastric intubation [frequency of administration not specified] to groups of 15 male and 15 female rats for 15 months. A control group of 15 male and 15 female rats were given distilled water intragastrically. Squamous colorectal metaplasia was observed in 29/29 rats in the high-dose group and 11/30 in the low-dose group. Colorectal tumours were found only in the high-dose group (8/29, 5 adenocarcinomas, 4 adenomas).

Eight-week-old male Fischer 344 rats were maintained on a diet containing 10% degraded carrageenan (from *Eucheuma spinosum*, degraded by acid hydrolysis; sulphate content about 30%; molecular weight 20 000-40 000). Thirty-nine animals received this ration for two months (group 1), 42 animals for six months (group 2), and 42 animals for nine months (group 3), respectively. Forty-six additional animals, referred to as controls, received the same diet without carrageenan, as did all other groups following cessation of carrageenan feeding. No mortality had occurred by 18 months following the start of the carrageenan feeding, when all animals were sacrificed. A 100% incidence of colorectal squamous metaplasia was found in all treated groups. Tumours were also reported in 5/39 animals in group 1 (3 squamous-cell carcinomas, 1 adenoma, 1 anaplastic carcinoma), 8/42 in group 2 (6 squamous-cell carcinomas, 1 adenocarcinoma, 1 adenoma) and 17/42 in group 3 (14 squamous-cell carcinomas, 4 adenocarcinomas). Colorectal changes were detected in none of the control rats (Oohashi *et al.*, 1981).

3.2 Other relevant biological data

(a) Experimental systems

The biological and toxicological properties of carrageenan have been reviewed (Di Rosa, (1972).

Carrageenan varies in structure and composition, depending on its source, and has been studied in both native and degraded forms. [The relevance of the latter is the suggestion that carrageenan may be degraded in the gut (Pittman *et al.*, 1976). No evidence bearing on the degradation of carrageenan during food preparation was available to the Working Group.]

Toxic effects

A. Native carrageenan

Several studies in which native carrageenan was administered to animals (guinea-pigs, rabbits, rats, mice, pigs, rhesus monkeys) in drinking-water (e.g., 0.5-2% for up to 14 weeks) or in the diet (e.g., 2-5% for 12 weeks) showed no ill effect (Maillet *et al.*, 1970; Abraham *et al.*, 1972; Benitz *et al.*, 1972, 1973; Poulsen, 1973). However, in one study

(Grasso *et al.*, 1973) pin-point caecal and colonic ulcerations were found in guinea-pigs given 5% native carrageenan in the diet for 3-5 weeks.

I.v. injection of 15 mg/kg bw carrageenan (derived from *Gigartina acicularis*) caused death in 2/3 dogs within 24 hours (Houck *et al.*, 1957). In rabbits, the lowest single i.v. doses that were lethal within 24 hours were 1-5 mg/kg bw *lambda* carrageenan and 3-15 mg/kg bw *kappa* carrageenan, both of which were isolated from *Chondrus crispus* (Anderson & Duncan, 1965).

Renal and hepatic function were compared in groups of seven rats for a period of 14 days following a single i.p. injection of 125 mg/kg bw purified *kappa*, *lambda* or *iota* carrageenan. *Kappa* carrageenan was clearly nephrotoxic, as shown by a progressive marked increase in serum creatinine and urea levels and in urinary N-acetyl-β-D-glucosaminidase activity. It was also hepatotoxic, as evidenced by elevated serum aspartate aminotransferase activity two to seven days after administration and by decreased circulating albumin concentrations. *Lambda* and *iota* carrageenan had no clear effect on these urinary or serum enzyme activities (Thomson & Whiting, 1981).

Carrageenan induces acute inflammatory responses in rats (oedema) (Winter *et al.*, 1962; Van Arman *et al.*, 1965; Di Rosa & Sorrentino, 1968; Di Rosa, 1972); this reaction has been used as a model system in which potential anti-inflammatory drugs are studied (discussed in Di Rosa, 1972). It also induces granulomatous lesions when injected subcutaneously into guinea-pigs (Robertson & Schwartz, 1953). It induces inflammation (pneumonia) in the lungs of rabbits and cats (Trenchard *et al.*, 1972), mice (Velo & Spector, 1973) and rats (Wachtlová *et al.*, 1975) as well as granulomatous lesions in rats (Bowers *et al.*, 1980) following its intratracheal or intralobular administration.

Suppressive effects on humoral- and cell-mediated immunity in experimental animals of the parenteral administration of carrageenans have been reviewed (Thomson *et al.*, 1979).

B. Degraded carrageenan

Degraded carrageenan, especially the C16 product with an average molecular weight of 20 000 derived from *Eucheuma spinosum*, caused ulceration of the caecum in guinea-pigs due to its accumulation in macrophage lysosomes when administered at a concentration of 2% in drinking-water for two weeks (Abraham *et al.*, 1974). It also caused haemorrhage and ulceration of the colon in rhesus monkeys when given at concentrations of 0.5-2% in the drinking-water (Benitz *et al.*, 1973).

Experiments with oral administration of several fractions of degraded *kappa*, *lambda* and *iota* carrageenans of different molecular weights to guinea-pigs indicated that caecal ulceration in this species is caused only by *iota* carrageenan of a certain range of molecular weights, administered in drinking-water. *Kappa* and *lambda* fractions of molecular weights of 8500-314 000 and 20 800-275 000, respectively, and *iota* fractions of 5000, 8700 and 145 000 produced no effect when given at a concentration of 1% in drinking-water for two weeks. *Iota* fractions of molecular weights of 21 000-107 000 given in the same way produced erosion and ulceration of the caecum. When given at 2% in the diet for 10 weeks, *iota* fractions of 21 000 and 39 000 molecular weights produced epithelial thinning of the caecum, but no ulceration (Engster & Abraham, 1976).

Effects on reproduction and prenatal toxicity

In a three-generation reproduction study, groups of 40 male and 40 female Osborne-Mendel rats of each generation were fed diets containing 0.5, 1.0, 2.5 or 5.0% calcium *kappa* and *lambda* carrageenan for 12 weeks before mating and thereafter. No effect was detected with respect to fertility, average litter size, average number of live born animals, viability, or survival of offspring (Collins *et al.*, 1977a). Developmental effects were studied in approximately 170 pregnant animals from each of the F_2 and F_3 generations. No external, skeletal or soft-tissue anomaly was correlated with treatment (Collins *et al.*, 1977b).

Groups of 21-26 pregnant female Syrian hamsters received 10, 40, 100 or 200 mg/kg bw sodium or calcium *kappa* and *lambda* carrageenan by oral intubation on days 6-10 of gestation, and further groups of eight animals received degraded *iota* carrageenan C16. No compound-related external, soft-tissue or skeletal abnormality was observed (Collins *et al.*, 1979).

Absorption, distribution, excretion and metabolism

Native carrageenan is absorbed to a very small extent, if at all, but degraded carrageenan is absorbed to an extent varying with its average molecular weight (Hawkins & Yaphe, 1965; Anderson & Soman, 1966; Dewar & Maddy, 1970; Grasso *et al.*, 1975; Pittman *et al.*, 1976). [There are no adequate data demonstrating that native carrageenan is absorbed.] Some evidence indicates that carrageenan of high molecular weight is changed during passage through the gut (Pittman *et al.*, 1976). The authors interpreted the changes as a reduction in molecular weight.

Degraded carrageenans are taken up and stored in the lysosomes of intestinal macrophages of guinea-pigs (Abraham *et al.*, 1974) and in macrophages and in Kuppfer cells of the rhesus monkey (Abraham *et al.*, 1972; Mankes & Abraham, 1975).

Mutagenicity and other short-term tests

No data on the activity of native carrageenan in short-term tests were available to the Working Group.

Degraded carrageenan was not mutagenic to *Salmonella typhimurium* TA98 or TA100, in the presence or absence of a rat liver activation system, nor to Chinese hamster V79 cells (8-azaguanine resistance). Degraded carrageenan also showed no positive result in the transformation assay with cryopreserved primary hamster embryo cells (Wakabayashi, 1981). [The Working Group noted the low frequency of transformed foci in positive controls.]

(b) *Humans*

Toxic effects

Six patients suffering from malignant disease of the colon were given 5 g degraded carrageenan daily for 10 days before colectomy was performed. Samples of normal sections of colon obtained at surgery showed no sign of ulceration, nor was degraded carrageenan detected by either histochemical or analytical investigation (Grasso *et al.*, 1973).

Effects on reproduction and prenatal toxicity

No data were available to the Working Group.

Absorption, distribution, excretion and metabolism

No data were available to the Working Group.

Mutagenicity and chromoşomal effects

No data were available to the Working Group.

3.3 Case reports and epidemiological studies of carcinogenicity in humans

No data were available to the Working Group.

4. Summary of Data Reported and Evaluation

4.1 Experimental data

Native (undegraded) carrageenan was tested for carcinogenicity in rats and hamsters by administration in the diet; no evidence of carcinogenicity was found. In female rats treated with azoxymethane or *N*-nitrosomethylurea together with native carrageenan in the diet, a greater incidence of colorectal cancers was observed than with treatment by azoxymethane or *N*-nitrosomethylurea alone. Degraded carrageenan was tested in rats by administration in the diet, in the drinking-water and by oral intubation, in four experiments; colorectal cancers were induced in each study.

Native carrageenan has not been tested in short-term assays. Degraded carrageenan was not mutagenic in bacteria or in mammalian cells *in vitro*. The data were *inadequate* to evaluate the activity of degraded carrageenan in short-term tests.

Native or degraded carrageenan had no reproductive or teratogenic effect in rats or hamsters.

4.2 Human data

Carrageenan-containing seeweeds have been used since at least two hundred years, and isolated carrageenan has been used as a food additive since 1937. Carrageenan is used in the manufacture of food, drug and cosmetic products and in multiple industrial applications, resulting in wide human exposure.

No data were available to assess the teratogenicity or chromosomal effects of this compound in humans.

No case report or epidemiological study on the carcinogenicity of native or degraded carrageenan was available to the Working Group.

4.3 Evaluation

The available data do not provide evidence that native (undegraded) carrageenan is carcinogenic to experimental animals. In the absence of epidemiological data, no evaluation of the carcinogenicity of native carrageenan to humans could be made.

Experiments in rats with doses of degraded carrageenan comparable to those used to test native carrageenan provide *sufficient evidence*[1] for the carcinogenicity of degraded carrageenan in rats. No data on humans were available.

5. References

Abraham, R., Golberg, L. & Coulston, F. (1972) Uptake and storage of degraded carrageenan in lysosomes of reticuloendothelial cells of the rhesus monkey, *Macaca mulatta. Exp. mol. Pathol.*, *17*, 77-93

Abraham, R., Fabian, R.J., Golberg, L. & Coulston, F. (1974) Role of lysosomes in carrageenan-induced cecal ulceration. *Gastroenterology*, *67*, 1169-1181

Anderson, W. (1967) Carrageenan. Structure and biological activity. *Can. J. pharm. Sci.*, *2*, 81-90

Anderson, W. & Duncan, J.G.C. (1965) The anticoagulant activity of carrageenan. *J. Pharm. Pharmacol.*, *17*, 647-654

Anderson, W. & Soman, P.D. (1966) The absorption of carrageenans. *J. Pharm. Pharmacol.*, *18*, 825-827

Benitz, K.-F., Abraham, R., Golberg, L. & Coulston, F. (1972) Carrageenan: An ulcerogenic agent? (Abstract no. 18). *Toxicol. appl. Pharmacol.*, *22*, 282

Benitz, K.-F., Golberg, L. & Coulston, F. (1973) Intestinal effects of carrageenans in the rhesus monkey (*Macaca mulatta*). *Food Cosmet. Toxicol.*, *11*, 565-575

Boyd, J.R., ed. (1982) *Facts and Comparisons*, St Louis, MO, Facts and Comparisons Division, J.B. Lippincott Company, pp. 321a, 323c

Bowers, R.R., Houston, F., Clinton, R., Lewis, M. & Ballard, R. (1980) A histological study of the carrageenan-induced granuloma in the rat lung. *J. Pathol.*, *132*, 243-253

Cater, D.B. (1961) The carcinogenic action of carrageenin in rats. *Br. J. Cancer.*, *15*, 607-614

CECA SA (undated) *The Carrageenans*, Velizy Villacoublay, France, Département des Algues et Colloides

---

[1]In the absence of adequate data on humans, it is reasonable, for practical purposes, to regard chemicals for which there is sufficient evidence of carcinogenicity in animals as if they presented a carcinogenic risk to humans.

Collins, T.F.X., Black, T.N. & Prew, J.H. (1977a) Long-term effects of calcium carrageenan in rats. I. Effects on reproduction. *Food Cosmet. Toxicol.*, *15*, 533-538

Collins, T.F.X., Black, T.N. & Prew, J.H. (1977b) Long-term effects of calcium carrageenan in rats. II. Effects on foetal development. *Food Cosmet. Toxicol.*, *15*, 539-545

Collins, T.F.X., Black, T.N. & Prew, J.H. (1979) Effects of calcium and sodium carragee-nans and iota-carrageenan on hamster foetal development. *Food Cosmet. Toxicol.*, *17*, 443-449

Cottrell, I.W. & Baird, J.K. (1980) *Gums*. In: Kirk, R.E. & Othmer, D.F., eds, *Encyclopedia of Chemical Technology*, 3rd ed., Vol. 12, New York, John Wiley & Sons, pp. 5l-53, 64-66

Craigie, J.S. & Leigh, C. (1978) *Carrageenans and agars*. In: Hellebust, J.A. & Craigie, J.S., eds, *Handbook of Phycological Methods: Physiological and Biochemical Methods*, London, Cambridge University Press, pp. 109-131

Dewar, E.T. & Maddy, M.L. (1970) Faecal excretion of degraded and native carrageenan by the young rat. *J. Pharm. Pharmacol.*, *22*, 791-793

Di Rosa, M. (1972) Biological properties of carrageenan. *J. Pharm. Pharmacol.*, *24*, 89-102

Di Rosa, M. & Sorrentino, L. (1968) The mechanism of the inflammatory effect of carrageenin. *Eur. J. Pharmacol.*, *4*, 340-342

Engster, M. & Abraham, R. (1976) Cecal response to different molecular weights and types of carrageenan in the guinea pig. *Toxicol. appl. Pharmacol.*, *38*, 265-282

FAO/WHO (1974) Toxicological evaluation of certain food additives with a review of general principles and of specifications. *WHO tech. Rep. Ser. No. 539*, pp. 21-22, 37

Grasso, P., Sharratt, M., Carpanini, F.M.B. & Gangolli, S.D. (1973) Studies on carrageenan and large-bowel ulceration in mammals. *Food Cosmet. Toxicol.*, *11*, 555-564

Grasso, P., Gangolli, S.D., Butterworth, K.R. & Wright, M.G. (1975) Studies on degraded carrageenan in rats and guinea-pigs. *Food Cosmet. Toxicol.*, *13*, 195-201

Guiseley, K.B. (1968) *Seaweed colloids*. In: Kirk, R.E. & Othmer, D.F., eds, *Encyclopedia of Chemical Technology*, 2nd ed., Vol. 17, New York, John Wiley & Sons, pp. 774-784

Hawkins, W.W. & Yaphe, W. (1965) Carrageenan as a dietary constituent for the rat: faecal excretion, nitrogen absorption, and growth. *Can. J. Biochem.*, *43*, 479-484

Houck, J.C., Morris, R.K. & Lazaro, E.J. (1957) Anticoagulant, lipemia clearing and other effects of anionic polysaccharides extracted from seaweed. *Proc. Soc. exp. Biol. Med.*, *96*, 528-530

Huebotter, E.E. & Gray, G.R. (1965) *Drilling fluids*. In: Kirk, R.E. & Othmer, D.F., eds, *Encyclopedia of Chemical Technology*, 2nd ed., Vol. 7, New York, John Wiley & Sons, pp. 299, 305-307

IARC (1976) *IARC Monographs on the Evaluation of Carcinogenic Risk of Chemicals to Man*, Vol. 10, *Some Naturally Occurring Substances*, Lyon, pp. 181-190

Idson, B. & Bachynsky, M.O. (1978) Natural raw materials in semi-solid dosage forms. *Drug Cosmet. Ind.*, February, 40-41

Informatics, Inc. (1972) *GRAS (Generally Recognized As Safe) Food Ingredients: Carrageenan*, PB-221206. Prepared for US Food & Drug Administration, Springfield, VA, National Technical Information Service, pp. 9-11, 30, 37

Maillet, M., Bonfils, S. & Lister, R.E. (1970) Carrageenan: Effects in animals. *Lancet, ii*, 414-415

Mankes, R. & Abraham, R. (1975) Lysosomal dysfunction in colonic submucosal macrophages of rhesus monkeys caused by degraded iota carrageenan. *Proc. Soc. exp. Biol. Med.*, *150*, 166-170

National Research Council (1981) *Food Chemicals Codex*, 3rd ed., Washington DC, National Academy Press, pp. 74, 75

Oohashi, Y., Ishioka, T., Wakabayashi, K. & Kuwabara, N. (1981) A study on carcinogenesis induced by degraded carrageenan arising from squamous metaplasia of the rat colorectum. *Cancer Lett.*, *14*, 267-272

Pittman, K.A., Golberg, L. & Coulston, F. (1976) Carrageenan: The effect of molecular weight and polymer type on its uptake, excretion and degradation in animals. *Food Cosmet. Toxicol.*, *14*, 85-93

Poulsen, E. (1973) Short-term peroral toxicity of undegraded carrageenan in pigs. *Food Cosmet. Toxicol.*, *11*, 219-227

Robertson, W. van B. & Schwartz, B. (1953) Ascorbic acid and the formation of collagen. *J. biol. Chem.*, *201*, 689-696

Rustia, M., Shubik, P. & Patil, K. (1980) Lifespan carcinogenicity tests with native carrageenan in rats and hamsters. *Cancer Lett.*, *11*, 1-10

Salminen, S. & Hallikainen, A. (1983) *The toxicity of carrageenan*. In: *Scandinavian Meeting of Food Toxicologists, Helsinki, 1982* (in press)

Swinyard, E.A. (1975) *Pharmaceutical necessities*. In: Osol, A., ed., *Remington's Pharmaceutical Sciences*, 15th ed., Easton, PA, Mack Publishing Co., pp. 1221, 1246

Thomson, A.W. & Whiting, P.H. (1981) A comparative study of renal and hepatic function in Sprague-Dawley rats following systemic injection of purified carrageenans (kappa, lambda and iota). *Br. J. exp. Pathol.*, *62*, 207-213

Thomson, A.W., Fowler, E.F., Pugh-Humphreys, R.G.P. (1979) Immunopharmacology of the macrophage-toxic agent carrageenan. *Int. J. Immunopharmacol.*, *I*, 247-261

Tong, H.-K., Lee, K.-H. & Wong, H.-A. (1980) The molecular weight and viscosity of the water-soluble polysaccharide(s) from *Eucheuma spinosum*. *Carbohydr. Res.*, *81*, 1-6

Towle, G.A. (1973) *Carrageenan.* In: Whistler, R.L., ed., *Industrial Gums*, New York, Academic Press, pp. 83-114

Trenchard, D., Gardner, D. & Guz, A. (1972) Role of pulmonary vagal afferent nerve fibres in the development of rapid shallow breathing in lung inflammation. *Clin. Sci., 42,* 251-263

US Department of Commerce (1980) *US Imports for Consumption and General Imports (FT246/Annual 1979)*, Washington DC, Bureau of the Census, p. I-54

US Environmental Protection Agency (1979) *Toxic Substances Control Act (TSCA) Chemical Substance Inventory*, Vol. II, *User Guide and Indices to the Initial Inventory. Substance Name Index*, Washington DC, Office of Toxic Substances, p. 344

US Environmental Protection Aency (1980) Protection of the environment. *US Code Fed. Regul., Title 40*, part 180.1001

US Food & Drug Administration (1978) *Voluntary Cosmetic Regulatory Program, Cosmetics Registration File, August 1978*, Washington DC

US Food & Drug Administration (1980) Food and drugs. *US Code Fed. Regul., Title 21*, part 172.620

Van Arman, C.G., Begany, A.J., Miller, L.M. & Pless, H.H. (1965) Some details of the inflammations caused by yeast and carrageenin (with appendix on kinetics of the reaction). *J. Pharmacol. exp. Ther., 150,* 328-334

Velo, G.P. & Spector, W.G. (1973) The origin and turnover of alveolar macrophages in experimental pneumonia. *J. Pathol., 109,* 7-19

Wachtlová, M., Chválová, M., Holusa, R. & Palecek, F. (1975) Carrageenin-induced experimental pneumonia in rats. *Physiol. bohemoslov., 24,* 263-268

Wade, A., ed. (1977) *Martindale, The Extra Pharmacopoeia*, 27th ed., London, The Pharmaceutical Press, pp. 919, 920

Wakabayashi, K. (1981) A study on carcinogenesis of degraded carrageenan, a polysaccharide-sulphate, derived from seaweeds (Jpn.). *Juntendo med. J., 27,* 159-171

Wakabayashi, K., Inagaki, T., Fujimoto, Y. & Fukuda, Y. (1978) Induction by degraded carrageenan of colorectal tumors in rats. *Cancer Lett., 4,* 171-176

Watanabe, K., Reddy, B.S., Wong, C.Q. & Weisburger, J.H. (1978) Effect of dietary undegraded carrageenan on colon carcinogenesis in F344 rats treated with azoxymethane or methylnitrosourea. *Cancer Res., 38,* 4427-4430

Whistler, R.L. & Zysk, J.R. (1978) *Carbohydrates.* In: Kirk, R.E. & Othmer, D.H., eds, *Encyclopedia of Chemical Technology*, 3rd ed., New York, John Wiley & Sons, pp. 544, 545, 554, 555

WHO (1974) Toxicological evaluation of some food additives including anticaking agents, antimicrobials, antioxidants, emulsifiers and thickening agents. *WHO/Food Additive Series, No. 5*, p. 386

Windholz, M., ed. (1976) *The Merck Index*, 9th ed., Rahway, NJ, Merck & Co., Inc., p. 238

Winter, C.A., Risley, E.A. & Nuss, G.W. (1962) Carrageenin-induced edema in hind paw of the rat as an assay for antiinflammatory drugs. *Proc. Soc. exp. Biol. Med.*, *111*, 544-547

CHOLESTEROL

This compound was considered by a previous working group, in October 1975 (IARC, 1976). Since that time, new data have become available, and these have been incorporated into the monograph and taken into consideration in the present evaluation.

1. Chemical and Physical Data

1.1 Synonyms and trade names

Chem. Abstr. Services Reg. No.: 57-88-5

Chem. Abstr. Name: Cholest-5-en-3-ol (3β)

IUPAC Systematic Name: Cholesterol

Synonyms: Cholest-5-en-3β-ol; Δ⁵-cholesten-3β-ol; 5-cholesten-3β-ol; 5,6-cholesten-3β-ol; cholesterin; cholesterine; (-)-cholesterol; cholesterol base H; cholesteryl alcohol; hydrocerin; 3β-hydroxycholest-5-ene; provitamin D

Trade Names: Cordulan; Dusoline; Dusoran; Dythol; Kathro; Lanol; Nimco Cholesterol Base H; Nimco Cholesterol Base No. 7l2; Super Hartolan; Tegolan

1.2 Structural and molecular formulae and molecular weight

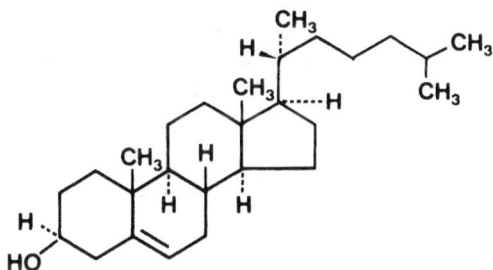

$C_{27}H_{46}O$

Mol. wt: 386.7

1.3 Chemical and physical properties of the pure substance

From Windholz (1976), unless otherwise specified

(a) *Description*: Pearly leaflets or plates recrystallized from dilute ethanol (monohydrate)

(b) *Melting-point*: 148.5°C (anhydrous)

(c) *Density*: 1.03 (monohydrate); d_{18}^{18} 1.052 (anhydrous)

(d) *Optical rotation*: $[\alpha]_D^{20}$ - 31.5° (in diethyl ether); $[\alpha]_D^{20}$ -39.5° (in chloroform)

(e) *Spectroscopy data*: Infra-red, mass and nuclear magnetic resonance spectroscopy data have been reported (NIH/EPA Chemical Information System, 1982).

(f) *Identity and purity test*: When sulphuric acid is added to a chloroform solution, it acquires a blood-red colour and the sulphuric acid shows a green fluorescence (US Pharmacopeial Convention, Inc., 1980).

(g) *Solubility*: Practically insoluble in water (about 2 mg/l); soluble in aqueous solutions of bile salts, benzene, chloroform (220 g/l), diethyl ether (360 g/l), ethanol (13 g/l at 20°C), fats, oils, petroleum ether and pyridine (665 g/l)

(h) *Stability*: On exposure to air, forms the α-epoxide, 1,4-chlolestadien-3-one and other products (Fioriti & Sims, 1967)

1.4 Technical products and impurities

Various national and international pharmacopoeias give specifications for the purity of cholesterol in pharmaceutical products. For example, it is available in the US as a USP grade with maxima of 0.3% moisture content and 0.1% residue on ignition, with a melting-point between 147°C and 150°C and a specific rotation between -38° and -34° (in 1,4-dioxane), and it must pass identification tests as well as solubility and acidity tests (US Pharmacopeial Convention, Inc., 1980).

In countries of the European Communities, cholesterol is available as a white powder or plates, with a melting-point of 145-150°C and a specific rotation of $[\alpha]_D^{20}$ = -40.5° to -38.5°, determined in a 2% w/v solution in chloroform (Council of Europe, 1969).

2. Production, Use, Occurrence and Analysis

2.1 Production and use

(a) *Production*

Cholesterol is the principal sterol of all higher animals. It was isolated from gallstones by Poulletier de la Salle in around 1760. Although progress was made toward elucidation of its structure in the nineteenth century (Kritchevsky, 1958), it was not until 1932 that advances in X-ray crystallography enabled determination of the final structure (Sabine, 1977). In the 1950s and 1960s, several routes of synthesis for cholesterol were reported (Woodward *et al.*, 1952; Cardwell *et al.*, 1953; Keana & Johnson, 1964).

Cholesterol is not produced commercially by synthetic methods: it is isolated from slaughterhouse wastes, such as the spinal cord of cattle, by extraction of the non-saponifiable matter with petroleum ether. It is also produced from wool grease (Windholz, 1976).

Because cholesterol is not a synthetic organic chemical, information on the number of US producers is sketchy, and no production data are published, although four US companies reported production in 1977 (NIH/EPA Chemical Information System, 1981). Separate data on US imports and exports of cholesterol are not reported; however, 10 US companies described importation of cholesterol in 1977, with total imports for six of the companies in the range of 10.9-109 thousand kg (NIH/EPA Chemical Information System, 1981).

Cholesterol has been made commercially in Japan since 1962. The two Japanese companies currently producing it made an estimated 20 thousand kg in 1981. Imports were negligible, and an estimated 5 thousand kg were exported.

Cholesterol is believed to be produced by three companies each in France and the United Kingdom and by one company in The Netherlands.

(b) *Use*

Cholesterol is widely used in pharmaceutical and dermal preparations as an emulsifying agent (e.g., in oils, creams, lotions and ointments). It is used in cosmetic preparations (e.g., cleansing and moisturizing creams, after-shave lotions, lipsticks, eye make-up, hair conditioners, shampoos and tanning creams). It is also a constituent of USP Hydrophilic Petrolatum (a soft paraffin containing 3% cholesterol) (US Pharmacopeial Convention, Inc., 1980) and similar ointment bases (e.g., wool alcohol, which contains 30% minimum cholesterol) used in pharmaceuticals and cosmetics. In addition, cholesterol is used as a raw material in the manufacture (*via* 7-dehydrocholesterol) of vitamin D_3 and a variety of steroids (Taub & Windholz, 1969) and of a variety of esters used as liquid crystals (DuPré, 1981).

Most of the estimated 15 thousand kg of cholesterol used in Japan in 1981 was used as an emulsifier in cosmetics. Minor amounts were used for synthesis of steroids and liquid crystals.

2.2 Occurrence

Cholesterol occurs either free or esterified with fatty acids in all body tissues of animals. Sites of high concentrations are the brain, spinal cord and fat tissue. Reported concentrations of cholesterol in several human tissues and body fluids are shown in Tables 1 (Sabine, 1977) and 2 (Lentner, 1981).

Table 1. Approximate distribution of cholesterol in a 70-kg man[a]

System	Weight (g)	Cholesterol		
		Concentration (% wet weight)	Amount (g)	Percentage of total body cholesterol
Brain and nervous system	1600	2.0	32.0	22
Connective tissue (including adipose) and body fluids	12 100	0.25	31.3	22
Muscle	30 000	0.1	30.0	21
Skin	4200	0.3-0.7	16.0	11
Blood	5400	0.2	10.8	8
Bone marrow	3000	0.25	7.5	5
Liver	1700	0.3	5.1	2
Alimentary tract	2500	0.15	3.8	3
Lungs	950	0.2	1.9	1
Kidneys	300	0.25-0.34	0.9	1
Adrenal glands	12	2.6-15	1.2	1
Other glands	100	0.2	0.2	
Heart	350	0.09-0.18	0.6	
Spleen	200	0.16-0.34	0.5	
Blood vessels	200	0.25	0.5	
Skeleton	7000	0.01	0.7	
			143.0	

[a]From Sabine (1977)

Table 2. Some reported concentrations of cholesterol in human body fluids

Tissue (units)	Mean
Urine (mg/day)	1.0
Hepatic bile (g/l)	1.79
Gallbladder bile (g/l)	3.90
Cerebrospinal fluid (mg/l)	4.63
Tears (mg/l)	150.0
Amniotic fluid (32-43 weeks) (mg/l)	57.4
Breast milk[a] (mg/l)	139.0

[a]Mature milk (15 days to 15 months *post partum*)

A bibliography has been published containing those literature citations from September 1974 to January 1982 which provide data on the cholesterol content of foods of animal origin (Food Sciences & Technology Abstracts, 1982). Because of the widespread occurrence of cholesterol in foods, no comprehensive listing is provided here. The concentrations of cholesterol in foods vary widely, even within classes of food. The following figures have been reported (Lentner, 1981): fats and oils, 0.01-5 g/kg; milk and dairy products, 0.02-1 g/kg; meat, 0.7-23 g/kg; poultry, 0.9-5.6 g/kg; egg yolk, 14 g/kg; and fish, 0.4-3 g/kg.

2.3 Analysis

A large number of analytical methods have been published regarding the extraction, separation and quantitation of cholesterol from biological materials. The preferred method of extraction (Folch *et al.*, 1957) of biological material makes use of chloroform:methanol (2:1 v/v), which readily removes all lipids. Separation of the lipids after hydrolysis is carried out by an array of chromatographic methods and systems. For quantitation, colorimetric measurement, gas-liquid chromatography, enzymatic determination, and isotope dilution with mass spectrometry have been used. Some typical methods for the analysis of cholesterol in food products and biological matrices are summarized in Table 3.

Table 3. Methods for the analysis of cholesterol[a]

Sample matrix	Sample preparation	Assay procedure[b]	Reference
Biological specimens	Inject finely divided specimen into a solution of cholesterol oxidase and esterase; measure the resulting hydrogen peroxide	Polarography	Clark et al. (1981)
	Mix with ethanolic ferric chloride; hydrolyse (ethanolic potassium hydroxide); centrifuge; treat with ethanolic ferric chloride, then sulphuric acid; extract the chromogen (dichloromethane)	UV	Clark et al. (1968)
	Mix with solution of standard (5α-cholestane), tetramethylammonium hydroxide and isopropanol; add ethyl acetate	GC/FID	MacGee et al. (1973)
	Mix with cholesterol esterase and oxidase; couple the resulting hydrogen peroxide oxidatively with 4-aminoantipyrine and phenol to yield chromogen	UV	Allain et al. (1974)
	Mix with cholesterol esterase and oxidase; catalytically oxidize homovanillic acid with the resulting hydrogen peroxide to highly fluorescent 2,2'-dihydroxy-3,3'-dimethoxy-biphenyl-5,5'-diacetic acid	FL	Huang et al. (1975)
	Mix with labelled cholesterol; hydrolyse esters (aqueous potassium hydroxide); isolate crude mixture; derivatize [bis(trimethylsilyl)acetamide]	ID/MS	Cohen et al. (1980)
Serum and high-density lipoprotein	Mix with cholesterol esterase and oxidase; use resulting hydrogen peroxide as a substrate for NAD^+ peroxidase	S	Avigad & Robertson (1981)

[a]Limits of detection are not given, because they are not applicable to this substance.

[b]Abbreviations: UV, ultra-violet detection; GC/FID, gas chromatography with flame-ionization detection; FL, fluorometric detection; ID/MS, isotope dilution with mass spectrometric detection; S, spectrophotometric analysis

3. Biological Data Relevant to the Evaluation of Carcinogenic Risk to Humans

3.1 Carcinogenicity studies in animals

(a) Oral administration

Mouse: Groups of 10-12 mice of the T.M. strain were maintained on a Rockland rat diet supplemented with cholesterol given in amounts of 50-100 mg daily, and were bred for three or more generations. Controls and offspring of treated groups were maintained on the same diet. Total numbers of 118 (60 males and 58 females) controls and 71 (36 males and 35 females) cholesterol-treated animals were evaluated. All mice lived for over 650 days. Of the 71 treated mice, 58 (81.6%) developed malignancies, *versus* 17.8% of the controls; lung adenocarcinomas occurred in 54 (76%) treated animals and 16 (13.5%) controls. Other malignancies found only in the treated animals were liver cancer, uterine cancer and four skin squamous-cell carcinomas (Szepsenwol, 1966). [The Working Group noted the high dose used; that there was no indication of equalization in the caloric content of the diets of treated and control groups; and that the experimental design does not permit an evaluation of the carcinogenicity of cholesterol.]

(b) Subcutaneous administration

Mouse: In a series of experiments in which stock, C57, MRC, $C_{57}xC_3H$, Swiss S, BALB/C, CBA and C_3H mice were injected subcutaneously with cholesterol in different solvents and after various forms of preparation, sarcomas were observed at the site of injection. The incidence of sarcomas varied from 0-28%; the variation was attributed by the authors to factors other than cholesterol (Hieger & Orr, 1954; Hieger, 1957, 1958, 1959, 1962).

(c) Other experimental systems

Various urinary or gall-bladder implant studies have been carried out using cholesterol pellets (Desforges *et al.*, 1950; Clayson *et al.*, 1958; Boyland *et al.*, 1964; Bryan *et al.*, 1964). The general outcome of such experiments is considered equivocal with regard to the carcinogenic potential of cholesterol.

(d) Co-carcinogenesis experiments

Mouse: Female DDD mice (20-30 animals/group) were fed a diet containing 1% cholesterol and 0.5% cholic acid, with or without N-hydroxy-2-acetylaminofluorene (0.05%) for 30 weeks. The results did not indicate that the cholesterol-cholic acid diet affected the carcinogenicity of N-hydroxy-2-acetylaminofluorene (Enomoto *et al.*, 1974).

Rat: Groups of 20 female inbred weanling Wistar rats received a standard diet, a cholesterol-free chemically defined diet (Vivonex) or Vivonex with added cholesterol (6-9 mg/rat/day). Half of the animals of each group were treated subcutaneously with 1,2-dimethylhydrazine (40 mg/kg bw) in saline, once weekly for 13 weeks; the other animals in each group were maintained on the respective diets and were injected with saline, to serve as non-carcinogen controls. The caloric intake per adult rat was comparable among the various groups. At 56 weeks, all the rats treated with 1,2-dimethylhydrazine had adenocarcinomas of the colon. The rats fed the cholesterol-free Vivonex diet showed a significant increase in time to tumour appearance (p < 0.001) and survival (p = 0.001) as compared with the carcinogen-injected group fed a standard diet. A statistically signifi-cant decrease in time to tumour appearance (p < 0.001) and survival (p = 0.008) as well as an increased incidence of metastasis was found when the cholesterol-treated rats were compared with the rats fed the cholesterol-free Vivonex diet (Cruse et al., 1978). [The Working Group noted that no information was available about the group of rats administered the standard diet plus cholesterol.]

Ninety female Sprague-Dawley rats, 22 days of age, were subdivided into three equal groups: group 1 received a cholesterol-free semisynthetic diet (SD), while two other groups (groups 2 and 3) were maintained on the same diet supplemented with 1.5% cholesterol and 0.5% bile salts (CB). Between the ages of 48 and 52 days, all animals received SD and at the age of 50 days a single gavage of 5 mg 7,12-dimethyl-benz[a]anthracene (DMBA) dissolved in 0.5 ml corn oil. Starting at the age of 52 days, group 2 was again fed CB, while groups 1 and 3 received SD. The CB diet induced a three-fold increase in serum cholesterol levels, as compared with SD (p < 0.001). There was no statistically significant difference in the incidence of mammary tumours among the three groups (69-73%) at the termination of the experiments four months after the administration of DMBA (Klurfeld & Kritchevsky, 1981).

Hamster: Male golden hamsters were given 13-15-mg cholesterol pellets as implants in the gall-bladder and N-nitrosodiethyl- or N-nitrosodimethylamine (NDEA or NDMA) in their drinking-water one day later at dose levels of 0.15 mg/l NDEA and 0.02 mg/l NDMA. The experiments were terminated at 22 weeks; no difference was observed in the incidences of liver tumours among the various groups. However, the incidence of carcinoma of the gall-bladder was 13/19 in hamsters treated with both NDMA and a cholesterol pellet and only 1/16 in those with no cholesterol pellet but NDMA. No carcinoma of the gall-bladder was observed in hamsters that received cholesterol implants alone or in combination with NDEA or NDEA alone (Kowalewski & Todd, 1971). [The Working Group noted that no control group was treated with pellets other than cholesterol, and that the duration of the experiment was short.]

3.2 Other relevant biological data

Reviews are available on cholesterol metabolism (Havel et al., 1980; Stanbury et al., 1983) as well as on the relationship of dietary cholesterol to serum concentration, cholesterol gallstone disease, familial hypercholesterolaemia and atherosclerosis in humans (Goldstein et al., 1975; Gurll & DenBesten, 1978; McGill, 1979; Berwick et al., 1980; Goldstein & Brown, 1983).

(a) *Experimental systems*

Toxic effects

No data were available to the Working Group.

Effects on reproduction and prenatal toxicity

Studies with ^{14}C-cholesterol have shown that 20-70% of cholesterol found in foetuses of rats, rabbits, guinea-pigs and monkeys was of maternal origin (Chevallier, 1964; Connor & Lin, 1967; Pitkin et al, 1972).

In groups of 5-7 pregnant Holtzmann and Snell-Supplee albino rats given daily s.c. injections of 5, 10 and 15 mg cholesterol on days 8-14 of pregnancy, cleft palate abnormalities were produced in 27, 52 and 57% of the offspring, respectively. No cleft palate occurred in controls (Buresh & Urban, 1964, 1967; Chase et al., 1971).

After daily s.c. administration of 20 mg cholesterol to pregnant Sprague-Dawley rats, a general reduction in foetal size was seen, and 112/286 pups had gross oral clefts. However, no histologically detectable cleft anomaly was observed in foetuses removed from rats injected with 6 mg cholesterol (Ursick et al., 1972).

Absorption, distribution, excretion and metabolism

The biochemistry of cholesterol has been extensively reviewed (Lehninger, 1975; Havel et al., 1980).

Cholesterol is distributed universally in all animal tissues. It can be derived either from intestinal absorption of dietary cholesterol or from synthesis *de novo* within the body (Dietschy & Wilson, 1968, 1970; Siperstein, 1970).

The metabolism of cholesterol, which is similar in most mammals, including man, is described in section 3.2b.

Cholesterol introduced into the caecum of rats is changed to lithocholic and isolithocholic acids, which are partly excreted in the faeces. In the guinea-pig, the gut bacteria can metabolize cholesterol to oestradiol and oestrone, which are excreted in the urine (Goddard & Hill, 1974).

Cholesterol is oxidized to its α-epoxide ($5\alpha,6\alpha$-epoxycholestan-3β-ol) by enzyme systems in liver (Aringer & Eneroth, 1974) and brain (Martin & Nicholas, 1973). Cholesterol α-epoxide is found together with the isomeric β-epoxide ($5\beta,6\beta$-epoxycholestan-3β-ol) in a ratio of 1:1-4 as normal constituents of various mammalian tissues (Sevanian et al., 1979; Watabe et al., 1980), including those of man (Assmann et al., 1975). The formation of cholesterol α and β epoxides has been shown to occur in the presence of rat liver microsomal lipid hydroperoxides (Watabe et al., 1982). The capacity of cholesterol to undergo auto-oxidation is also well established (Bergström & Samuelsson, 1961; Smith et al., 1967).

Mutagenicity and other short-term tests

Pure cholesterol at doses of up to 10 µg/ml did not transform Syrian golden hamster embryo cells (Pienta, 1980). No enhancement of soft agar growth of baby Syrian hamster kidney 21 clone 13 cells was found, with or without exogenous metabolic activation (Styles, 1978).

Cholesterol α-epoxide, a product of the autoxidation of cholesterol, was not mutagenic to *Salmonella typhimurium* TA1535, TA1537, TA1538, TA98 or TA100 (Ansari et al., 1982). Air-aged commercial samples of cholesterol were mutagenic towards *S. typhimurium* TA1537, TA1538 and TA98, but no activity was observed with strains TA100 or TA1535

(Smith *et al.*, 1979; Ansari *et al.*, 1982). The observed mutagenicity was associated with polar cholesterol autoxidation products generated during oxidation of the sterol B-ring and of the side-chain, and did not require metabolic activation for mutagenic activity (Ansari *et al.*, 1982). Cholesterol was not mutagenic to *S. typhimurium* TA1535, TA1536, TA1537, TA1538, TA98 or TA100 (Cotruvo *et al.*, 1977). Pure crystalline steroid was converted to a mutagen after heating at 70°C in air or after exposure to ^{60}Co γ-radiation (Smith *et al.*, 1979). Cholesterol α-epoxide damaged chromosomes and initiated DNA repair synthesis in cultured human fibroblasts (Parsons & Goss, 1978), and it transformed cultured hamster embryo cells (Kelsey & Pienta, 1979). Cholestan-3β,5α,6β-triol, a metabolite of cholesterol α-epoxide, also induced transformation in cultured hamster embryo cells (Kelsey & Pienta, 1981).

(b) Humans

Toxic effects

Substantial epidemiological evidence has established a graduated increase in risk of coronary heart disease · associated with increasing levels of total and low-density lipoprotein cholesterol in the blood (Pooling Project Research Group, 1978; Grundy *et al.*, 1982). This risk of developing peripheral vascular disease (due to non-coronary atherosclerosis) is also increased by raised blood cholesterol levels. By contrast, the risk of cholesterol gallstone formation may be increased by a serum-cholesterol-lowering diet (Sturdevant *et al.*, 1973).

Effects on reproduction and prenatal toxicity

No data were available to the Working Group.

Absorption, distribution, excretion and metabolism

Cholesterol serves three major functions in man: (1) it is a required structural component of the plasma membrane of all cells; (2) it is a precursor of steroid hormones; and (3) it is a precursor of bile acids. Five major classes of lipoprotein serve to transport and regulate the supply of cholesterol to different body tissues: chylomicrons, very-low-density lipoproteins (VLDL), intermediate-density lipoproteins (IDL), low-density lipoproteins (LDL) and high-density lipoproteins (HDL). Cholesterol can exist either in the unesterified form or as an ester of a long-chain fatty acid. The former, often termed 'free cholesterol' to distinguish it from esterified cholesterol, is the metabolically active form of the sterol (Havel *et al.*, 1980).

The fraction of dietary cholesterol absorbed is dependent on the intake; after reaching a plateau, the amount absorbed decreases with increased dietary intake. Most people in western societies ingest between 500 and 800 mg/day and absorb from 300 to 400 mg/day (Montgomery *et al.*, 1980).

While virtually all nucleated mammalian cells can synthesize cholesterol (Bloch, 1965), quantitatively the most important tissues in man are the liver and the intestine (Dietschy & Wilson, 1970). These two tissues together probably account for more than 95% of the total cholesterol produced in the body each day. On a low cholesterol diet, the liver of an adult man of average size synthesizes about 0.9 g cholesterol per day (Havel *et al.*, 1980).

Cholesterol is metabolized in the liver, the main metabolic pathway being conversion to the two primary bile acids, cholic acid and chenodeoxycholic acid. These, after conjugation with either glycine or taurine, pass into the intestine *via* the bile, where they may be further metabolized by bacterial enzymes to yield the secondary bile acids, deoxycholic acid and lithocholic acid. Cholesterol is also converted to other neutral sterols; in the liver, reduction yields cholestanol (Elliott & Hyde, 1971). In the intestine, the main metabolites produced by bacterial enzymes are coprostanol (a stereoisomer of cholestanol) and cholestanone (Hill, 1980). Although both bile acids and neutral sterols undergo enterohepatic recirculation, there is a net loss daily of about 250 mg cholesterol as bile acids and about 500 mg as neutral sterols (Havel *et al.*, 1980).

In the adrenal cortex, testes and ovaries, cholesterol serves as the precursor for synthesis of steroid hormones. Cholesterol is converted *via* pregnenolone to progesterone, which in turn is the precursor of androgens (e.g., testosterone and androsterone), oestrogens (e.g., oestrone and oestradiol), and of the adrenal corticosteroids (e.g., cortisol, corticosterone and aldosterone) (Lehninger, 1975).

In the skin, there is evidence that cholesterol can be oxidized photochemically by irradiation with ultra-violet light (240-440 nm) to cholesterol α-epoxide (Black & Lo, 1971). A hydrolysis product of cholesterol α-epoxide, cholestane-3β,5α,6β-triol, is excreted in increased amounts in the faeces of patients with colonic cancer (Reddy & Wynder, 1977).

Various intestinal metabolites of cholesterol, such as the neutral steroids and the hydrolysis products of cholesterol and epoxide, are excreted in increased amounts in the faeces of patients with colonic cancer (Reddy & Wynder, 1977).

Cholesterol α-oxide, coprostanol and cholest-4-en-3-one have each been isolated and identified in serum (Gray *et al.*, 1971). The latter compound is believed to be an intermediate in the formation of cholestanol from cholesterol (Rosenfeld *et al.*, 1967). The concentration of cholesterol α-oxide found in normal serum is very low; however, in the serum of hypercholesterolaemic patients (cholesterol levels in the range 316-454 mg/100 ml), the concentrations were found to range from 250-3205 μg/100 ml serum (Gray *et al.*, 1971).

Mutagenicity and chromosomal effects

No data were available to the Working Group.

3.3 Case reports and epidemiological studies of carcinogenicity in humans

Several problems of a general nature apply in evaluating the possible causal association between cholesterol and human cancer.

Firstly, cholesterol is an integral part of the diet, and differences in dietary intake of cholesterol between individuals or population groups are thus likely to be accompanied by other dietary differences. This is illustrated by the strong correlation between cholesterol intake and the intake of other nutrients, e.g., fat, protein (Liu *et al.*, 1979). Thus, dietary cholesterol cannot be studied, within the observational research setting, as an isolated variable; and, further, the combined and perhaps interactive effects of various dietary constituents in carcinogenesis, while little understood, must be recognized (Armstrong et al., 1982).

Secondly, cholesterol is a natural component of virtually all tissues, with many biological or metabolic functions (see section 3.2b). The disturbance of such functions might influence various aspects of carcinogenesis, as has been discussed with regard to the influence of cholesterol on the fluidity of cell membranes and the functioning of immunocompetent cells (Oliver, 1981). In studies of faecal cholesterol in relation to bowel cancer, the closely-related metabolites of both cholesterol and bile acids must also be considered.

Thirdly, it would be difficult to reconcile observations of an association between a reduced level of a compound (cholesterol) and cancer risk with the assumption that the compound is 'carcinogenic'. In fact, the major current interest is in the possible increase in human cancer risk associated with low serum cholesterol.

The evaluation of this particular association, between low serum cholesterol and cancer risk, is further complicated by the possible influence of the late (pre-clinical) stages of carcinogenesis upon cholesterol metabolism, leading perhaps to a reduction in blood cholesterol levels, and thus making it difficult to distinguish between cause and effect. This possible effect has been widely discussed by various investigators and is referred to in the ensuing text as the 'undetected cancer effect' (UCE). Further, the covariation between serum cholesterol levels and other substances, believed to influence carcinogenesis (e.g., retinols) is largely unknown, and it must therefore be considered whether low serum cholesterol is merely an indication of one or several other factors as yet unidentified, that influence carcinogenesis.

Human studies relevant to the question of cholesterol and cancer, therefore, collectively embrace cholesterol in three distinct contexts; first, dietary cholesterol - which influences, to a degree that appears to vary between individuals, the concentration of cholesterol in the blood and faeces; second, blood cholesterol - which reflects the dynamic equilibrium between intestinal absorption, hepatic and intestinal synthesis and metabolism, transfer to peripheral tissues and clearance into the bile; and third, faecal cholesterol - which reflects diet, intestinal functioning and bile composition. While dietary cholesterol is appropriately construed as 'exogenous' cholesterol, cholesterol levels in both blood and faeces represent an unspecifiable combination of exogenous and endogenously synthesized cholesterol. Epidemiological studies of levels of cholesterol in the diet, blood and faeces in relation to cancer risk are therefore considered separately.

The studies summarized below describe cancer risk in relation to exposure to exogenous cholesterol by ingestion in foodstuffs, and in relation to endogenous cholesterol in blood and faeces. No case report or epidemiological study on other exogenous exposures was available.

(a) *Case reports*

No case report on exposure to exogenous cholesterol and cancer was available.

(b) *Epidemiological studies*

Dietary Cholesterol

1. Descriptive studies

Most of the initial epidemiological indications of associations of diet with cancer resulted from population-based correlation analyses in which international data on estimates of food consumption were correlated with cancer mortality or morbidity data (e.g., Drasar & Irving, 1973; Armstrong & Doll, 1975; Knox, 1977). The quality of such data is necessarily limited and varies between countries. In such studies, those cancers prominent in western populations, especially those of the colon, breast, endometrium and prostate, show consistently positive correlations with dietary fat and meat. Overall, populations with high dietary fat intakes are at high risk of developing these cancers, particularly colon cancer.

Liu *et al.* (1979) carried out an international correlation analysis of colon cancer mortality in relation to dietary cholesterol, fat and fibre. Food consumption estimates for 1954-1965 (FAO) were correlated with mortality data for 1967-1973 for the 20 industriali-zed countries studied. The partial positive correlation of high dietary cholesterol with colon cancer was highly statistically significant when dietary fat and fibre intake were controlled for.

In Hawaii, Kolonel *et al.* (1981) compared the diets of large random samples of people aged 45 years or more within the five main ethnic groups. Multiple regression analysis of the ten ethnic-sex-specific dietary profiles (assessed at interview by estimated weekly intake of 83 food items) and the corresponding incidence rates of 15 selected cancer sites showed that the only cancer sites that had a specific, statistically significant association with dietary cholesterol were lung and larynx (positive in each case): breast cancer and endometrial cancer were positively correlated with both unsaturated and saturated fat, and prostate cancer with saturated fat.

Studies of Japanese migrants to the US have indicated that an increase in dietary fat, dietary cholesterol and blood cholesterol levels (Marmot *et al.*, 1975) accompany an increased risk of cancers of the colon, pancreas and prostate (Haenszel & Kurihara, 1968).

2. Analytical studies

Because of the widely-recognized methodological difficulties in obtaining valid estimates of individual dietary intake in analytical epidemiological research, few such studies have attempted to estimate specifically the intake of dietary cholesterol. The difficulty is compounded in case-control studies, which have usually sought to measure past diet because it has presumedly greater etiological relevance than present diet. Only reports of analytical studies of breast cancer in women and of large-bowel cancer were available to the Working Group.

Miller *et al.* (1978) conducted a population-based case-control study in Canada, comparing the diets of 400 women with breast cancer and 400 individually matched neighbourhood controls. Diets were estimated on the basis of a dietary history question-naire, 24-hour recall and a four-day diary. While total fat intake was moderately positively associated with breast cancer, both pre- and post-menopausally, the intake of dietary cholesterol (controlling for other nutrients) was only weakly (relative risk = 1.3) associated with breast cancer risk.

In a subsequent case-control study in Canada (Lubin *et al.*, 1981), 577 women, aged 30-80, were compared with an age-stratified random sample of population controls. A simple, eight-item food frequency questionnaire was used. Age-adjusted relative risks were calculated for each food item across four levels of consumption and for the derived nutrients cholesterol, animal fat and animal protein. Cholesterol intake showed a weak, statistically insignificant relationship (relative risk = 1.2) with breast cancer risk, whereas various other nutrients showed significantly positive associations.

Jain *et al.* (1980) reported a population-based case-control study of colo-rectal cancer in Canada. The 348 cases of colon cancer and 194 cases of rectal cancer were compared with age- and sex-matched sets of hospital controls and community controls. Usual intake of major nutrients was estimated from a food-frequency dietary history questionnaire. The investigators reported that a high intake of cholesterol was associated with increased risk of colo-rectal cancer (relative risk = 1.8 for men and 1.6 for women). Multivariate analysis, including controlling for other major nutrients, indicated that a statistically significant stepwise increase in risk of colo-rectal cancer was associated with increasing cholesterol intake for people of each sex.

Blood Cholesterol

1. Descriptive studies

There are few descriptive studies of mean serum cholesterol and cancer risk in different populations. Studies of Japanese migrants have been summarized above. Seventh Day Adventists (Walden *et al.*, 1964) and Mormons (Enstrom, 1980) in California have serum cholesterol levels lower than those of the general US population, and both groups have mortality rates for all combined cancers and colon cancer below that of the general US population (Phillips, 1975; Lyon *et al.*, 1977).

2. Analytical studies

There are two basic categories of analytical studies - experimental and observational. In this particular context, experimental studies investigate changes in cancer risk resulting from dietary or pharmacological interventions which result in a lowering of serum cholesterol levels. Observational studies, on the other hand, are concerned with the risk of cancer in individuals in relation to their naturally-occurring levels of serum cholesterol.

(i) Experimental studies

Seven experimental human studies have been reported in which the effect of lowering blood cholesterol by dietary or drug intervention upon subsequent cancer risk has been assessed. Each study was originally designed to assess the effect of the intervention upon risk of coronary heart disease. These studies are summarized in Table 4.

Table 4. Summary of intervention trials (experimental) of cholesterol-lowering[a]

Study and author(s)	Years of follow-up	Study subjects	Study design	Achieved difference in serum cholesterol	Method of analysis	Results	Comments
Los Angeles Veterans' Administration Hospital Study Pearce & Dayton (1971)	1959-1967 (8 years)	846 male residents in veterans' home	Randomly allocated to two different dietary regimes (high P:S ratio[b] vs conventional)	Mean serum cholesterol 12.7% lower in experimental group	Comparison of numbers of cancer deaths	31 cancer deaths in experimental group vs 17 in control group (p = 0.06)	No such difference occurred among the 'better adherers' to the 2 diets (6 vs 7)
Finnish Mental Hospital Study, Turpeinen (1979)	1959-1971 (12 years)	4000 male patients	Two hospital populations, crossover design (2 x 6-year periods): experimental (high P:S) and control diets	Mean serum cholesterol 15% lower in experimental group	Comparison of cancer mortality rates	No difference (actual data not presented)	
United States Coronary Drug Project, Coronary Drug Project Research Group (1975)	1966-1969 to 1974 (av., 6.2 years)	Males with proven myocardial infarct. from 53 clinical centres: niacin, 1119; clofibrate, 1103; controls, 2789	Random allocation to drug therapies	Mean serum cholesterol 6.5-9.9% lower in treated groups	Comparison of numbers of cancer deaths	Clofibrate, 10 cancers (0.9%); niacin, 9 (0.8%); controls, 24 (0.9%)	

Table 4. (contd)

Study and author(s)	Years of follow-up	Study subjects	Study design	Achieved difference in serum cholesterol	Method of analysis	Results	Comments
Clofibrate Trial, Committee of Principal Investigators (1980)	1965-1979 (av., 9.6 years, comprising 5.3 years active treatment and 4.3 years follow-up)	Three groups of (approx.) 5000 males, aged 30-59: Group I (clofibrate) and Group II (placebo) each had high serum cholesterol; Group III (placebo) had low serum cholesterol	Groups I and II chosen by random allocation of subjects in upper tertile of blood cholesterol	Mean serum cholesterol in Group I (225 mg/dl) 9% lower than in Group II (247 mg/dl). Group III = 181 mg/dl	Age-standardized cancer death rates	I = 2.6 II = 2.1 III = 2.0	The similar cancer mortality in Groups II and III indicates lack of influence of blood cholesterol. Cancer excess in Group I attributable to clofibrate per se

a Ederer et al. (1971) reviewed data from 5 prospective studies, including the first two listed above. The pooled results indicated no relationship between a lowered blood cholesterol and risk of subsequent cancer.

b Ratio of polyunsaturated fats to saturated fats

Trials of lowering blood cholesterol by diet

The first report of an inverse relationship between serum cholesterol and cancer risk was from an eight-year cardiovascular disease prevention trial on men at the Wadsworth Veterans Administration Hospital, Los Angeles (Pearce & Dayton, 1971). The 846 participants were randomly assigned to either a cholesterol-lowering diet or a control diet. A difference of 12.7% in mean serum cholesterol was achieved between the groups. Although fatal atherosclerotic events were more common in controls (70 *versus* 48, $p < 0.05$), a marked increase of fatal cancers occurred in the low-cholesterol group (31 *versus* 17, $p = 0.06$) (relative risks of cancer incidence and mortality, 1.28 and 1.36, respectively) (Ederer *et al.*, 1971)). This cancer excess, first apparent after three years (16 *versus* 8), increased in a cumulative fashion during the subsequent five years of follow-up. However, among the minority of subjects who closely adhered to their allocated diet, six (6.1%) of the cholesterol-lowering group and seven (5.5%) of the control group died from cancer. [The Working Group noted the apparent paradox wherein the greatest difference in cancer risk occurred among those sub-sets of study subjects who might be presumed to have differed least in their diets. However, no data are available to confirm this presumption.]

Ederer *et al.* (1971) analysed pooled data from five dietary trials of cardiovascular disease prevention performed during the 1960s, comprising the above-mentioned Los Angeles Veterans Trial, three other studies employing randomization of individuals (in Oslo, London and Minnesota), and the Finnish Mental Hospital study referred to below. The pooled data from the four studies, other than the Los Angeles Veterans Trial, indicated that the relative risks of cancer incidence and mortality were lower (0.75 and 0.62, respectively) in the serum cholesterol-lowering diet group than in the control group, though not at a statistically significant level. [This data subset represents the appropriate independent data with which to evaluate the finding of Pearce and Dayton (1971).] For all five studies combined, the cancer incidence and mortality rates were not significantly different between the treatment and control groups.

In a report of an extension of the Finnish Mental Hospital study, in which 4000 institutionalized men were followed for 12 years *via* a cross-over design (Turpeinen, 1979), the patients on a cholesterol-lowering diet achieved a 15% decrease in serum cholesterol relative to those on the control diet. The total mortality rate was 11% lower in the cholesterol-lowering diet group; however, differences in the cancer mortality rates between the treatment and control groups 'were small and showed no consistent pattern'.

Trials of lowering blood cholesterol by drugs

The Coronary Drug Project Research Group (1975) reported a coronary prevention trial of cholesterol-lowering by drug therapy in men aged 30-64 with a history of proven myocardial infarction. Groups that received niacin (n = 1119) and clofibrate (n = 1103) [see IARC, 1980] experienced significant cholesterol lowering in comparison with the control group, which received a placebo. Though case numbers were small, cancer mortality was not significantly different among the niacin (0.8%), clofibrate (0.9%) and placebo (0.9%) groups during an average of 6.2 years of treatment.

In a trial of primary prevention of coronary heart disease by clofibrate, based in three European centres (Edinburgh, Budapest and Prague), three groups were studied, each comprising approximately 5000 men aged 30-59 at entry and free of manifest heart or other major disease (Committee of Principal Investigators, 1978). Group I, comprising men with serum cholesterol in the upper third of the cholesterol distribution and who received clofibrate for an average of 5.3 years, achieved a 9% lowering of serum cholesterol, compared with Group II, which consisted of men with high serum cholesterol receiving a placebo. Group III consisted of men with low serum cholesterol who also received a placebo. After 9.6 years of follow-up (Committee of Principal Investigators, 1980), the total mortality rate was significantly higher in the clofibrate group (Group I) than in the high-cholesterol control group (Group II). However, no single cause of mortality, including cancer, accounted for this increase. Detailed analysis of the data, while suggesting an increased overall hazard of mortality with specific use of clofibrate as a cholesterol-lowering agent [see IARC, 1980], also indicated that the attained low cholesterol levels *per se* are not associated with increased total mortality or cancer mortality risk. The men in Group III, with a mean serum cholesterol of 181 mg/dl, demonstrated lower age-adjusted mortality rates from all causes and virtually identical cancer mortality rates in comparison with the men in Group II, with a mean cholesterol of 247 mg/dl. [Of relevance to the discussion below is the observation of fewer deaths in the low cholesterol group from cancers of the 'liver, gallbladder, intestines'.]

[Overall, of the three reports on dietary trials and the two drug trials of blood cholesterol lowering, only one (the Los Angeles Veterans study) indicated an increased cancer risk associated with the lowering of cholesterol *per se*. However, since in that study the non-adhering subgroups within the two randomized groups who differed least in their subsequent diets showed the greatest difference in their cancer risk, interpretation is difficult.]

(ii) Observational studies

In reports of ten prospective studies (all originally designed to study the etiology of cardiovascular disease) and of one case-control study, an inverse relationship between serum cholesterol, as measured at entry into the study, and cancer has been evident. It should be noted that although the prospective studies were not originally designed to measure or study cancer incidence or mortality, in principle there is no impediment to their subsequently being used as sources of data for such a purpose.

The studies reporting an inverse relationship are considered first in this section; subsequently, the six prospective studies and one case-control study in which no such relationship was found are considered. Summaries of the fifteen reports of prospective studies appear in Table 5. A recently published report (Feinleib, 1982) of a workshop held in the US in May 1981 summarized unpublished data from nine other prospective studies, six of which showed no relation between blood cholesterol and total cancer mortality, while three showed an inverse relationship. [Since only selected data were included, in the absence of details of study design and data analysis, no evaluation was possible.]

Studies showing an inverse relationship to cancer risk

Rose *et al.* (1974) pooled the results of six prospective studies of heart disease in men: The 'Seven Countries' study, the Framingham study, the Chicago Gas Company study, the London Whitehall study, the Minnesota Businessmen study, and the Western Electric Company study. They found that the 90 subjects who had thus far died from colon cancer during these studies had mean blood cholesterol levels, measured at entry, about 5-7 mg/dl below the expected value (p < 0.05). Further, the extent of this deviation was similar in those dying within four years of screening and in those dying later; overall, there was little indication of any general tendency for serum cholesterol to correlate with the interval from initial screening to death (r = -0.0051). These figures were interpreted

Table 5. Summary of observational (follow-up) studies of the relationship between serum cholesterol levels and cancer risk

a. Studies showing an inverse relationship

Study and author(s)	Study subjects	Age at entry	Mean serum cholesterol of study population	No. of years follow-up	Outcome measure	Cancers showing inverse relationship	Other factors controlled in analysis	Comments
Six pooled studies, Rose et al. (1974)	[36 211 males]	35-64	NR[a]	5-23	Deaths; case-control analysis	Colon (n = 90)	NR	Cholesterol decrement in cases unrelated to time lapse after entry
Whitehall study, Rose & Shipley (1980)	17 718 males	40-64	[197]	7.5	Deaths; mortality rates and case-control analysis	Total cancer (353), lung (143), stomach (35) and colon (28)	NR	Detailed analysis by single year of follow-up suggests that low cholesterol levels reflect UCE[b]
Paris prospective study of coronary heart disease, Cambien et al. (1980)	7603 males	43-52	223 (in survivors)	6.5	Deaths; case-control analysis	All cancers except bronchus and lung (total = 134)	NR	Inverse relationship declined with increasing time lapse after entry
Framington study, Williams et al. (1981)	2236 males 2873 females	35-64	Males, 235[c] Females, 240[c]	24 (1948-1972)	Incidence; rates	Males: colon (n = 88) and all other sites combined (n = 603)	Age, alcohol, cigarettes, education, systolic blood pressure, rel. weight	Inverse relationship in males only. Risk increase predominantly at serum cholesterol < 190 mg/dl and evident throughout follow-up period
Honolulu heart study, Kagan et al. (1981)	8006 males	45-68	218 (alive)	9 (1965-1974)	Deaths; mortality rates and case-control analysis	Total cancer, colon, lung (total = 185)	Age, systolic blood pressure, cigarettes, alcohol, rel. weight	Cases prevalent at intake or incident in first 2 years were excluded. Greatest risk at cholesterol < 180 mg/dl
Honolulu heart study, Stemmermann et al. (1981)	8006 males	45-68	218 non-cancer cases	14 (1965-1980)	Incidence; rates and case-control analysis	Colon only (especially right-sided)	Age, systolic blood pressure, cigarettes, alcohol, rel. weight	Lack of association of other sites that suggests prior findings (Kagen et al., 1980) reflected UCE

Table 5. (contd)

Study and author(s)	Study subjects	Age at entry	Mean serum cholesterol of study population	No. of years follow-up	Outcome measure	Cancers showing inverse relationship	Other factors controlled in analysis	Comments
Puerto Rico Heart Health Program, Garcia-Palmieri et al. (1981)	9824 males	45-64	196 (rural) and 205 (urban) non-cancer cases	8	Deaths; mortality rates	Total cancer in rural males (total = 179)	Relative weight, heart rate, physical activity, haematocrit, education, cigarettes	Predominant risk increase at serum cholesterol < 165. No site-specific data
New Zealand Maoris, Beaglehole et al. (1980)	391 males 311 females	25-74	[Males, 225] [Females, 212]	11	Deaths; mortality rates	Total cancer (total = 30)	Age, systolic blood pressure, rel. weight	UCE precluded by omitting deaths in first 2 years
Evans County, Georgia, Kark et al. (1980)	947 (white) males, 537 (black) males, 972 (white) females, 646 (black) females	15-74	[206-229]	12-14	Incidence; case-control analysis	All except pancreas, ovary and basal-cell (total = 127 incident cases during years 1-14)	Age, race, sex, rel. weight, social class, smoking	Inverse relationship statistically significant in males only. Low serum cholesterol and low serum vitamin A correlated
Yugoslavia cardiovascular disease study, Kozarevic et al. (1981)	11 121 males	35-62	198	7	Deaths; mortality rates and case-control analysis	Colo-rectal cancer (total cancers = 224)	Obesity, systolic blood pressure, cigarettes, age, bowel medical history, education	Total cancer mortality inversely related - but not statistically significant
Malmö study, Peterson et al. (1981)	10 000 males	47-50	NR	2.5	Deaths; proportional mortality analysis	Total cancer (n = 28)	None	Small numbers, from preliminary data analysis

b. Studies showing no relationship

Study and author(s)	Study subjects	Age at entry	Mean serum cholesterol of study population	No. of years follow-up	Outcome measure	Cancers showing inverse relationship	Other factors controlled in analysis	Comments
Norwegian workers, Westlund & Nicolaysen (1972)	3751 males	40-49	270	10	Incidence; rates and case-control analysis	All cancers (total = 89)	Blood pressure, rel. weight	No exclusion of cancer cases occurring early in study

Table 5. (contd)

Study and author(s)	Study subjects	Age at entry	Mean serum cholesterol of study population	No. of years follow-up	Outcome measure	Cancers showing inverse relationship	Other factors controlled in analysis	Comments
Updated analysis of three Chicago-based studies, Dyer et al. (1981)d,e,f	d. 1233 males e. 1899 males f. 6890 males 5750 females	40-59 40-55 45-64	234 (survivors) 247 (survivors) 213 (survivors)	18 17 5	Deaths; rates and case-control analysis (all three studies)	d. All cancers (total = 99) e. Sarcoma, leukaemia, Hodgkin's disease inversely associated (total = 78) f. All cancers (total = 116)	Age, systolic blood pressure, cigarettes, rel. weight (all three studies)	
Israel ischaemic heart disease study, Yaari et al. (1981)	10 059 males	40-65	209	7	Deaths; rates and case-control analysis	All cancers (total = 110)	Age, history of myocardial infarction, dietary fat, anxiety index, serum uric acid, rel. weight	Inverse relationship of borderline significance with total cancer mortality (p = 0.09)
Johns Hopkins' medical students study, Thomas et al. (1982)	1018 males	18-37	234	20-33	Incidence; mainly retrospective analysis	All cancers (total = 30)	Age, smoking, rel. weight	

a Not reported

b Undetected cancer effect, i.e., the likelihood that incipient cancer cases, undiagnosed at entry into study, will have a lowered blood cholesterol as a metabolic consequence of the cancer process

c Estimated from grouped data

d Chicago People's Gas Company study

e Chicago Western Electric Company study

f Chicago Heart Association Detection Project in Industry

as indicating that the presence of pre-existing cancer at the time of entry into the study, with its possible metabolic consequences, could not explain the lowered blood cholesterol levels. [The notion of the metabolic consequences of pre-existing (but undiagnosed) cancer, as a cause of low serum cholesterol in those individuals at the time of their entry into the study, is referred to subsequently as the 'undetected cancer effect', or UCE. See also introductory remarks to section 3.3.]

Rose and Shipley (1980) reviewed the (updated) London Whitehall study, one of the six studies included in the report of Rose et al. (1974). This study examined the mortality from coronary heart disease and total mortality of 17 718 male London civil servants, initially aged 40 to 64, with 7.5 years of follow-up. The non-coronary heart disease mortality was inversely related to plasma cholesterol, measured at entry, over the entire cholesterol range. Cancer mortality was the primary cause of this inverse relationship, with cancer deaths accounting for 58% of all non-coronary heart disease deaths. Cancer mortality was 66% higher in those with lowest plasma cholesterol levels than in those with the highest levels. Site-specific analyses demonstrated an association between low plasma cholesterol and cancers of the lung (143 deaths), stomach (35 deaths) and colon (28 deaths). The inverse relationship between plasma cholesterol and cancer mortality was most evident during the first one to two years; the authors concluded that it was probably a reflection of the UCE, implying that cancer caused low plasma cholesterol rather than that low cholesterol caused cancer.

In the Paris Prospective Study of Coronary Heart Disease (Cambien et al., 1980), 7603 French male government employees, aged 43 to 52, were followed for an average of 6.6 years. The mean serum cholesterol, measured at entry into the study, was 212 mg/dl in the 134 persons who subsquently died of cancer, which was statistically significantly lower (p = 0.01) than the figure of 223 mg/dl in the survivors. Those who died of lung cancer had higher mean initial cholesterol levels than did survivors (233 versus 223). Among the cancer cases, the later an individual died after entering into the study, the higher his initial serum cholesterol level tended to have been (p < 0.02); initial mean serum cholesterol in cancer cases dying at least seven years after entry into the study was not lower than that in the survivors. Further, in the 81% of those individuals who died from cancer and had also had follow-up cholesterol measurements, there had been a mean decrease of 5 mg/dl in serum cholesterol after an average of three years of follow-up. [These findings are consistent with the UCE notion.]

Updated analysis of the Framingham Study data (Williams et al., 1981), with up to 24 years follow-up of 5209 [2336 male and 2873 female] subjects, demonstrates, in men, a significant inverse association of serum cholesterol levels at entry into the study with the incidence of colon cancer and of cancer of all sites other than the colon. No such relationship was found in women. Colon cancer rates in men with initial serum cholesterol values of less than 190 mg/dl were approximately three times as great as those in men with higher initial serum cholesterol levels. This inverse relationship was not attributable to the UCE since, first, of the 88 cases of colon cancer detected during follow-up, only five occurred during the first four years of follow-up; and, second, the excess cancer among those with initially low serum cholesterol was cumulative throughout the entire follow-up period. Multivariate analysis, allowing for effects of age, alcohol, cigarettes, education, systolic blood pressure and relative weight, did not eliminate the possibility of the inverse relationship in men. The authors comment that the observed inverse association may also reflect effects of competing risks from other fatal diseases. This possibility was evaluated (Feinleib, 1981) with an actuarial life-table analysis of cancer mortality within the cohort, which showed that the overall cancer mortality excess in the men with low cholesterol, over the 20-year period, occurred whether deaths from coronary heart disease were included or excluded.

In the Honolulu Heart Study (Kagan *et al.*, 1981), 8006 Japanese-American men aged 45-68 were followed for nine years. Serum cholesterol level at entry into the study was inversely related to total cancer mortality and to mortality from cancers of the oeso-phagus, colon, liver, lung and malignancies of the lymphatic and haematopoietic systems. When deaths in the first two years of follow up were excluded from the analysis (to take into account the UCE), the inverse relationship remained significant for total cancer, colon cancer, lung cancer and malignancies of the lymphatic and haematopoietic system. When cases of cancer present at intake were eliminated from the calculations, the inverse relationship persisted only for total cancers and colon cancer. Total cancer mortality rates in men with serum cholesterol values of less than 180 mg/dl were approximately twice as great as those in men with serum cholesterol levels of 180-269 mg/dl, and four times higher than in men with serum cholesterol levels greater than 269 mg/dl. This negative trend was statistically significant. Multivariate analysis, including age, systolic blood pressure, cigarettes, alcohol, and relative weight did not eliminate this inverse relationship with total cancer mortality. The relationship was strongest for colon cancer.

Stemmermann *et al.* (1981), in a subsequent five-year extension of this Honolulu study, found that the incidence of colon cancer was inversely associated with serum cholesterol measured at entry into the study (p = 0.057). The authors suggested that the lack of such an association with other site-specific cancer incidence (particularly stomach and lung) indicates that the inverse association observed earlier in the follow-up (see above) may reflect the UCE. However, for colon cancer, the inverse association persisted in cases diagnosed 5-9.9 years after entry, although not in those diagnosed 10-14 years after intake. [Indeed, the progressive diminution of the effect across the 0-4.9, 5-9.9, 10-14 year categories is consistent with the UCE.]

Garcia-Palmieri *et al.* (1981) found, in an eight-year follow-up study in Puerto Rico of 9824 men aged 45-64, that serum cholesterol at entry was inversely related to total cancer mortality in the group living in rural areas. The risk of mortality was particularly increased in men with initial serum cholesterol levels of less than 165 mg/dl. Multivariate analysis, including relative weight, heart rate, physical activity, haematocrit and education, eliminated any statistically significant relationship in the urban group, but this was maintained in the rural residents. Initial serum cholesterol did not vary with proximity of time of death to commencement of follow-up [thereby making the UCE a less likely explanation]. No data are presented for specific cancers in relation to serum cholesterol.

In a study of 630 male and female New Zealand Maoris, aged 25 to 74 years, followed for up to 11 years, Beaglehole *et al.* (1980) reported an increased cancer death rate (observed:expected = 1.9) in individuals with initially low serum cholesterol levels (< 197 mg/dl). This relationship, examined only for men and women combined, persisted when deaths within two years of intake were excluded (p < 0.001). However, the number of individuals followed in this study was small, and only 30 cancer deaths occurred overall.

In a 12-14-year follow-up study of 3102 male and female individuals aged 15 to 74 in Evans County, Georgia, USA (Kark *et al.*, 1980), the initial mean serum cholesterol level, measured at entry, in 166 individuals who subsequently developed cancer was 6.7 mg/dl lower than that in age- and sex-matched controls. The initial mean cholesterol level was 8 mg/dl lower in the 'incident' group of 127 cancer cases, i.e., those cases who did not develop cancer within one year of the beginning of the study. This inverse relationship was statistically significant and was evident in both the 1-6-year and 7-13-year periods of follow-up, but only in men. Colon, uterus, liver, skin (squamous-cell) and prostate cancer were associated with the lowest mean cholesterol levels; pancreas, ovary and basal-cell cancers were associated with increases in mean cholesterol level. Age, race, sex, weight, social class and smoking were all controlled for in the analysis.

Because of the possibility of positive confounding between low serum cholesterol and low serum vitamin A, the latter factor was also examined. Serum cholesterol and vitamin A (retinol) levels were strongly correlated in this population (age-adjusted Pearson partial correlation coefficient = 0.4 in whites), and retinol levels were lower in cases than in controls (Kark et al., 1982). Independent data (Smith & Hoggard, 1981) from 102 healthy New Zealand adults showed a statistically significant correlation between serum low-density lipoprotein cholesterol and serum retinol (r = 0.30 in men, 0.27 in women).

In a follow-up study of 11 121 men, aged 35-62, in Yugoslavia, Kozarevic et al. (1981) have shown an inverse relationship between initial serum cholesterol and total mortality. This relationship was reported to be statistically significant after adjustment, by multiple logistic regression, for relative weight, systolic blood pressure, cigarette smoking, age, history of intestinal parasitism, and socioeconomic status (i.e., educational level). While total cancer mortality was not inversely related to serum cholesterol, colorectal cancer was (although the data were not tabulated).

Preliminary data (mean follow-up, 2.5 years) from a prospective study of 10 000 men, initially aged 47-50, in Malmö, Sweden, showed an inverse relationship between serum cholesterol and cancer mortality (Peterson et al., 1981). Twenty-three of 28 cancer deaths occurred in the 60% of individuals with the lowest serum cholesterol levels. [However, the short period of follow-up precludes any discounting of the UCE.]

In a matched case-control study of colon cancer in Caucasian patients at the Mount Sinai Hospital, New York, Miller et al. (1981) found that, overall, patients with colon cancer had initial serum cholesterol levels lower than those of controls. In 133 pairs matched by age and sex, mean serum cholesterol levels at entry into the study were 188 mg/dl for cases and 213 mg/dl for controls (p < 0.001). Following stratification by tumour stage, significant differences in serum cholesterol levels persisted between cases with advanced tumours and controls (p < 0.001) but not between cases with early tumours and controls, although the same trend was noted. Matching of 130 early tumours to advanced tumours showed that women, but not men, had a significantly lower serum cholesterol level with advancing disease. The authors conclude that, at least in women, the findings support the concept of an UCE.

Studies not showing a relationship to overall cancer risk

Westlund and Nicolaysen (1972) reported on the 10-year mortality and morbidity experience of 3751 Norwegian male workers, aged 40 to 49. The serum cholesterol levels, measured at entry into the study, of the 89 men who subsequently developed cancer (271 mg/dl) did not differ from those who did not develop cancer (269 mg/dl). [However, it should be noted that very few men had low initial serum cholesterol levels, indicating little variation within the study population. No attempt was made to exclude from the analysis men who had pre-existing cancer at the beginning of the study.]

Dyer et al. (1981) examined the data from three prospective studies of cardiovascular disease in the US. Serum cholesterol at entry into the study was examined in relation to death from cancer and from other non-cardiovascular causes for: 1233 white men, aged 40-59, followed for 18 years from the Chicago People's Gas Company study; 1899 white men, aged 40-55, followed for 17 years from the Chicago Western Electric Company study; and 6890 white men and 5750 white women, aged 45-64, followed for an average of five years from the Chicago Heart Association Detection Project in Industry. In none of the studies was there a significant association between initial serum cholesterol level and subsequent mortality from total cancer. When cancer deaths were examined by site, there was a significant inverse association between serum cholesterol and deaths from sarcoma, leukaemia and Hodgkin's disease in the Western Electric men. Serum cholesterol level was not related to lung cancer, colorectal cancer, oral cancer, pancreatic cancer, or to all other cancers combined in any of the three studies, either in men or in women. There was, however, the suggestion of a positive association with breast cancer in women.

In 10 059 adult male civil servants and municipal employees, aged 40 to 65, and followed up for seven years in the Israel Ischaemic Heart Disease study (Yaari et al., 1981), an inverse relationship was found between lower levels of serum cholesterol measured at entry and total mortality (n = 465). This association disappeared when multivariate logistic regression analysis was performed, adjusting for age, history of myocardial infarction, cigarette smoking, percentage of saturated fat in the dietary fat, index of anxiety, serum uric acid and relative weight. No clear-cut association between total serum cholesterol and cancer mortality (n = 110) was demonstrated, although multivariate analysis indicated an inverse relationship of 'borderline significance' (p = 0.09). High-density lipoprotein cholesterol levels were not related to cancer risk.

Thomas et al. (1982) followed up 1018 men from the time they entered medical school (Johns Hopkins University) for periods of 20-33 years. The 30 who subsequently developed cancer had not had low initial serum cholesterol levels. Indeed, the number of cancer cases among the 20% of men with the highest cholesterol levels was twice that expected. The four subjects who developed cancer less than five years after entering the study had the lowest initial cholesterol levels [consistent with the UCE].

Malarkey et al. (1977), in a small case-control study of 24-hour-preoperative endocrine profiles of women with benign and with malignant breast disease, found no difference in initial serum cholesterol.

In summary, among published observational studies indicating an inverse relationship between initial serum cholesterol and cancer, there were reports of nine large populations followed for at least five years. Two of them (Framingham and Evans County - both of which investigated cancer incidence) demonstrate an inverse relationship between total cancer risk and initial serum cholesterol that cannot be attributed to the UCE. In each study, the relationship was present in men only. This relationship was consistently strong for colon cancer. In the remaining reports of the five other studies, only male subjects were included. In two of those studies (Honolulu and Yugoslavia), an inverse relationship with colon cancer is evident which cannot be explained by the UCE, while the inverse relationship with total cancer may largely reflect the UCE (Honolulu), or is not presented very clearly (Yugoslavia). In the Puerto Rican study, the inverse relationship is evident for total cancer mortality, after multivariate adjustment, and is not obviously attributable to the UCE. Site-specific data are not available. In each of the other two studies (Whitehall and Paris), the data indicate that the UCE accounts for the apparent inverse relationship between initial serum cholesterol and cancer risk.

The moderately consistent finding from these studies that serum cholesterol is inversely associated with risk of cancer of the colon in men warrants special consideration. In view of the hypothesis that bile constituents (acidic and/or neutral) and their intracolonic degradation products influence colon carcinogenesis (Armstrong *et al.*, 1982), it may be that those individuals with a metabolic predisposition towards low serum cholesterol also have a raised secretion of bile (containing bile acids and cholesterol), or a higher excretion of non-absorbed cholesterol in faeces, and are therefore at increased risk of colon cancer (McMichael & Potter, 1980; Laskarzewski *et al.*, 1982). (Quite independently, those same individuals, and others, might undergo an increased risk of colon cancer if they ingest more dietary cholesterol, some of which passes, unabsorbed, through the bowel.)

The prospective data from the New Zealand Maori and from the Malmö studies are insufficient for firm inferences to be drawn. The one relevant case-control study (Miller *et al.*, 1981) showed an inverse relationship between cancer and serum cholesterol and clearly supports the UCE proposition.

Six published prospective studies (one in Norway, four in the US and one in Israel) show no apparent relationship between serum cholesterol and total cancer risk, although some inverse relationships specific to sarcoma and lymphoproliferative neoplasms were seen in one of the US cohorts.

Faecal Excretion of Cholesterol and Cholesterol Metabolites

Those few studies that have examined faecal cholesterol levels in relation to cancer risk are concerned exclusively with cancer of the large bowel. It should be noted that faecal cholesterol (amount and concentration) reflects *both* dietary intake and biliary excretion. The extent of intra-colonic bacterial degradation of cholesterol exerts an additional influence (see section 3.2b). Most authors have thus paid more attention to the faecal excretion and concentration of total neutral sterols than to cholesterol *per se*.

1. Descriptive studies

Hill *et al.* (1971) found that the concentration of cholesterol, total neutral sterols and faecal bile acids were higher in English, Scottish and US populations at high risk of colon cancer than in low-risk populations in Japan, India and Uganda. [The non-random samples are small, ranging from 11 to 26 persons per area.]

Small groups of Americans on a mixed western diet (17 persons), American vegetarians (12), American Seventh-Day Adventists (11), Japanese (17) and Chinese (11) at different risks of colon cancer were examined (Reddy & Wynder, 1973). Daily excretion of cholesterol was inversely related to colon cancer risk, whereas there was a positive association between colon cancer and the excretion of total neutral sterols. In the same study, there was an association between colon cancer risk and the excretion of bile acids. [Faecal concentrations of cholesterol, neutral sterols and bile acids were not reported.]

In a comparison between samples of populations at high risk of colon cancer in New York (20 subjects) and those at low risk in Kuopio, Finland (15 subjects), the daily excretion of faecal cholesterol and its metabolites was highest in the low-incidence area. No difference in faecal concentration was observed between the two areas (Reddy *et al.*,

1978). Similarly, no difference was observed in faecal cholesterol concentration between socio-economic groups in Hong Kong with a two-fold variation in colon cancer risk (Crowther et al., 1976). In both studies, the differences in faecal bile acid concentration followed the colon cancer gradient.

In two comparative studies of random samples of the population in Denmark (high-risk) and Finland (low-risk), there was an inverse association between colon cancer and faecal concentration of neutral sterols; in one of the studies, the three-fold risk gradient for large-bowel cancer also paralleled the faecal bile acid concentration (IARC Intestinal Microecology Group, 1977; Jensen et al., 1982).

2. Analytical studies

Reddy and Wynder (1977), in the US, compared the faecal composition of 31 colon cancer cases, 13 patients with adenomatous polyps, 9 patients with other bowel diseases, and 34 healthy controls. They found the faecal concentrations of cholesterol, cholesterol metabolites and bile acids to be higher in the colon cancer cases and in patients with adenomatous polyps than in the controls.

In a similar case-control study in the US of 15 colon cancer cases, 16 patients with non-gastrointestinal cancer and 23 controls, there was no difference in concentration of faecal cholesterol, total sterol concentration or bile acid concentration between the groups (Moskovitz et al., 1979).

Four further case-control studies did not report specifically on faecal cholesterol. Hill et al. (1975) found increased concentrations of faecal neutral sterols (and bile acids) in 14 patients with colon cancer compared with 41 controls, as did Reddy et al. (1975) in a comparison of 12 colon cancer cases with 15 control subjects. Mudd et al. (1980) found no difference in faecal bile acid concentration between colon cancer cases and controls, while Murray et al. (1980), comparing 37 patients and 36 controls, found significantly lower mean concentrations in the cancer cases. Neutral sterols in the faeces were not examined. [The relevance of studying faecal constituents in patients with bowel diseases is open to question in view of the possible influences of the disease on the parameters measured and on the diet of the patients.]

4. Summary of Data Reported and Evaluation

4.1 Experimental data

Cholesterol was tested for carcinogenicity in mice by administration in the diet, by subcutaneous administration and by bladder implantation. These studies were all inadequate for evaluation. Cholesterol was also tested in combination with various carcinogens, but the results are insufficient to assess the co-carcinogenic potential of this compound.

Cholesterol, when free of oxidation products, was not mutagenic in bacteria and did not cause cell transformation. The data were *inadequate* to evaluate the activity of cholesterol in short-term tests.

Cholesterol induced cleft palate in rats.

4.2 Human data

Cholesterol and cholesterol derivatives are widely distributed in human tissues and in the human diet. Cholesterol is used in a multitude of pharmaceutical and cosmetic preparations.

As in the preceding presentation of epidemiological data, the evidence is summarized according to the three contexts in which cholesterol has been measured, i.e., in the diet, the blood and the faeces.

Few epidemiological studies of cancer have examined dietary cholesterol specifically, although many have examined total saturated fat intake. At the population level, cancers of the colon and female breast (and, to a lesser extent, the prostate, endometrium, ovary, pancreas and rectum) are strongly positively correlated with estimated per-caput intake of dietary saturated fat and, where studied, cholesterol. In the few case-control studies that have estimated individual dietary cholesterol intake, cancers of the breast and colon-rectum have tended to be positively associated with dietary total fat, saturated fat and cholesterol. Although there is moderately consistent, albeit limited, evidence of an association between high dietary intake of cholesterol and cancers of the colon, breast and, less convincingly, some other cancers, a causal relationship cannot be inferred from these epidemiological data. In particular, there is a difficulty in distinguishing between any effect of cholesterol and the effects of other dietary factors with which cholesterol is positively or negatively correlated.

With respect to serum cholesterol, the findings from seven cholesterol-lowering intervention trials (five by diet, two by drugs) indicate no alteration in cancer risk consequent upon a reduction in individual serum cholesterol. However, long-term observational follow-up studies have shown either an inverse relationship between individual serum cholesterol (measured at entry into the study) and subsequent total cancer risk (mortality or incidence) or no such relationship. The lack of consistency of these studies, and the partial attributability of the observed inverse relationships to a presumed cholesterol-lowering effect of subclinical cancer (the 'undetected cancer effect'), preclude any conclusion that there is an increased general cancer risk consequent upon low serum cholesterol.

It seems clear that serum cholesterol does not have a strong or direct relationship with human carcinogenesis in general, of the kind it apparently has with coronary heart disease. The inverse relationship with total cancer risk, when present, is not strong, is not graded (but, instead, tends to occur in stepwise fashion below concentrations of 180-190 mg/dl), and applies predominantly to men. For cancer of the colon, specifically, the prospective observational studies show a moderately consistent inverse association with serum cholesterol.

No data were available to assess the teratogenicity or chromosomal effects of this compound in humans.

4.3 Evaluation[1]

No evaluation of the carcinogenicity of cholesterol to experimental animals could be made.

---

[1]The pattern of associations between cholesterol and human cancer risk contains some apparent contradictions. Depending on whether cholesterol is measured in the diet, blood or faeces, its association with cancer risk may tend to be either positive or negative. Because the biological significance, in relation to carcinogenesis, of cholesterol in each of these basically different contexts is not sufficiently understood, it is not yet possible to reconcile these apparently divergent findings.

There is *inadequate evidence*[1] from epidemiological studies that cholesterol as such is carcinogenic to humans.

There is *limited evidence*[1] to indicate that raised dietary intake of cholesterol by individuals is associated with an increased risk of breast and colo-rectal cancer.

There is strong evidence that a low serum cholesterol level attained by dietary or pharmacological means is not *per se* associated with an increased risk of cancer.

There is *limited evidence*[1] that, within the populations studied, those male individuals with relatively low serum concentrations have an increased risk of colon cancer; the data pertaining to women were inadequate for evaluation. There is *inadequate evidence*[1] that a low serum cholesterol level increases the risk of cancer at sites other than the colon.

The available epidemiological and experimental studies do not permit an evaluation of the carcinogenicity to humans of cholesterol *per se*.

5. References

Allain, C.C., Poon, L.S., Chan, C.S.G., Richmond, W. & Fu, P.C. (1974) Enzymatic determination of total serum cholesterol. *Clin. Chem.*, *20*, 470-475

Ansari, G.A.S., Walker, R.D., Smart, V.B. & Smith, L.L. (1982) Further investigations of mutagenic cholesterol preparations. *Food Cosmet. Toxicol.*, *20*, 35-41

Aringer, L. & Eneroth, P. (1974) Formation and metabolism *in vitro* of 5,6-epoxides of cholesterol and β-sitosterol. *J. Lipid Res.*, *15*, 389-398

Armstrong, B. & Doll, R. (1975) Environmental factors and cancer incidence and mortality in different countries, with special reference to dietary practices. *Int. J. Cancer*, *15*, 617-631

Armstrong, B.K., McMichael, A.J. & MacLennan, R. (1982) *Diet*. In: Schottenfeld, D. & Fraumeni, J.F., Jr, eds, *Cancer Epidemiology and Prevention*, Philadelphia, W.B. Saunders Co., pp. 419-433

Assmann, G., Fredrickson, D.J., Sloan, H.R., Fales, H.M. & Highest, R.J. (1975) Accumulation of oxygenated steryl esters in Wolman's disease. *J. Lipid Res.*, *16*, 28-38

Avigad, G. & Robertson, B. (1981) A coupled NAD^+-peroxidase spectrophotometric assay for cholesterol. *Clin. Chem.*, *27*, 2035-2037

Beaglehole, R., Foulkes, M.A., Prior, I.A.M. & Eyles, E.F. (1980) Cholesterol and mortality in New Zealand Maoris. *Br. med. J.*, *i*, 285-287

---

[1]See preamble, p. 17.

Bergström, S. & Samuelsson, B. (1961) *The autoxidation of cholesterol.* In: Lundberg, O., ed., *Autoxidation and Antioxidants.* Vol. 1, New York, Interscience, pp. 233-248

Berwick, D.M., Cretin, S. & Keeler, E.B. (1980) *Cholesterol, Children and Heart Disease. An Analysis of Alternatives*, New York/Oxford, Oxford University Press, pp. 28-38

Black, H.S. & Lo, W.-B. (1971) Formation of a carcinogen in human skin irradiated with ultraviolet light. *Nature, 234,* 306-308

Bloch, K. (1965) The biological synthesis of cholesterol. *Science, 150,* 19-28

Boyland, E., Busby, E.R., Dukes, C.E., Grover, P.L. & Manson, D. (1964) Further experiments on implantation of materials into the urinary bladder of mice. *Br. J. Cancer, 18,* 575-581

Bryan, G.T., Brown, R.R. & Price, J.M. (1964) Mouse bladder carcinogenicity of certain tryptophan metabolites and other aromatic nitrogen compounds suspended in cholesterol. *Cancer Res., 24,* 596-602

Buresh, J.J. & Urban, T.J. (1964) The teratogenic effect of the steroid nucleus in the rat. *J. dent. Res., 43,* 548-554

Buresh, J.J. & Urban, T.J. (1967) Cholesterol induced palatal clefts in the rat. *Arch. oral Biol., 12,* 1221-1228

Cambien, F., Ducimetiere, P. & Richard, J. (1980) Total serum cholesterol and cancer mortality in a middle-aged population. *Am. J. Epidemiol., 112,* 388-394

Cardwell, H.M.E., Cornforth, J.W., Duff, S.R., Holtermann, H. & Robinson, R. (1953) Experiments on the synthesis of substances related to the sterols. LI. Completion of the synthesis of androgenic hormones and of the cholesterol group of sterols. *J. chem. Soc.,* 361

Chase, P.F., Urban,T.J. & Buresh, J.J. (1971) Ether-induced cleft palates in rats (Abstract no. 2). *J. dent. Res., 50,* 700

Chevallier, F. (1964) Transfer and synthesis of cholesterol in rats during their growth (Fr.). *Biochim. biophys. Acta, 84,* 316-339

Clark, B.R., Rubin, R.T. & Arthur, R.J. (1968) A new micro method for determination of cholesterol in serum. *Anal. Biochem., 24,* 27-33

Clark, L.C., Jr, Duggan, C.A., Grooms, T.A., Hart, L.M. & Moore, M.E. (1981) One-minute electrochemical enzymic assay for cholesterol in biological materials. *Clin. Chem., 27,* 1978-1982

Clayson, D.B., Jull, J.W. & Bonser, G.M. (1958) The testing of *ortho* hydroxy-amines and related compounds by bladder implantation and a discussion of their structural requirements for carcinogenic activity. *Br. J. Cancer, 12,* 222-230

Cohen, A., Hertz, H.S., Mandel, J., Paule, R.C., Schaffer, R., Sniegoski, L.T., Sun, T., Welch, M.J. & White, E.V. (1980) Total serum cholesterol by isotope dilution/mass spectrometry: A candidate definitive method. *Clin. Chem., 26,* 854-860

Committee of Principal Investigators (1978) A co-operative trial in the primary prevention of ischaemic heart disease using clofibrate. *Br. Heart J.*, *40*, 1069-1118

Committee of Principal Investigators (1980) WHO cooperative trial on primary prevention of ischaemic heart disease using clofibrate to lower serum cholesterol: mortality follow-up. *Lancet*, *ii*, 379-385

Connor, W.E. & Lin, D.S. (1967) Placental transfer of cholesterol-4-^{14}C in rabbit and guinea pig fetus. *J. Lipid Res.*, *8*, 558-564

Coronary Drug Project Research Group (1975) Clofibrate and niacin in coronary heart disease. *J. Am. med. Assoc.*, *231*, 360-381

Cotruvo, J.A., Simmon, V.F. & Spanggord, R.J. (1977) Investigation of mutagenic effects of products of ozonation reactions in water. *Ann. N.Y. Acad. Sci.*, *298*, 124-140

Council of Europe (1969) *European Pharmacopoeia*, Vol. 1, Paris, Maisonneuve, p. 147

Crowther, J.S., Drasar, B.S., Hill, M.J., MacLennan, R., Magnin, D., Peach, S. & Teoh-Chan, C.H. (1976) Faecal steroids and bacteria and large bowel cancer in Hong Kong by socio-economic groups. *Br. J. Cancer,*, *34*, 191-198

Cruse, J.P., Lewin, M.R., Ferulano, G.P. & Clark, C.G. (1978) Co-carcinogenic effects of dietary cholesterol in experimental colon cancer. *Nature*, *276*, 822-825

Desforges, G., Desforges, J. & Robbins, S.L. (1950) Carcinoma of the gallbladder. An attempt at experimental production. *Cancer*, *3*, 1088-1096

Dietschy, J.M. & Wilson, J.D. (1968) Cholesterol synthesis in the squirrel monkey: Relative rates of synthesis in various tissues and mechanisms of control. *J. clin. Invest.*, *47*, 166-174

Dietschy, J.M. & Wilson, J.D. (1970) Regulation of cholesterol metabolism. *New Engl. J. Med.*, *282*, 1128-1238

Drasar, B.S. & Irving, D. (1973) Environmental factors and cancer of the colon and breast. *Br. J. Cancer*, *27*, 167-172

DuPré, D.B. (1981) *Liquid crystals*. In: Kirk, R.E. & Othmer, D.F., eds, *Encyclopedia of Chemical Technology*, 3rd ed., Vol. 14, New York, John Wiley & Sons, pp. 408-4l0, 427

Dyer, A.R., Stamler, J., Paul, O., Shekelle, R.B., Schoenberger, J.A., Berkson, D.M., Lepper, M., Collette, P., Shekelle, S. & Lindberg, H.A. (1981) Serum cholesterol and risk of death from cancer and other causes in three Chicago epidemiological studies. *J. chronic Dis.*, *34*, 249-260

Ederer, F., Leren, P., Turpeinen, O. & Frantz, I.D., Jr (1971) Cancer among men on cholesterol-lowering diets. Experience from five clinical trials. *Lancet*, *ii*, 203-206

Elliott, W.H. & Hyde, P.M. (1971) Metabolic pathways of bile acid synthesis. *Am. J. Med.*, *51*, 568-579

Enomoto, M., Naoe, S., Harada, M., Miyata, K., Saito, M. & Noguchi, Y. (1974) Carcinogenesis in extrahepatic bile duct and gallbladder - Carcinogenic effect of N-hydroxy-2-acetamidofluorene in mice fed a 'gallstone-inducing' diet. *Jpn. J. exp. Med.*, *44*, 37-54

Enstrom, J.E. (1980) *Health and dietary practices and cancer mortality among California Mormons.* In: Cairns, J., Lyon, J.L. & Skolnick, M., eds, *Cancer Incidence in Defined Populations (Banbury Report 4)*, Cold Spring Harbor, NY, Cold Spring Harbor Laboratory, pp. 69-92

Feinleib, M. (1981) On a possible inverse relationship between serum cholesterol and cancer mortality. *Am. J. Epidemiol.*, *114*, 5-10

Feinleib, M. (1982) Summary of a workshop on cholesterol and noncardiovascular disease mortality. *Prev. Med.*, *11*, 360-367

Fioriti, J.A. & Sims, R.J. (1967) Autoxidation products from cholesterol. *J. Am. Oil Chem. Soc.*, *44*, 221-224

Folch, J., Lees, M. & Stanley, G.H.S. (1957) A simple method for the isolation and purification of total lipides from animal tissues. *J. biol. Chem.*, *226*, 497-509

Food Sciences & Technology Abstracts (1982) *Cholesterol in Foods and Its Effects on Animals and Humans. September 1974-January 1982 (PB 82-861345)*, Springfield, VA, National Technical Information Services

Garcia-Palmieri, M.R., Sorlie, P.D., Costas, R., Jr & Havlik, R.J. (1981) An apparent inverse relationship between serum cholesterol and cancer mortality in Puerto Rico. *Am. J. Epidemiol.*, *114*, 29-40

Goddard, P. & Hill, M.J. (1974) The *in vivo* metabolism of cholesterol by gut bacteria in the rat and guinea-pig. *J. Steroid Biochem.*, *5*, 569-572

Goldstein, J.L. & Brown, M.S. (1983) *Familial hypercholesterolemia.* In: Stanbury, J.B., Wynaarden, J.B., Fredrickson, D.S., Goldstein, J.L. & Brown, M.S., eds, *The Metabolic Basis of Inherited Disease*, 5th ed., New York, McGraw Hill, pp. 672-712

Goldstein, J.L., Dana, S.E., Brunschede, G.Y. & Brown, M.S. (1975) Genetic heterogeneity in familial hypercholesterolemia: Evidence for two different mutations affecting functions of low-density lipoprotein receptor. *Proc. natl Acad. Sci. USA*, *72*, 1092-1096

Gray, M.F., Lawrie, T.D.V & Brooks, C.J.W. (1971) Isolation and identification of cholesterol α-oxide and other minor sterols in human serum. *Lipids*, *6*, 836-843

Grundy, S.M., Bilheimer, D., Blackburn, H., Brown, W.V., Kwiterovich, P.O., Jr, Mattson, F., Schonfeld, G. & Weidman, W.H. (1982) Rationale of the diet-heart statement of the American Heart Association. Report of nutrition committee. *Circulation*, *65*, 839A-854A

Gurll, N. & DenBesten, L. (1978) Animal models of human cholesterol gallstone disease: A review. *Lab. Animal Sci.*, *28*, 428-432

Haenszel, W. & Kurihara, M. (1968) Studies of Japanese migrants. I. Mortality from cancer and other diseases among Japanese in the United States. *J. natl Cancer Inst.*, *40*, 43-68

Havel, R.J., Goldstein, J.L. & Brown, M.S. (1980) *Lipoproteins and lipid transport.* In: Bondy, P.K. & Rosenberg, L.E., eds, *Metabolic Control and Disease*, 8th ed., Philadelphia, W.B. Saunders Co., pp. 393-494

Hieger, I. (1957) Cholesterol as a carcinogen. *Proc. R. Soc. (Lond.), Ser. B, 147*, 84-89

Hieger, I. (1958) Cholesterol carcinogenesis. *Br. med. Bull., 14*, 159-160

Hieger, I. (1959) Carcinogenesis by cholesterol. *Br. J. Cancer, 13*, 439-451

Hieger, I. (1962) Cholesteral as carcinogen. I. Sarcoma induction by cholesterol in a sensitive strain of mice. II. Croton oil a complete carcinogen. *Br. J. Cancer, 16*, 716-721

Hieger, I. & Orr, S.F.D. (1954) On the carcinogenic activity of purified cholesterol. *Br. J. Cancer, 8*, 274-290

Hill, M.J. (1980) Bacterial metabolism and human carcinogenesis. *Br. med. Bull., 36*, 89-94

Hill, M.J., Crowther, J.S., Drasar, B.S., Hawksworth, G., Aries, V. & Williams, R.E.O. (1971) Bacteria and aetiology of cancer of large bowel. *Lancet, i*, 95-100

Hill, M.J., Drasar, B.S., Williams, R.E.O., Meade, T.W., Cox, A.G., Simpson, J.E.P. & Morson, B.C. (1975) Faecal bile-acids and *Clostridia* in patients with cancer of the large bowel. *Lancet, i*, 535-539

Huang, H.-S., Kuan, J.-C.W. & Guilbault, G.G. (1975) Fluorometric enzymatic determination of total cholesterol in serum. *Clin. Chem., 21*, 1605-1608

IARC (1976) *IARC Monographs on the Evaluation of Carcinogenic Risk of Chemicals to Man*, Vol. 10, *Some Naturally Occurring Substances*, Lyon, pp. 99-111

IARC (1980) *IARC Monographs on the Evaluation of the Carcinogenic Risk of Chemicals to Humans*, Vol. 24, *Some Pharmaceutical Drugs*, Lyon, pp. 39-58

IARC Intestinal Microecology Group (1977) Dietary fibre, transit-time, faecal bacteria, stroids, and colon cancer in two Scandinavian populations. *Lancet, ii*, 207-211

Jain, M., Cook, G.M., Davis, F.G., Grace, M.G., Howe, G.R. & Miller, A.B. (1980) A case-control study of diet and colo-rectal cancer. *Int. J. Cancer, 26*, 757-768

Jensen, O.M., MacLennan, R. & Wahrendorf, J. (1982) Diet, bowel function, fecal characteristics, and large bowel cancer in Denmark and Finland. *Nutr. Cancer, 4*, 5-19

Kagan, A., McGee, D.L., Yano, K., Rhoads, G.G. & Nomura, A. (1981) Serum cholesterol and mortality in a Japanese-American population. The Honolulu heart program. *Am. J. Epidemiol., 114*, 11-20

Kark, J.D., Smith, A.H. & Hames, C.G. (1980) The relationship of serum cholesterol to the incidence of cancer in Evans County, Georgia. *J. chronic Dis.*, *33*, 311-322

Kark, J.D., Smith, A.H. & Hames, C.G. (1982) Serum retinol and the inverse relationship between cholesterol and cancer. *Br. med. J.*, *284*, 152-154

Keana, J.F.W. & Johnson, W.S. (1964) Racemic cholesterol. *Steroids*, *4*, 457-462

Kelsey, M.I. & Pienta, R.J. (1979) Transformation of hamster embryo cells by cholesterol-α-epoxide and lithocholic acid. *Cancer Lett.*, *6*, 143-149

Kelsey, M.I. & Pienta, R.J. (1981) Transformation of hamster embryo cells by neutral sterols and bile acids. *Toxicol. Lett.*, *9*, 177-182

Klurfeld, D.M. & Kritchevsky, D. (1981) Serum cholesterol and 7,12-dimethylbenz[a]anthracene-induced mammary carcinogenesis. *Cancer Lett.*, *14*, 273-278

Knox, E.G. (1977) Foods and diseases. *Br. J. prev. soc. Med.*, *31*, 71-80

Kolonel, L.N., Hankin, J.H., Lee, J., Chu, S.Y., Nomura, A.M.Y. & Hinds, M.W. (1981) Nutrient intakes in relation to cancer incidence in Hawaii. *Br. J. Cancer*, *44*, 332-339

Kowalewski, K. & Todd, E.F. (1971) Carcinoma of the gallbladder induced in hamsters by insertion of cholesterol pellets and feeding dimethylnitrosamine. *Proc. Soc. exp. Biol. Med.*, *136*, 482-486

Kozarevic, D., McGee, D., Vojvodic, N.,Gordon, T., Racic, Z., Zukel, W. & Dawber, T. (1981) Serum cholesterol and mortality. The Yugoslavia Cardiovascular Disease Study. *Am. J. Epidemiol.*, *144*, 21-28

Kritchevsky, D. (1958) *Cholesterol*, New York, John Wiley & Sons Inc., pp. 1, 2

Laskarzewski, P., Khoury, P., Morrison, J.A., Kelly, K., Mellies, M. & Glueck, C.J. (1982) Cancer, cholesterol, and lipoprotein cholesterols. *Prev. Med.*, *11*, 253-268

Lehninger, A.L. (1975) *Biochemistry*, 2nd ed., New York, Worth, pp. 679-685

Lentner, C., ed. (1981) *Geigy Scientific Tables*, 8th ed., Vol. 1, *Units of Measurements, Body Fluids, Composition of the Body, Nutrition*, West Caldwell, NJ, Medical Education Division, Ciba-Geigy Corporation, pp. 92, 98, 143-145, 157, 163, 174, 184, 191, 201, 202, 214, 220, 222, 223, 241, 254-260

Liu, K., Stamler, J., Moss, D., Garside, D., Persky, V. & Soltero, I. (1979) Dietary cholesterol, fat, and fibre, and colon-cancer mortality. *Lancet*, *ii*, 782-785

Lubin, J.H., Burns, P.E., Blot, W.J., Ziegler, R.G., Lees, A.W. & Fraumeni, J.F., Jr (1981) Dietary factors and breast cancer risk. *Int. J. Cancer*, *28*, 685-689

Lyon, J.L., Gardner, J.W., Klauber, M.R. & Smart, C.R. (1977) Low cancer incidence and mortality in Utah. *Cancer*, *39*, 2608-2618

MacGee, J., Ishikawa, T., Miller, W., Evans, G., Steiner, P. & Glueck, C.J. (1973) A micromethod for analysis of total plasma cholesterol using gas-liquid chromatography. *J. Lab. clin. Med.*, *82*, 656-662

Malarkey, W.B., Schroeder, L.L., Stevens, V.C., James, A.G. & Lanese, R.R. (1977) Twenty-four-hour preoperative endocrine profiles in women with benign and malignant breast disease. *Cancer Res.*, *37*, 4655-4659

Marmot, M.G., Syme, S.L., Kagan, A., Kato, H., Cohen, J.B. & Belsky, J. (1975) Epidemiologic studies of coronary heart disease and stroke in Japanese men living in Japan, Hawaii, and California: Prevalence of coronary and hypertensive heart disease and associated risk factors. *Am. J. Epidemiol.*, *102*, 514-525

Martin, C.M. & Nicholas, H.J. (1973) Metabolism of cholesteryl palmitate by rat brain *in vitro*; formation of cholesterol epoxides and cholestan-3β,5α,6β-triol. *J. Lipid Res.*, *14*, 618-624

McGill, H.C., Jr (1979) The relationship of dietary cholesterol to serum cholesterol concentration and to atherosclerosis in man. *Am. J. clin. Nutr.*, *32*, 2664-2702

McMichael, A.J. & Potter, J.D. (1980) Reproduction, endogenous and exogenous sex hormones, and colon cancer: A review and hypothesis. *J. natl Cancer Inst.*, *65*, 1201-1207

Miller, A.B., Kelly, A., Choi, N.W., Matthews, V., Morgan, R.W., Munan, L., Burch, J.D., Feather, J., Howe, G.R. & Jain, M. (1978) A study of diet and breast cancer. *Am. J. Epidemiol.*, *107*, 499-509

Miller, S.R., Tartter, P.I., Papatestas, A.E., Slater, G. & Aufses, A.H., Jr (1981) Serum cholesterol and human colon cancer. *J. natl Cancer Inst.*, *67*, 297-300

Montgomery, R., Dryer, R.L., Conway, T.W. & Spector, A.A. (1980) *Biochemistry: A Case-Oriented Approach*, 3rd ed., Saint Louis, MO, C.V. Mosby Company, pp. 446-463

Moskovitz, M., White, C., Barnett, R.N., Stevens, S., Russell, E., Vargo, D. & Floch, M.H. (1979) Diet, fecal bile acids, and neutral sterols in carcinoma of the colon. *Dig. Dis. Sci.*, *24*, 746-751

Mudd, D.G., McKelvey, S.T.D., Norwood, W., Elmore, D.T. & Roy, A.D. (1980) Faecal bile acid concentrations of patients with carcinoma or increased risk of carcinoma in the large bowel. *Gut*, *21*, 587-590

Murray, W.R., Blackwood, A., Trotter, J.M., Calman, K.C. & MacKay, C. (1980) Faecal bile acids and clostridia in the aetiology of colorectal cancer. *Br. J. Cancer*, *41*, 923-928

NIH/EPA Chemical Information System (1981) *TSCA Plant and Production Data Base*, Washington DC, CIS Project, Information Services Corporation

NIH/EPA Chemical Information System (1982) *Infra-Red Spectral Search System, Mass Spectral Search System*, and *C^{13} Nuclear Magnetic Resonance Search System*, Washington DC, CIS Project, Information Sciences Corporation

Oliver, M.F. (1981) Serum cholesterol - The knave of hearts and the joker. *Lancet*, *ii*, 1090-1095

Parsons, P.G. & Goss, P. (1978) Chromosome damage and DNA repair induced in human fibroblasts by UV and cholesterol oxide. *Aust. J. exp. biol. Med. Sci.*, *56*, 287-296

Pearce, M.L. & Dayton, S. (1971) Incidence of cancer in men on a diet high in polyunsaturated fat. *Lancet*, *i*, 464-467

Peterson, B., Trell, E. & Sternby, N.H. (1981) Low cholesterol level as risk factor for noncoronary death in middle-aged men. *J. Am. med. Assoc.*, *245*, 2056-2057

Phillips, R.L. (1975) Role of life-style and dietary habits in risk of cancer among Seventh-Day Adventists. *Cancer Res.*, *35*, 3513-3522

Pienta, R.J. (1980) *Transformation of Syrian hamster embryo cells by diverse chemicals and correlation with their reported carcinogenic and mutagenic activities.* In: de Serres, F.J. & Hollaender, A., eds, *Chemical Mutagens. Principles and Methods for Their Detection*, Vol. 6, New York, Plenum, pp. 175-202

Pitkin, R.M., Connor, W.E. & Lin, D.S. (1972) Cholesterol metabolism and placental transfer in the pregnant rhesus monkey. *J. clin. Invest.*, *51*, 2584-2592

Pooling Project Research Group (1978) Relationship of blood pressure, serum cholesterol, smoking habit, relative weight and ECG abnormalities to incidence of major coronary events: Final report of the pooling project. *J. chronic Dis.*, *31*, 201-306

Reddy, B.S. & Wynder, E.L. (1973) Large-bowel carcinogenesis: Fecal constituents of populations with diverse incidence rates of colon cancer. *J. natl Cancer Inst.*, *50*, 1437-1442

Reddy, B.S. & Wynder, E.L. (1977) Metabolic epidemiology of colon cancer. Fecal bile acids and neutral sterols in colon cancer patients and patients with adenomatous polyps. *Cancer*, *39*, 2533-2539

Reddy, B.S., Mastromarino, A. & Wynder, E.L. (1975) Further leads on metabolic epidemiology of large bowel cancer. *Cancer Res.*, *35*, 3403-3406

Reddy, B.S., Hedges, A., Laakso, K. & Wynder, E.L. (1978) Fecal constituents of a high-risk North American and a low-risk Finnish population for the development of large bowel cancer. *Cancer Lett.*, *4*, 217-222

Rose, G. & Shipley, M.J. (1980) Plasma lipids and mortality: A source of error. *Lancet*, *i*, 523-526

Rose, G., Blackburn, H., Keys, A., Taylor, H.L., Kannel, W.B., Paul, O., Reid, D.D. & Stamler, J. (1974) Colon cancer and blood-cholesterol. *Lancet*, *i*, 180-183

Rosenfeld, R.S., Zumoff, B. & Hellman, L. (1967) Conversion of cholesterol injected into man to cholestanol via a 3-ketonic intermediate. *J. Lipid Res.*, *8*, 16-23

Sabine, J.R. (1977) *Cholesterol*, New York/Basel, Marcel Dekker Inc., pp. 7, 29-32

Sevanian, A., Mead, J.F. & Stein, R.A. (1979) Epoxides as products of lipid autoxidation in rat lungs. *Lipids*, *14*, 634-643

Siperstein, M.D. (1970) *Regulation of cholesterol biosynthesis in normal and malignant tissues*. In: Horecker, B.L. & Stadtman, E.R., eds, *Current Topics in Cellular Regulation*, Vol. 2, New York, Academic Press, pp. 65-100

Smith, A.H. & Hoggard, B.M. (1981) Retinol, carotene, and the cancer/cholesterol association (Letter). *Lancet*, *i*, 1371-1372

Smith, L.L., Matthews, W.S., Price J.C., Bachmann, R.C. & Reynolds, B. (1967) Thin-layer chromatographic examination of cholesterol autoxidation. *J. Chromatogr.*, *27*, 187-205

Smith, L.L., Smart,V.B. & Ansari, G.A.S. (1979) Mutagenic cholesterol preparations. *Mutat. Res.*, *68*, 23-30

Stanbury, J.B., Wyngaarden, J.B., Fredrickson, D.S., Goldstein, J.L. & Brown, M.S. (1983) *The Metabolic Basis of Inherited Disease*, 5th ed., New York, McGraw Hill

Stemmermann, G.N., Nomura, A.M.Y., Heilbrun, L.K., Pollack, E.S. & Kagan, A. (1981) Serum cholesterol and colon cancer incidence in Hawaiian Japanese men. *J. natl Cancer Inst.*, *67*, 1179-1182

Sturdevant, R.A.L., Pearce, M.L. & Dayton, S. (1973) Increased prevalence of cholelithiasis in men ingesting a serum-cholesterol-lowering diet. *New Engl. J. Med.*, *288*, 24-27

Styles, J.A. (1978) Mammalian cell transformation *in vitro*. *Br. J. Cancer*, *37*, 931-936

Szepsenwol, J. (1966) Carcinogenic effect of cholesterol in mice. *Proc. Soc. exp. Biol. Med.*, *121*, 168-171

Taub, D. & Windholz, T.B. (1969) *Steroids*. In: Kirk, R.E. & Othmer, D.F., eds, *Encyclopedia of Chemical Technology*, 2nd ed., Vol. 18, New York, John Wiley & Sons, pp. 835-837, 896

Thomas, C.B., Duszynski, K.R. & Shaffer, J.W. (1982) Cholesterol levels in young adulthood and subsequent cancer: A preliminary note. *Johns Hopkins med. J.*, *150*, 89-94

Turpeinen, O. (1979) Effect of cholesterol-lowering diet on mortality from coronary heart disease and other causes. *Circulation*, *59*, 1-7

Ursick, J.A., Israelsen, L.D. & Shaw, D.H. (1972) Cholesterol side-chain degradation and cleft palate development in the rat. *J. dent. Res.*, *51*, 1421-1425

US Pharmacopeial Convention, Inc. (1980) *The US Pharmacopeia*, 20th rev., Rockville, MD, pp. 148, 149, 604

Walden, R.T., Schaefer, L.E., Lemon, F.R., Sunshine, A. & Wynder, E.L. (1964) Effect of environment on the serum cholesterol-triglyceride distribution among Seventh-Day Adventists. *Am. J. Med.*, *36*, 269-276

Watabe, T., Isobe, M. & Kanai, M. (1980) Cholesterol diet increases plasma and liver concentrations of cholesterol epoxides and cholestanetriol. *J. Pharmacobio-Dyn.*, *3*, 553-556

Watabe, T., Isobe, M. & Tsubaki, A. (1982) Epoxidation of cholesterol by hepatic microsomal lipid hydroperoxides. *Biochem. biophys. Res. Commun.*, *108*, 724-730

Westlund, K. & Nicolaysen, R. (1972) Ten-year mortality and morbidity related to serum cholesterol. *Scand. J. clin. Lab. Invest.*, *30, Suppl. 127*, 3-24

Williams, R.R., Sorlie, P.D., Feinleib, M., McNamara, P.M., Kannel, W.B. & Dawber, T.R. (1981) Cancer incidence by levels of cholesterol. *J. Am. med. Assoc.*, *245*, 247-252

Windholz, M., ed. (1976) *The Merck Index*, 9th ed., Rahway, NJ, Merck & Co., Inc., p. 283

Woodward, R.B., Sondheimer, F., Taub, D., Heusler, K. & McLamore, W.M. (1952) The total synthesis of steroids. *J. Am. chem. Soc.*, *74*, 4223

Yaari, S., Goldbourt, U., Even-Zohar, S. & Neufeld, H.N. (1981) Associations of serum high density lipoprotein and total cholesterol with total, cardiovascular, and cancer mortality in a 7-year prospective study of 10,000 men. *Lancet*, *i*, 1011-1014

CINNAMYL ANTHRANILATE

This substance was considered by a previous Working Group, in June 1977 (IARC, 1978). Since that time, new data have become available, and these have been incorporated into the monograph and taken into consideration in the present evaluation.

1. Chemical and Physical Data

1.1 Synonyms and trade names

Chem. Abstr. Services Reg. No.: 87-29-6

Chem. Abstr. Name: Benzoic acid, 2-amino-, 3-phenyl-2-propenyl ester

IUPAC Systematic Name: Cinnamyl anthranilate

Synonyms: Anthranilic acid, cinnnamyl ester; cinnamyl alcohol anthranilate; cinnamyl 2-aminobenzoate; cinnamyl *ortho*-aminobenzoate; 3-phenyl-2-propen-1-yl anthranilate; 3-phenyl-2-propenyl anthranilate

1.2 Structural and molecular formulae and molecular weight

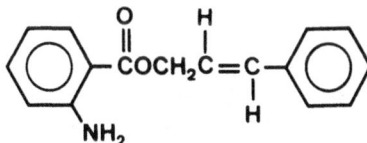

$C_{16}H_{15}NO_2$ Mol. wt: 253.3

1.3 Chemical and physical properties of the substance

Data are given for the technical product and are from National Research Council (1972) and Furia and Bellanca (1975), unless otherwise specified

  (a) *Description*: Brownish or reddish-yellow powder, with a characteristic fruity flavour

  (b) *Melting-point*: 63-64.5°C (National Cancer Institute, 1980)

  (c) *Density*: 1.18 at 15.5°C

  (d) *Spectroscopy data*: Infra-red, ultra-violet and nuclear magnetic resonance spectra have been reported (National Cancer Institute, 1980).

  (e) *Solubility*: Insoluble in water; soluble in chloroform, diethyl ether and 95% ethanol (50 g/l)

  (f) *Stability*: Sensitive to oxidation and hydrolysis

  (g) *Reactivity*: Reacts with various aldehydes, forming highly coloured compounds (Bedoukian, 1967)

1.4 Technical products and impurities

The *Food Chemicals Codex* in the US specified that formulations of cinnamyl anthranilate contain a minimum of 96% active ingredient and have a melting-point >60°C (National Research Council, 1972).

2. Production, Use, Occurrence and Analysis

2.1 Production and use

  (a) *Production*

Cinnamyl anthranilate can be made by esterification of anthranilic acid or isatoic anhydride with cinnamyl alcohol (Furia & Bellanca, 1975; Opdyke, 1975). It is believed that isatoic anhydride is used in commercial production of this chemical.

Cinnamyl anthranilate was first produced commercially in the US in 1939 (US Tariff Commission, 1940). Separate data on US production and sales were last reported in 1974 and 1977, respectively, when the three producing companies made and sold 454 kg (US International Trade Commission, 1976, 1978). Only one US company is believed to be producing cinnamyl anthranilate now. Separate data on US imports and exports of cinnamyl anthranilate are not published.

Cinnamyl anthranilate has been produced in Japan since 1950. Production in 1981 by the only producing company is estimated to have been about 300 kg.

Cinnamyl anthranilate is not produced commercially in western Europe.

(b) *Use*

Cinnamyl anthranilate is a synthetic flavouring agent used in mixtures to imitate grape or cherry flavour. It is added to a variety of food products (e.g., beverages, ice cream, sweets, baked goods, gelatins, puddings, and chewing gums) at levels ranging from 1.7 to 730 mg/kg (National Cancer Institute, 1980). It is also used as a fragrance in soaps, detergents, creams, lotions and perfumes at levels of 0.00l-0.4% (Opdyke, 1975).

In 1974, the Council of Europe authorized use of cinnamyl anthranilate as an artificial flavour at levels of up to 25 mg/kg (Opdyke, 1975). This compound is approved for use in the US as a synthetic flavouring substance and adjuvant provided it is used in the minimum quantity required to produce its intended effect (US Food & Drug Administration, 1980); however, the US Food and Drug Administration (1982) is considering a proposed regulation that would prohibit the use of cinnamyl anthranilate in human food and ingestible cosmetics. The World Health Organization (1981) has recommended that cinnamyl anthranilate not be used in food.

2.2 Occurrence

Cinnamyl anthranilate is not known to occur as a natural product.

2.3 Analysis

Cinnamyl anthranilate can be assayed by a method based on ester hydrolysis (National Research Council, 1972). Bulk samples of food-grade cinnamyl anthranilate have been analysed for purity by thin-layer chromatography and high-performance liquid chromatography (National Cancer Institute, 1980). A method has been described for determining the content of this compound in food products by steam distillation followed by paper chromatography and examination under ultra-violet light; it has a limit of detection of 1 μg (Jorysch & Marcus, 1961).

3. Biological Data Relevant to the Evaluation of Carcinogenic Risk to Humans

3.1 Carcinogenicity studies in animals

(a) Oral administration

Mouse: Groups of 50 male and 50 female B6C3F1 mice, six weeks old, were fed 15 or 30 g/kg cinnamyl anthranilate in the diet for 103 weeks (96% pure; at least five nonidentified impurities were found by thin-layer chromatography and two by high-performance liquid chromatography). The doses were selected on the basis of a subchronic experiment. Fifty male and 50 female mice of the same strain served as matched controls. Survival rates at the end of the study (105 to 107 weeks) in the control, low-dose and high-dose groups were 88, 82 and 80% of males and 78, 82 and 74% of females. Dose-related reductions in mean body weight gain were noted in both sexes. A significant dose-related increase (p < 0.001, Cochran-Armitage) in the incidence of hepatocellular carcinomas was found in animals of both sexes: females - 1/50 (2%); 8/49 (16%) (p = 0.014); and 14/49 (29%) (p < 0.001) in the control, low- and high-dose groups, respectively; males - 6/48 (13%), 7/50 (14%) and 12/47 (26%) [p = 0.047]. When the liver-cell carcinomas were grouped with the liver adenomas (males: 8/48 controls; 23/50 low-dose; 25/47 high-dose; females: 2/50 controls; 14/49 low-dose; 19/49 high-dose), there was a significant dose-related increase in their incidences in males and females (p < 0.001, Cochran-Armitage test for trend; p = 0.002 (low-dose males) and p < 0.001 by the Fisher exact test). A few metastases were seen in the lungs of high-dose females (National Cancer Institute, 1980).

Rat: Two groups of 50 male and 50 female Fischer 344 rats, seven weeks of age, were fed 15 or 30 g/kg cinnamyl anthranilate (same sample as used above) in the diet for 103 weeks. Fifty male and 50 female Fischer 344 rats served as controls. The dietary levels were selected on the basis of a subchronic study. Dose-related reductions in mean body weight gain were seen throughout the study. Surviving animals were sacrificed at 105 to 107 weeks, at which time 64, 80 and 80% of the males and 78, 88 and 92% of the females were still alive in the control, low- and high-dose groups, respectively. There was an increased incidence of mineralization and inflammation of the kidneys of treated rats. A non-statistically significant increase in the incidence of kidney tumours was observed in high-dose male rats (4/49, 2 adenocarcinomas and 2 adenomas); there was also a non-statistically significant increase in the incidence of acinar-cell pancreatic tumours (3/45, 1 carcinoma and 2 adenomas). No such tumour was observed in matched controls (National Cancer Institute, 1980). [The Working Group noted that the incidences of kidney and acinar-cell pancreatic tumours in historical male controls of the Bioassay Testing Programme were 0.05-0.16% (Goodman *et al.*, 1979).]

(b) Intraperitoneal administration

Mouse: Cinnamyl anthranilate was tested in a screening study using the induction of lung tumours as an endpoint. In the first series, groups of 15 male and 15 female A/He mice, six to eight weeks old, were given thrice weekly i.p. injections of cinnamyl anthranilate [purity unspecified] dissolved in tricaprylin, as 24 doses of 500 mg/kg bw (the maximal tolerated dose, as found in subchronic experiments) or 100 mg/kg bw (total doses, 12 and 2.4 g/kg bw, respectively). A control group of 25 females received i.p. injections of the vehicle by the same schedule. Lung tumours [type not specified] were found in 10 high-dose females, 11 high-dose males, 7 low-dose females, 10 low-dose males and 45% control females [absolute numbers not given]. The numbers of tumours/mouse were 0.59 $\pm$ 0.13 in control females, 2.14 $\pm$ 0.70 (p < 0.05) in high-dose females, and 2.69 $\pm$ 0.75 (p < 0.05) in high-dose males. Comparison was apparently [not specified in the text] made only with the female groups (Stoner *et al.*, 1973).

In the second series, cinnamyl anthranilate was reassayed in 15 females and 15 males under similar experimental conditions, except that redistilled tricaprylin was used as the vehicle. The control group consisted of 80 females and 80 males. Numbers of tumours/mouse were 0.85 $\pm$ 0.23 (p < 0.01) in high-dose females, 1.40 $\pm$ 0.36 (p < 0.001) in high-dose males, 0.54 $\pm$ 0.15 (p < 0.05) in low-dose females, and 0.47 $\pm$ 0.12 (statistically not significant) in low-dose males. In controls, the numbers of tumours per mouse were 0.20 $\pm$ 0.02 in females and 0.24 $\pm$ 0.03 in males (Stoner et al., 1973).

3.2 Other relevant biological data

(a) Experimental systems

Toxic effects

No adequate data were available to the Working Group.

Effects on reproduction and prenatal toxicity

No data were available to the Working Group. In the chicken embryo test, no effect on structural or functional development was observed in embryos or hatched chicks with doses of up to 10 mg/egg (Verrett et al., 1980).

Absorption, distribution, excretion and metabolism

No data were available to the Working Group.

Mutagenicity and other short-term tests

Cinnamyl anthranilate was not mutagenic to Salmonella typhimurium strains TA1535, TA1537, TA1538, TA98 or TA100 when tested in the presence or absence of a metabolic activation system prepared from non-induced or induced rats, mice or hamsters (Dunkel & Simmon, 1980).

(b) Humans

No data were available to the Working Group.

3.3 Case reports and epidemiological studies of carcinogenicity in humans

No data were available to the Working Group.

4. Summary of Data Reported and Evaluation

4.1 Experimental data

Cinnamyl anthranilate was tested for carcinogenicity in mice and rats by administration in the diet and in mice by intraperitoneal injection. In mice, a dose-related increase in the incidence of hepatocellular tumours was found following its oral administration and an increased incidence of lung tumours following its intraperitoneal injection. The study in rats could not be evaluated.

Cinnamyl anthranilate was not mutagenic to *Salmonella typhimurium*. The data were *inadequate* to evaluate the activity of this compound in short-term tests.

No data were available to evaluate the teratogenicity of this compound to experimental animals.

4.2 Human data

Cinnamyl anthranilate has been used since at least 1939, but its use during the last few years has diminished. Its consumption as a flavouring agent and to a lesser extent as a fragrance in cosmetics are sources of exposure for the general population.

No data were available to evaluate the teratogenicity or chromosomal effects of this compound in humans.

No case report or epidemiological study of the carcinogenicity of cinnamyl anthranilate was available to the Working Group.

4.3 Evaluation

There is *limited evidence*[1] for the carcinogenicity of cinnamyl anthranilate in experimental animals. In the absence of epidemiological data, no evaluation of the carcinogenicity of cinnamyl anthranilate to humans could be made.

5. References

Bedoukian, P.Z. (1967) *Perfumery and Flavoring Synthetics*, 2nd rev. ed., Amsterdam, Elsevier, pp. 41-47

Dunkel, V.C. & Simmon, V.F. (1980) *Mutagenic activity of chemicals previously tested for carcinogenicity in the National Cancer Institute bioassay programme.* In: Montesano, R., Bartsch, H. & Tomatis, L., eds, *Molecular and Cellular Aspects of Carcinogen Screening Tests (IARC Scientific Publications No. 27)*, Lyon, International Agency for Research on Cancer, pp. 283-302

Furia, T.E. & Bellanca, N., eds (1975) *Fenaroli's Handbook of Flavor Ingredients*, 2nd ed., Vol. 2, Cleveland, OH, CRC Press, Inc., p. 94

Goodman, D.G., Ward, J.M., Squire, R.A., Chu, K.C. & Linhart, M.S. (1979) Neoplastic and nonneoplastic lesions in aging F344 rats. *Toxicol. appl. Pharmacol.*, *48*, 237-248

---

[1]See preamble, p. 18.

IARC (1978) *IARC Monographs on the Evaluation of the Carcinogenic Risk of Chemicals to Humans*, Vol. 16, *Some Aromatic Amines and Related Nitro Compounds - Hair Dyes, Colouring Agents and Miscellaneous Industrial Chemicals*, Lyon, pp. 287-291

Jorysch, D. & Marcus, S. (1961) Determination of anthranilates by paper chromatography. *J. Assoc. off. agric. Chem.*, *44*, 541-545

National Cancer Institute (1980) *Bioassay of Cinnamyl Anthranilate for Possible Carcino-genicity (Tech. Rep. Ser. No. 196, DHEW Publ. No. (NIH) 80-1752, No. (NTP) 80.10)*, Washington DC, US Government Printing Office

National Research Council (1972) *Food Chemicals Codex*, 2nd ed., Washington DC, National Academy of Sciences, pp. 199, 896, 897

Opdyke, D.L.J. (1975) Special Issue II. Monographs on fragrance raw materials. Cinnamyl anthranilate. *Food Cosmet. Toxicol.*, *13 Suppl.*, 751-752

Stoner, G.D, Shimin, M.B., Kniazeff, A.J., Weisburger, J.H., Weisburger, E.K. & Gori, G.B. (1973) Test for carcinogenicity of food additives and chemotherapeutic agents by the pulmonary tumor response in strain A mice. *Cancer Res.*, *33*, 3069-3085

US Food & Drug Administration (1980) Food and drugs. *US Code Fed. Regul.*, *Title 21*, Part 172.515, pp. 44, 45

US Food & Drug Administration (1982) Cinnamyl anthranilate; proposed prohibition of use in human food. *US Code Fed. Regul.*, *Title 21*, parts 172, 189; *Fed. Regist.*, *47*, 22545-22547

US International Trade Commission (1976) *Synthetic Organic Chemicals, US Production and Sales, 1974 (USITC Publication 776)*, Washington DC, US Government Printing Office, pp. 115, 117

US International Trade Commission (1978) *Synthetic Organic Chemicals, US Production and Sales, 1977 (USITC Publication 920)*, Washington DC, US Government Printing Office, pp. 193, 196

US Tariff Commission (1940) *Synthetic Organic Chemicals, US Production and Sales, 1939 (Report No. 140)*, Second Series, Washington DC, US Government Printing Office, pp. 39, 59

Verrett, M.J., Scott, W.F., Reynaldo, E.F., Alterman, E.K. & Thomas, C.A. (1980) Toxicity and teratogenicity of food additive chemicals in the developing chicken embryo. *Toxicol. appl. Pharmacol.*, *56*, 265-273

World Health Organization (1981) International Programme on Chemical Safety, IPCS, Toxicological Evaluation of Certain Food Additives. *WHO Food Add. Ser.*, *No. 16*, pp. 70-73

FURAZOLIDONE

1. Chemical and Physical Data

1.1 Synonyms and trade names

Chem. Abstr. Services Reg. No.: 67-45-8

Chem. Abstr. Name: 2-Oxazolidinone, 3-([(5-nitro-2-furanyl)methylene]amino)-

IUPAC Systematic Name: 3-[(5-Nitrofurfurylidene)amino]-2-oxazolidinone

Synonyms: N-(5-Nitro-2-furfurylidene)-3-amino-2-oxazolidone; 5-nitro-N-(2-oxo-3-oxazolidinyl)-2-furanmethanimine; nitrofurazolidone; nitrofurazolidonum

Trade Names: Bifuron; Corizium; Diafuron; Enterotoxon; Furaphen; Furaxon; Furaxone; Furazol; Furazolidon; Furazon; Furidon; Furovag; Furox; Furoxal; Furoxane; Furoxon; Furoxone; Furoxone Swine Mix; Furozolidine; Giardil; Giarlam; Medaron; Neftin; NF 180; NF 180 Custom Mix Ten; Nicolen; Nifulidone; Nifuran; Nitrofuroxon; Optazol; Ortazol; Puradin; Roptazol; Sclaventerol; Tikofuran; Topazone; Trichofuron; Tricofuron; Trifurox; Viofuragyn

1.2 Structural and molecular formulae and molecular weight

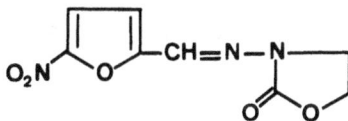

$C_8H_7N_3O_5$ Mol. wt: 225.2

1.3 Chemical and physical properties of the pure substance

From Windholz (1976), National Formulary Board (1970), and Wade (1977)

(a) *Description*: Yellow crystals

(b) *Melting-point*: 275°C (dec.)

(c) *Spectroscopy data*: Ultra-violet and infra-red spectra have been determined.

(d) *Solubility*: Practically insoluble in carbon tetrachloride, diethyl ether, ethanol and chloroform. Soluble in water at pH 6 (40 mg/l)

(e) *Stability*: Sensitive to light and decomposed by alkali

1.4 Technical products and impurities

In 1970, furazolidone was reported to be available in the US as a NF grade containing 97.0-103.0% active ingredient on a dried basis and with a maximum loss on drying at l00°C for 1 hour of 1% and a maximum residue on ignition of 0.05%. It was also reported to be available in combination with nifuroxime in powder and suppository formulations. The powder contained 0.09-0.11% furazolidone in a suitable, slightly acidified powder base, and the suppository contained 0.225-0.275% furazolidone (National Formulary Board, 1970). In 1979, it was reported that the products containing combinations of furazolidone and nifuroxime were no longer marketed in the US (US Food & Drug Administration, 1979).

In 1979, furazolidone was reported to be available in the UK as 100-mg tablets, as tablets containing 16 mg furazolidone with 110 mg nitrofurazone, and as tablets containing 250 mg furazolidone with 500 mg chloramphenicol; as capsules containing 20 mg furazolidone; as a suspension containing 5% or 7.5% furazolidone; and as a premix containing 4% or 20% furazolidone (The Pharmaceutical Society of Great Britain, 1979). In 1981, furazolidone was reported to be available in France as 100-mg tablets and as a suspension (344 mg/100 ml) in combination with methyl- and propyl-*para*-oxybenzoate (Anon., 1981).

Furazolidone is available for use in animal feeds as concentrates (221, 111 and 22 g/kg) in corn meal or ground rice hulls (Anon., 1979).

2. Production, Use, Occurrence and Analysis

2.1 Production and use

(a) Production

The synthesis of furazolidone was first described in a 1956 patent (Windholz, 1976). It can be made by the reaction of 5-nitro-2-furancarboxaldehyde (5-nitrofurfural) with 3-amino-2-oxazolidinone, which is made by the reaction of 2-hydrazinoethanol and diethyl carbonate (Ebetino, 1978). It is not known whether this method is used for commercial production.

Furazolidone was first produced commercially in the US in 1955 (US Tariff Commission, 1956). Since only one US company currently produces it, production data are not available (see preamble, p. 21). Separate data on US imports and exports of furazolidone are not available.

Furazolidone is produced by one company in Japan, which produced about 900 thousand kg in 1981. Japanese imports and exports of furazolidone in 1981 are estimated to have been 5-10 thousand kg and 700 thousand kg, respectively.

Furazolidone is believed to be produced by two companies in Spain and by one company each in Belgium and Italy. It is imported into France.

(b) *Use*

Furazolidone is an antiprotozoal and antibacterial agent. In 1975, it was reported to be the second-choice drug for the treatment of cholera (Goodman & Gilman, 1975). It is used in the treatment of gastro-enteritis and vaginal infections of bacterial origin and in conjunction with other nitro compounds in the local treatment of vaginal trichomoniasis or candidiasis and to combat protozoal infections such as African sleeping sickness, staphylococcal infection, cholera, salmonellosis, shigellosis, amoebiasis, giardiasis, thyroid fever and coccidiosis (Wade, 1977; Ebetino, 1978; Anon., 1981). Vaginal products containing furazolidone and nifuroxime are no longer marketed in the US, and the approval of the new drug application for these products was withdrawn in 1979 (US Food & Drug Administration, 1979).

Furazolidone is used in veterinary medicine as an antibacterial agent for a number of poultry diseases (e.g., coccidiosis, fowl typhoid, pullorum disease, histomoniasis, hexami-tiasis, synovitis, non-specific enteritis, and certain infections associated with the chronic respiratory disease complex). It is also used in the treatment of bacterial enteritis and infectious haemorrhagic enteritis of swine, enteritis and *Pasteurella* pneumonia in rabbits, and grey diarrhoea in mink (Siegmund, 1979). It is used alone or in combination with antibiotics to stimulate growth in poultry and swine (Anon., 1979).

In 1980, approval was given for use in the US of aerosol powders containing furazolidone on horses and ponies for preventing or treating bacterial infection of wounds, abrasions and lacerations (US Food & Drug Administration, 1980a).

In the US, a tolerance of zero is established for residues of furazolidone in the uncooked edible tissues of swine (US Food & Drug Administration, 1980b).

The estimated 200 thousand kg of furazolidone used in Japan in 1981 are believed to have been as a veterinary drug for swine and aquatic animals. It is not used in chicken.

2.2 Occurrence

Furazolidone is not known to occur as a natural product. No data were available to the Working Group on its persistence in the edible tissues of food-producing animals.

2.3 Analysis

Typical methods for the analysis of furazolidone are summarized in Table 1.

Table 1. Methods for the analysis of furazolidone

Sample matrix	Sample preparation	Assay procedure[a]	Limit of detection	Reference
Pharmaceutical pre-parations	Extract (dimethyl forma-mide); filter; dilute (water)	UV	not given	Elsayed et al. (1980)
	Extract (dimethyl forma-mide); dilute (water); add 1% aqueous sodium hydroxide	UV	not given	Biswas & Ghosh (1980)
	Extract (acetone-water); evaporate; redissolve (dimethylformamide-5% tetraethylammonium bromide)	HPLC/UV	7 mg/kg	Smallidge et al. (1981)
Human plasma and urine	Extract (chloroform); cen-trifuge; evaporate; dissolve (acetonitrile-water)	HPLC/UV	2 ng/ml	Guinebault et al. (1981)
Animal liver and kidney	Extract (ethyl acetate-anhy-drous sodium sulphate); evaporate; redissolve (ace-tonitrile); heat to 40°C; cool; filter	HPLC/UV	50 µg/kg	Ernst & Van Der Kaaden (1980)
Animal feeds	Extract (acetone)	TLC/UV	50 mg/kg	Cieri (1978)
	Extract (petroleum ether); evaporate; redissolve (ace-tone)	HPTLC/S	10 ng	Rauter (1979)
	Extract (acetone); evapo-rate; purify (aluminium oxide column)	HPLC/UV	60 µg/kg	Schweighardt & Leibetseder (1979)
Turkey tissues	Extract (dichloromethane); evaporate; liquid partition (hexane-0.01M acetic acid, then dichloromethane); evaporate; dissolve (30% methyl sulphoxide-0.01M acetic acid)	HPLC/UV	0.5 µg/kg	Winterlin et al. (1981)
	Extract (methanol); evapo-rate; redissolve (methanol-0.01M aqueous sodium acetate)	HPLC/UV	2 µg/kg	Hoener et al. (1979)

[a]Abbreviations: UV, ultra-violet spectrometry; HPLC/UV, high-performance liquid chromatography with ultra-violet spectrometric detection; TLC/UV, thin-layer chromatography with ultra-violet spectrometric detection; HPTLC/S, high-performance thin-layer chromatography with spectrometric determination

3. Biological Data Relevant to the Evaluation of Carcinogenic Risk to Humans

3.1 Carcinogenicity studies in animals

[The Working Group was aware that one study in mice and six studies in rats have been carried out on the carcinogenicity of furazolidone (US Department of Health, Education, & Welfare, 1976a,b; National Academy of Sciences, 1981). See 'General Remarks on the Substances Considered', p. 39.]

3.2 Other relevant biological data

(a) *Experimental systems*

Toxic effects

The oral LD_{50} of furazolidone is 2.3 g/kg bw in rats (Goldenthal, 1971) and about 4.5 g/kg bw in mice (Rogers *et al.*, 1956).

Daily oral doses of 100 mg/kg bw furazolidone to Donryu rats for seven days induced cytotoxic effects on the testes and atrophy and degeneration of the seminiferous tubules within one week (Miyaji *et al.*, 1964).

The chronic oral toxicity of furazolidone was investigated in both rats (0.03, 0.1, or 0.3% in the diet for 35 days) and dogs (7.5 or 25 mg/kg bw for up to 6 months). Toxicity was manifested as central nervous system symptoms and effects on spermatogenesis (Rogers *et al.*, 1956).

Given orally to rats furazolidone decreased liver and brain monoamine oxidase activity. This effect was dose-dependent and lasted for approximately 21 days. A saturated solution of furazolidone did not affect rat liver monoamine oxidase activity *in vitro*. It was thus postulated that a metabolite was responsable for the in-vivo activity (Stern *et al.*, 1967).

Effects on reproduction and prenatal toxicity

An oral dose of 1.0 g/kg bw furazolidone interrupted pregnancy in 5/5 and 9/10 mice treated on days 7 and 1 of gestation, respectively, but in only 2/6 animals when given on day 10. Animals in all litters had lower than normal body weight; no congenital abnormality was detected (Jackson & Robson, 1957).

Absorption, distribution, excretion and metabolism

After a single oral dose of 100 mg/kg bw to rats, only 3% of the dose was recovered in the faeces as unmetabolized compound (Paul *et al.*, 1960).

In-vitro metabolism of furazolidone by milk xanthine oxidase and rat liver homogenate yielded approximately equal amounts (30%) of 2,3-dihydro-3-cyano-methyl-2-hydroxyl-5-nitro-1a,2-di(2-oxo-oxazolidin-3-yl)iminomethylfuro[2,3b]furan, and 3-(4-cyano-2-oxobuty-lideneamino)-2-oxazolidone. The latter was also isolated from the urine of rabbits given an oral dose of furazolidone (Tatsumi et al., 1978, 1981).

Mutagenicity and other short-term tests

The mutagenicity of nitrofurans, including furazolidone, has been reviewed (Klemencic & Wang, 1978). Furazolidone is active without exogenous metabolic activation in the *Bacillus subtilis rec* assay (Ohta et al., 1980) and in an *Escherichia coli* DNA repair test (Ebringer & Bencová, 1980). It caused induction of prophage (Waterbury & Freedman, 1964).

Furazolidone is a strong, direct-acting mutagen in *Salmonella typhimurium* strain TA100, a weak mutagen in TA98, and non-mutagenic in TA1535, TA1537 and TA1538 (Byeon et al., 1976; Ebringer & Bencová, 1980; Ohta et al., 1980). It was mutagenic without metabolic activation to *E. coli* WP2 and to its *uvr*A-derivative by reversion from trp⁻ to trp⁺ (McCalla & Voutsinos, 1974; Klemencic & Wang, 1978; Lu et al., 1979).

3-(4-Cyano-2-oxobutylideneamino)-2-oxazolidone, a metabolite of furazolidone, was not mutagenic to *S. typhimurium* TA100 (Tatsumi et al., 1978).

Furazolidone induced loss of chloroplasts in *Euglena gracilis* (Ebringer et al., 1976).

It induced sex-linked recessive lethal mutations in *Drosophila melanogaster* (Blijleven et al., 1977; Kramers, 1982).

Furazolidone causes chromosomal aberrations, and a weak but dose-dependent induction of sister chromatid exchange in phytohaemagglutinin-stimulated human peripheral lymphocytes (Cohen & Sagi, 1979). [The Working Group noted, however, that the weak induction of sister chromatid exchanges might be attributed to the observed anti-mitotic effects of the compound in combination with exposure of the cells to bromodeo-xyuridine.] In an earlier study (Tonomura & Sasaki, 1973), employing similar conditions, the drug had no effect on either chromosomal damage in human lymphocytes or unscheduled DNA synthesis in human fibroblasts. Furazolidone induced unscheduled DNA synthesis in primary cultures of adult rat hepatocytes (Probst et al., 1981).

(b) *Humans*

Toxic effects

Allergic contact eczema has been reported in subjects handling animal feed containing furazolidone (Scharfenberg, 1967; Jirásek & Kalenskyé, 1975).

After use of furazolidone as a drug, acute nausea, emesis, occasional diarrhoea, abdominal pain and intestinal bleeding were observed (Wade, 1977; Cohen, 1978); hepatic damage, as evidenced by biochemical tests (Lo"wenberg, 1970), and peripheral neuropathy were also seen (Manor et al., 1975).

It also causes haemolytic anaemia associated with a deficiency of erythrocytic glucose-6-phosphate dehydrogenase (Wade, 1977; Cohen, 1978).

Effects on reproduction and prenatal toxicity

No data were available to the Working Group.

Absorption, distribution, excretion and metabolism

An oral dose of furazolidone was poorly absorbed from the gut and extensively metabolized in the intestine. When furazolidone was given *per os* to volunteers (400 mg per day for 21 days), plasma levels ranged between 60-200 ng/ml. Only small amounts of free, unchanged furazolidone were found in the urine (Wade, 1977; Guinebault *et al.*, 1981).

Mutagenicity and chromosomal effects

No data were available to the Working Group.

3.3 Case reports and epidemiological studies of carcinogenicity in humans

No data were available to the Working Group.

4. Summary of Data Reported and Evaluation

4.1 Experimental data

Data on the carcinogenicity of furazolidone were reported only in secondary sources and therefore could not be evaluated. (See 'General Remarks on the Substances Considered', p. 39.)

Furazolidone has been shown to induce DNA damage and mutations in bacteria and mutations in fungi and insects. It caused unscheduled DNA synthesis in mammalian cells *in vitro* and yielded conflicting results when tested for chromosomal anomalies in human cells *in vitro*. There is *sufficient evidence* that furazolidone is active in short-term tests.

Furazolidone induced abortion in mice. The data were inadequate to evaluate other prenatal effects.

4.2 Human data

Furazolidone has been produced commercially since 1955. It is used in human and veterinary medicine as an antibacterial and antiprotozoal agent.

No data were available to assess the teratogenicity or chromosomal effects of this compound in humans.

No case report or epidemiological study of the carcinogenicity of furazolidone was available to the Working Group.

4.3 Evaluation

No evaluation of the carcinogenicity of furazolidone to experimental animals could be made. In the absence of epidemiological data, no evaluation of the carcinogenicity of furazolidone to humans could be made.

5. References

Anon. (1979) *1980 Feed Additive Compendium*, Minneapolis, MN, The Miller Publishing Co., pp. 218-224

Anon. (1981) *Dictionnaire Vidal*, 57th ed., Paris, Office de Vulgarisation Pharmaceutique, p. 521

Biswas, A. & Ghosh, S. (1980) Spectrophotometric method of analysis of furazolidone in pharmaceutical preparations. *Indian J. pharm. Sci.*, *42*, 60-62

Blijleven, W.G.H., Kortselius, M.J.H. & Kramers, P.G.N. (1977) Mutagenicity testing of H-193, AF-2 and furazolidone in *Drosophila melanogaster*. *Mutat. Res.*, *56*, 95-100

Byeon, W.-H., Hyun, H.H. & Lee, S.Y. (1976) Mutagenicity of nitrofuran, nitroimidazole and nitrothiazole derivatives on *Salmonella*/microsome system. *Korean J. Microbiol.*, *14*, 151-158

Cieri, U.R. (1978) Quantitative thin layer chromatographic determination of furazolidone and nitrofurazone in animal feeds. *J. Assoc. off. anal. Chem.*, *61*, 92-95

Cohen, S.M. (1978) *Toxicity and carcinogenicity of nitrofurans*. In: Bryan, G.T., ed., *Carcinogenesis - A Comprehensive Survey*, Vol. 4, *Nitrofurans: Chemistry, Metabolism, Mutagenesis and Carcinogenesis*, New York, Raven Press, pp. 171-231

Cohen, M.M. & Sagi, M. (1979) The effect of nitrofurans on mitosis, chromosome breakage and sister-chromatid exchanges in human peripheral lymphocytes. *Mutat. Res.*, *59*, 139-142

Ebetino, F.F. (1978) *Antibacterial agents, nitrofurans*. In: Kirk, R.E. & Othmer, D.F., eds, *Encyclopedia of Chemical Technology*, 3rd ed., Vol. 2, New York, John Wiley & Sons, pp. 791-794

Ebringer, L. & Bencová, M. (1980) Mutagenicity of nitrofuran drugs in bacterial systems. *Folia Microbiol.*, *25*, 388-396

Ebringer, L., Jurásek, A., Konícek, J., Koníckova, M., Lahitová, N. & Trubacík, S. (1976) Mutagenic action of nitrofurans on *Euglena gracilis* and *Mycobacterium phlei*. *Antimicrob. Agents Chemother.*, *9*, 682-689

Elsayed, L., Hassan, S.M., Kelani, K.M. & El-Fatatry, H.M. (1980) Simultaneous spectrophotometric determination of nifuroxime and furazolidone in pharmaceutical preparations. *J. Assoc. off. anal. Chem.*, *63*, 992-995

Ernst, G.F. & Van Der Kaaden, A. (1980) High-performance liquid chromatographic analysis of furazolidone in liver and kidney. *J. Chromatogr.*, *198*, 526-528

Goldenthal, E.I. (1971) A compilation of LD_{50} values in newborn and adult animals. *Toxicol. appl. Pharmacol.*, *18*, 185-207

Goodman, L.S. & Gilman, A., eds (1975) *The Pharmacological Basis of Therapeutics*, 5th ed., New York, The Macmillan Company, pp. 1100-1101

Guinebault, P.R., Broquaire, M., Thebault, J.J., Larribaud, J., Trocherie, S. & Braithwaite, R.A. (1981) *Determination of nifuroxazide and furazolidone in biological fluids. Application to the comparative study of their intestinal absorption* (Fr.) In: Aiache, J.M. & Hirtz, J., eds, *Premier Congrès Européen de Biopharmacie et de Pharmacocinétique* [*First European Congress on Biopharmacy and Pharmacokinetics*], Paris, Documentation Technique, pp. 151-158

Hoener, B.-A., Lee, G. & Lundergan, W. (1979) High pressure liquid chromatographic determination of furazolidone in turkey tissue. *J. Assoc. off. anal. Chem.*, *62*, 257-261

Jackson, D. & Robson, J.M. (1957) The action of furazolidone on pregnancy. *J. Endocrinol.*, *15*, 355-359

Jirásek, L. & Kalenskyé, J. (1975) Allergic contact eczema from feeding mixtures in animal production (Czech.). *Cech. Dermatol.*, *50*, 217-225

Klemencic, J.M. & Wang, C.Y. (1978) *Mutagenicity of nitrofurans.* In: Bryan, G.T., ed., *Carcinogenesis - A Comprehensive Survey*, Vol. 4, *Nitrofurans: Chemistry, Metabolism, Mutagenesis and Carcinogenesis*, New York, Raven Press, pp. 99-130

Kramers, P.G.N. (1982) Studies on the induction of sex-linked recessive lethal mutations in *Drosophila melanogaster* by nitroheterocyclic compounds. *Mutat. Res.*, 209-236

Löwenberg, A. (1970) Hepatic damage due to the use of furazolidone (Dutch). *Ned. Tijdschr. Geneesk.*, *114*, 1404-1405

Lu, C., McCalla, D.R. & Bryant, D.W. (1979) Action of nitrofurans on *E. coli.* Mutation and induction and repair of daughter-strand gaps in DNA. *Mutat. Res.*, *67*, 133-144

Manor, Y., Steiner, Z. & Klejman, A. (1975) Peripheral neuropathy due to furazolidone (Heb.). *Harefuah*, *89*, 120-121

McCalla, D.R. & Voutsinos, D. (1974) On the mutagenicity of nitrofurans. *Mutat. Res.*, *26*, 3-16

Miyaji, T., Miyamoto, M. & Ueda, Y. (1964) Inhibition of spermatogenesis and atrophy of the testis caused by nitrofuran compounds. *Acta pathol. jpn.*, *14*, 261-273

National Academy of Sciences (1981) *Aromatic Amines: An Assessment of the Biological and Environmental Effects. Report of the Committee on Amines, Board on Toxicology and Environmental Health Hazards, Assembly of Life Sciences*, National Research Council, Washington DC, National Academy Press, pp. 288-319

National Formulary Board (1970) *National Formulary XIII*. 13th ed., American Pharmaceutical Association, Washington D.C., pp. 323-324

Ohta, T., Moriya, M., Kaneda, Y., Watanabe, K., Miyazawa, T., Sugiyama, F. & Shirasu, Y. (1980) Mutagenicity screening of feed additives in the microbial system. *Mutat. Res.*, *77*, 21-30

Paul, M.F., Paul, H.E., Bender, R.C., Kopko, F., Harrington, C.M., Ells, V.R. & Buzard, J.A. (1960) Studies on the distribution and excretion of certain nitrofurans. *Antibiot. Chemother.*, *10*, 287-302

The Pharmaceutical Society of Great Britain (1979) *The Pharmaceutical Codex*, 11th ed., London, The Pharmaceutical Press, pp. 376-377

Probst, G.S., McMahon, R.E., Hill, L.E., Thompson, C.Z., Epp, J.K. & Neal, S.B. (1981) Chemically-induced unscheduled DNA synthesis in primary rat hepatocyte cultures. A comparison with bacterial mutagenicity using 218 compounds. *Environ. Mutagenesis*, *3*, 11-32

Rauter, H. (1979) Determination of furazolidone in feeds with high-performance thin-layer chromarography (Ger.). *Landwirtsch. Forsch.*, *32*, 232-236

Rogers, G.S., Belloff, G.B., Paul, M.F., Yurchenco, J.A. & Gever, G. (1956) Furazolidone, a new antimicrobial nitrofuran. A review of laboratory and clinical data. *Antibiot. Chemother.*, *6*, 231-242

Scharfenberg, B. (1967) Chicken feed containing nitrofuran as occupational eczmatogen (Ger.). *Dermatol. Wschr.*, *153*, 60-63

Schweighardt, H. & Leibetseder, J. (1979) Quantitative dosage of furazolidone with high-performance liquid chromatography (HPLC) in feeds (Ger.). *Wien tieraerztl. Mschr.*, *66*, 325-329

Siegmund, O.H., ed. (1979) *The Merck Veterinary Manual*, 5th ed., Rahway, NJ, Merck & Co., Inc., pp. 506-507

Smallidge, R.L., Rowe, N.W., Wadgaonkar, N.D. & Stringham, R.W. (1981) High performance liquid chromatographic determination of furazolidone in feed and feed premixes. *J. Assoc. off. anal. Chem.*, *64*, 1100-1104

Stern, I.J., Hollifield, R.D., Wilk, S. & Buzard, J.A. (1967) The anti-monoamine oxidase effects of furazolidone. *J. Pharmacol. exp. Ther.*, *156*, 492-499

Tatsumi, K., Ou, T., Yamada, H., Yoshimura, H., Koga, H. & Horiuchi, T. (1978) Isolation and identification of the metabolite of *N*-(5-nitro-2-furfurylidene)-3-amino-2-oxazolidone (furazolidone). *J. pharm. Dyn.*, *1*, 256-261

Tatsumi, K., Yamada, H., Yoshimura, H. & Kawazoe, Y. (1981) Metabolism of furazolidone by milk xanthine oxidase and rat liver 9000g supernatant: Formation of a unique nitrofuran metabolite and an aminofuran derivative. *Arch. Biochem. Biophys.*, *208*, 167-174

Tonomura, A. & Sasaki, M.S. (1973) Chromosome aberrations and DNA repair synthesis in cultured human cells exposed to nitrofurans. *Jpn. J. Genet.*, *48*, 291-294

US Department of Health, Education, & Welfare (1976a) Furazolidone (NF-180): Notice of opportunity for hearing on proposal to withdraw approval of certain new animal drug applications. *Fed. Regist.*, *41*, 19907-19921

US Department of Health, Education, & Welfare (1976b) Furazolidone, nihydrazone, furaltadone, nitrofurazone: Withdrawal of proposals and notice of proposed rule making. *Fed. Regist.*, *41*, 34884-34921

US Food & Drug Administration (1979) Tricofuron vaginal powder and suppositories. *Fed. Regist.*, *44*, 2017

US Food & Drug Administration (1980a) Ophthalmic and topical dosage form of new animal drugs not subject to certification; furazolidone aerosol powder. *US Code Fed. Regul., Title 21*, part 524; *Fed. Regist.*, *45*, 49543-49544

US Food & Drug Administration (1980b) Food and drugs. *US Code Fed. Regul., Title 21*, part 556.290

US Tariff Commission (1956) *Synthetic Organic Chemicals, US Production and Sales, 1955 (Report No. 198)*, Second Series, Washington DC, US Government Printing Office, p. 112

Wade, A., ed. (1977) *Martindale, The Extra Pharmacopoeia*, 27th ed., London, The Pharmaceutical Press, pp. 78-79

Waterbury, W.E. & Freedman, R. (1964) Induction of phage formation by nitrofurans. *Can. J. Microbiol.*, *10*, 932-934

Windholz, M., ed. (1976) *The Merck Index*, 9th ed., Rahway, NJ, Merck & Co., Inc., p. 554

Winterlin, W., Hall, G. & Mourer, C. (1981) Ultra trace determination of furazolidone in turkey tissues by liquid partitioning and high performance liquid chromatography. *J. Assoc. off. anal. Chem.*, *64*, 1055-1059

FUSARENON X

This substance was considered by a previous Working Group, in February 1976 (IARC, 1976). Since that time new data have become available, and these have been incorporated into the monograph and taken into consideration in the present evaluation.

1. Chemical and Physical Data

1.1 Synonyms and trade names

Chem. Abstr. Services Reg. No.: 23255-69-8

Chem. Abstr. Name: Trichothec-9-en-8-one, 4-(acetyloxy)-12,13-epoxy-3,7,15-trihydroxy(3α,4β,7β)-

IUPAC Systematic Name: 12,13-Epoxy-3α,4β,7β,15-tetrahydroxytrichothec-9-en-8-one 4-acetate or (2R,3R,4S,5S,5aR,6R,9aR,10S)-2,3,4,5,5a,9a-Hexahydro-3,4,6-trihydroxy-5a-(hydroxymethyl)-5,8-dimethylspiro[2,5-methano-1-benzoxepin-10-2′-oxirane]-7(6H)-one 4-acetate

Synonyms: Fusarenon; fusarenone X; nivalenol-4-0-acetate; 3,7,15-trihydroxy-4-acetoxy-8-oxo-12,13-epoxy-Δ⁹-trichothecene; 3,7,15-trihydroxyscirp-4-acetoxy-9-en-8-one

1.2 Structural and molecular formulae and molecular weight

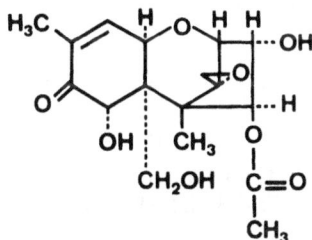

$C_{17}H_{22}O_8$ Mol. wt: 354.1

1.3 Chemical and physical properties of the pure substance

From Ueno *et al.* (1969) and Tatsuno *et al.* (1969), unless otherwise specified

(*a*) *Description*: Transparent bipyramid crystals

(*b*) *Melting-point*: 9l-92°C

(*c*) *Optical rotation*: $[\alpha]_D^{25}$ + 58° (l% in methanol); $[\alpha]_D^{24}$ + 56°.1 (in ethanol) (Saito & Ohtsubo, 1974)

(*d*) *Spectroscopy data*: λ_{max} 220 nm (in methanol) (A_1^1 = 184); infra-red, nuclear magnetic resonance and mass spectra have been reported (Cole & Cox, 1981)

(*e*) *Solubility*: Soluble in chloroform, ethyl acetate, methanol and water; insoluble in *n*-hexane and *n*-pentane

(*f*) *Stability*: Stable in solid state; hydrolysed by bases to nivalenol

(*g*) *Reactivity*: Reacts with acetic anhydride to give tetraacetylnivalenol

1.4 Technical products and impurities

No technical product containing fusarenon X is available.

2. Production, Use, Occurrence and Analysis

2.1 Production and use

(*a*) *Production*

Fusarenon X was first isolated in 1968 (Tatsuno *et al.*, 1968; Tsunoda *et al.*, 1968) from grains polluted by *Fusarium nivale* Fn-2B. Its structure was established in 1969 (Tatsuno *et al.*, 1969; Ueno *et al.*, 1969).

Fusarenon X is not produced commercially.

(*b*) *Use*

Fusarenon X is not used commercially.

2.2 Occurrence

Fusarenon X is formed by fungi such as *Fusarium nivale*, *F. episphaeria*, *F. oxysporum* and *Gibberella zeae* (Smalley & Strong, 1974; Ueno *et al*., 1972a, 1973).

Strains such as *F. nivale* and *G. zea* have occasionally been isolated from scabbed wheat grains in Japan (Tsunoda, 1970; Ueno *et al*., 1972b). In one study in Japan, 20% of mouldy wheat and barley samples examined were found to be contaminated by such fungi (Tsuruta, 1974).

2.3 Analysis

The isolation and analysis of fusarenon X is complicated due, in part, to the large number of compounds with closely related structures (all produced by *Fusarium* species) and to the fact that the fusarenon X molecule contains only a weak chromophore. Some general methods of analysis for fusarenon X have been reviewed (Smalley & Strong, 1974).

Typical methods for the analysis of fusarenon X are summarized in Table 1.

Table 1. Methods for the analysis of fusarenon X

Sample matrix	Sample preparation	Assay procedure[a]	Limit of detection	Reference
Cereals, grains and foodstuffs	Extract (aqueous methanol); purify in two steps (Amberlite XAD-4 and Florisil columns)	TLC	20-50 µg/kg	Kamimura *et al*. (1981)
	(For GLC) derivatize (trimethylsilylimidazole)	GLC/FID GLC/ECD	100 µg/kg 2 µg/kg	
Corn, peanuts, rice (polished and rough) and wheat	Extract (20% sulphuric acid/4% potassium chloride/acetonitrile); defat (isooctane); transfer to chloroform; clean up (silica gel column)	TLC/FL	300 µg/kg	Takeda *et al*. (1979)

[a]Abbreviations: TLC, thin-layer chromatography; GLC/FID, gas-liquid chromatography with flame-ionization detection; GLC/ECD, gas-liquid chromatography with electron capture detection; TLC/FL, thin-layer chromatography with fluorescence detection

3. Biological Data Relevant to the Evaluation of Carcinogenic Risk to Humans

3.1 Carcinogenicity studies in animals

(a) Oral administration

Rat: A group of 20 male eight-week old Donryu rats was given 0.4 mg/kg bw fusarenon X [purity unspecified] weekly by oral intubation for 50 weeks. Twelve rats survived 50 weeks, and 1 developed a hepatoma. No tumour occurred in 10 male controls during the experimental period of over 400 days (Saito & Ohtsubo, 1974). [The Working Group noted the incomplete reporting of the experiment.]

Groups of 25 or 49 male Donryu rats, six weeks old, weighing 100-130 g, were given diets containing either 3.5 or 7 mg/kg fusarenon X [purity unspecified] (isolated from a culture filtrate of *Fusarium nivale*) for two years; a third group of 26 animals was given 7 mg/kg diet for only one year. An adequate control group of 48 animals was also available. All animals were given a restricted volume of feed (15 g/day). Survivors were killed at 24 months. The mean body weights of the treated animals were in general lower than those of the respective controls, and a treatment-related effect on survival was noted: after 18 months of treatment, 50% of the controls were alive, compared with 15/49 (31%) and 4/25 (16%) in the low- and high-dose groups, respectively; survival at that time in the group receiving the 7 mg/kg diet for one year was 9/52 (17%). The major cause of death was chronic bronchopneumonia. No increase in the incidence of tumours was noted in treated rats (Saito *et al.*, 1980). [The Working Group noted the poor survival of the treated animals.]

(b) Subcutaneous administration

Mouse: Two groups of 16 or 18 DDD male mice [age unspecified] received 10 or 20 weekly s.c. injections of 2.5 mg/kg bw fusarenon X. A group of 11 mice served as controls. No increase in tumour incidence was noted in treated animals when compared with controls; one case of leukaemia was observed (Saito & Ohtsubo, 1974). [The Working Group noted the incomplete reporting of the experiment.]

Rat: Eighteen eight-week old male Donryu rats were given weekly s.c. injections of 0.4 mg/kg bw fusarenon X for 22 weeks; most of the rats survived more than one year, and 1 developed a lung adenoma. No tumour was seen in 10 controls (Saito & Ohtsubo, 1974). [The Working Group noted the incomplete reporting of the experiment.]

3.2 Other relevant biological data

(a) Experimental systems

The toxicology and pharmacology of fusarenon X have been reviewed (Ueno, 1971; Wilson, 1973; Saito & Ohtsubo, 1974; Ueno, 1977a,b; Matsuoka *et al.*, 1979).

Toxic effects

The oral, i.p., s.c. and i.v. LD_{50}s of fusarenon X in DDD mice and Wistar rats range from 3-5 mg/kg bw. The s.c. LD_{50} in newborn mice and guinea-pigs is about 0.1 mg/kg bw. I.p. administration of 0.5 mg/kg bw to an adult guinea-pig, 5 mg/kg bw i.p. to an adult cat and 1 mg/kg bw s.c. to a one-week-old cat were lethal (Ueno *et al.*, 1971).

The main acute toxic effects of fusarenon X in rats and mice are cellular destruction and karyorrhexis (destruction of the cell nucleus) in intestinal mucosa, spleen, lymph nodes, bone marrow, thymus, testes and ovary (Ueno *et al.*, 1971) . It also causes severe irritation of the skin (Ueno *et al.*, 1970).

At concentrations of 0.1-0.5 µg/ml, fusarenon X inhibits cell growth and protein and DNA synthesis in eukaryotic (HeLa) cells *in vitro* (Ohtsubo & Saito, 1970). It binds *in vitro* to active SH groups of creatine phosphokinase, lactate dehydrogenase and alcohol dehydrogenase, inhibiting their catalytic activities (Ueno & Matsumoto, 1975).

Effects on reproduction and prenatal toxicity

In studies in groups of 4-6 pregnant DDD mice, a single s.c. dose of 2.6 mg/kg bw fusarenon X [purity unspecified] injected on day 10 of gestation induced abortion in all dams on the following day; at doses of 0.6-1.6 mg/kg bw, abortion occurred less frequently (16-20%) and at longer intervals after injection. The weight and length of surviving foetuses from dams given 1.6 mg/kg bw on day 6 or 8 of gestation were significantly reduced as compared with those of controls. Embryonal implantation was inhibited in mice fed diets containing 5, 10 or 20 ppm fusarenon X ($\sim$ 25, 50 or 100 µg per animal per day) during early pregnancy or throughout. Feeding of diets containing 10 and 20 ppm fusarenon X for seven days during the middle of pregnancy caused abortion in 40 and 100% of the dams, respectively. No teratogenic effect was observed in these studies (Ito *et al.*, 1980).

Absorption, distribution, excretion and metabolism

Thirty minutes after a s.c. injection of 4 mg/kg bw ^{3}H-fusarenon X to mice, radioactivity was found in the liver, kidneys, intestine, stomach, spleen, bile and plasma. The highest radioactivity (corresponding to 3% of the dose) was found in the liver. The retention of radioactivity in the tissues and body fluids is short, and three hours after dosing no measureable radioactivity was detected. Twenty-five percent of the radioactivity is excreted in the urine within 12 hours. No intact fusarenon X could be recovered from the urine, indicating extensive metabolism (Ueno *et al.*, 1971).

Fusarenon X is deacetylated by rat and rabbit liver esterases to nivalenol (Ohta *et al.*, 1978).

Mutagenicity and other short-term tests

The genetic effects of mycotoxins, including fusarenon X, have been reviewed (Stark, 1980).

Fusarenon X had no effect in a *Bacillus subtilis rec* assay measuring DNA damage when tested at 20 and 100 µg/plate (Ueno & Kubota, 1976). It has been reported to be mutagenic to *Salmonella typhimurium* TA100 and TA98 without exogenous metabolic activation (Nagao *et al.*, 1976). However, Ueno *et al.* (1978) found no mutagenic activity of fusarenon X in *S. typhimurium* TA98 or TA100, either in the plate or preincubation test, at concentrations of up to 500 μg/plate.

Induction of petite mutations in *Saccharomyces cerevisiae* after exposure to fusarenon X has been reported (Ueno *et al.*, 1971).

In HeLa cells, a small change in the sedimentation pattern of single stranded DNA, indicating DNA breakage, was noted (Umeda *et al.*, 1972). No increase in mutations to 8-azaguanine resistance was found in C3H mouse mammary carcinoma cells (FM3A) treated with 0.1 to 1.0 μg/ml fusarenon X (Umeda *et al.*, 1977).

(*b*) *Humans*

Toxic effects

Splashing of a crude solution caused dermatitis of the hands and face in laboratory workers (Saito & Ohtsubo, 1974).

Effects on reproduction and prenatal toxicity

No data were available to the Working Group.

Absorption, distribution, excretion and metabolism

No data were available to the Working Group.

Mutagenicity and chromosomal effects

No data were available to the Working Group.

3.3 Case reports and epidemiological studies of carcinogenicity in humans

No data were available to the Working Group.

4. Summary of Data Reported and Evaluation

4.1 Experimental data

Fusarenon X was tested for carcinogenicity in male rats by administration in the diet and in male mice and male rats by subcutaneous injection. The studies were inadequate for evaluation.

Fusarenon X was found to be mutagenic to *Salmonella typhimurium* and caused petite mutations in yeast. No mutagenic activity was reported in mammalian cells *in vitro*. The data were *inadequate* to evaluate the activity of fusarenon X in short-term tests.

In the only available study, fusarenon X induced abortion in mice and was foetotoxic but not teratogenic to the surviving foetuses.

4.2 Human data

Fusarenon X is a naturally occurring mycotoxin first isolated in 1968. There is a risk of exposure to this toxin by consumption of fusarenon X-contaminated foods.

No data were available to evaluate the teratogenicity or chromosomal effects of this compound in humans.

No case report or epidemiological study of the carcinogenicity of fusarenon X was available to the Working Group.

4.3 Evaluation

No evaluation of the carcinogenicity of fusarenon X to experimental animals could be made. In the absence of epidemiological data, no evaluation of the carcinogenicity of fusarenon X to humans could be made.

5. References

Cole, R.J. & Cox, R.H. (1981) *Handbook of Toxic Fungal Metabolites*, New York, Academic Press, pp. 213-263

IARC (1976) *IARC Monographs on the Evaluation of Carcinogenic Risk of Chemicals to Man*, Vol. 11, *Cadmium, Nickel, Some Epoxides, Miscellaneous Industrial Chemicals and General Considerations on Volatile Anaesthetics*, Lyon, pp. 169-173

Ito, Y., Ohtsubo,K. & Saito, M. (1980) Effects of fusarenon-X, a trichothecene produced by *Fusarium nivale*, on pregnant mice and their fetuses. *Jpn. J. exp. Med.*, *50*, 167-172

Kamimura, H., Nishijima, M., Yasuda, K., Saito, K., Ibe, A., Nagayama, T., Ushiyama, H. & Naoi, Y. (1981) Simultaneous detection of several *Fusarium* mycotoxins in cereals, grains,and foodstuffs. *J. Assoc. off. anal. Chem.*, *64*, 1067-1073

Matsuoka, Y., Kubota, K. & Ueno, Y. (1979) General pharmacological studies of fusarenon-X, a trichothecene mycotoxin from *Fusarium* species. *Toxicol. appl. Pharmacol.*, *50*, 87-94

Nagao, M., Honda, M., Hamasaki, T., Natori, S., Ueno, Y., Yamasaki, M., Seino, Y., Yahagi, T. & Sugimura, I. (1976) Mutagenicity of mycotoxins on *Salmonella* (Jpn.). *Proc. Jpn. Assoc. Mycotoxicol.*, *3-4*, 41-43

Ohta, M., Matsumoto, H., Ishii, K. & Ueno, Y. (1978) Metabolism of trichothecene mycotoxins. II. Substrate specificity of microsomal deacetylation of trichothecenes. *J. Biochem.*, *84*, 697-706

Ohtsubo, K. & Saito, M. (1970) Cytotoxic effects of scirpene compounds, fusarenon-X produced by *Fusarium nivale*, dihydronivalenol and dihydrofusarenon-X, on HeLa cells. *Jpn. J. med. Sci. Biol.*, *23*, 217-225

Saito, M. & Ohtsubo, K. (1974) *Trichothecene toxins of* Fusarium *species*. In: Purchase, I.F.H., ed., *Mycotoxins*, Amsterdam, Elsevier Scientific Publishing Co., pp. 263-281

Saito, M., Horiuchi, T., Ohtsubo, K., Hatanaka, J. & Ueno, Y. (1980) Low tumor incidence in rats with long-term feeding of fusarenon-X, a cytotoxic trichothecene produced by *Fusarium nivale. Jpn. J. exp. Med.*, *50*, 293-302

Smalley, E.B. & Strong, F.M. (1974) *Toxic trichothecenes*. In: Purchase, I.F.H., ed., *Mycotoxins*, Amsterdam, Elsevier Scientific Publishing Co., pp. 199-228

Stark, A.-A. (1980) Mutagenicity and carcinogenicity of mycotoxins: DNA binding as a possible mode of action. *Ann. Rev. Microbiol.*, *34*, 235-262

Takeda, Y., Isohata, E., Amano, R. & Uchiyama, M. (1979) Simultaneous extraction and fractionation and thin layer chromatographic determination of 14 mycotoxins in grains. *J. Assoc. off. anal. Chem.*, *62*, 573-578

Tatsuno, T., Saito, M., Enomoto, M. & Tsunoda, H. (1968) Nivalenol, a toxic principle of *Fusarium nivale. Chem. pharm. Bull.*, *16*, 2519-2520

Tatsuno, T., Fujimoto, Y. & Morita, Y. (1969) Toxicological research on substances from *Fusarium nivale* III. The structure of nivalenol and its monoacetate. *Tetrahedron Lett.*, *33*, 2823-2826

Tsunoda, H. (1970) *Micro-organisms which deteriorate stored cereals and grains*. In: Herzberg, M., ed., *Proceedings of the Ist US-Japan Conference on Toxic Micro-organisms*, Washington DC, US Department of the Interior, pp. 143-162

Tsunoda, H., Toyazaki, N., Morooka, N., Nakano, N., Yoshiyama, H., Okubo, K. & Isoda, M. (1968) *Rep. Food Res. Inst. (Tokyo)*, *23*, 89-116

Tsuruta, O. (1974) Micro-organisms infection of domestic cereals. I. Parasitic fungi on wheat and barley. *Rep. Food Res. Inst. (Tokyo)*, *29*, 16-20

Ueno, Y. (1971) *Toxicological and biological properties of fusarenon-X, a cytotoxic mycotoxin of* Fusarium nivale Fn-2B. In: Purchase, I.F.H., ed., *Symposium on Mycotoxins in Human Health*, London, MacMillan, pp. 163-178

Ueno, Y. (1977a) Mode of action of trichothecenes. *Pure appl. Chem.*, *49*, 1737-1745

Ueno, Y. (1977b) *Tricothecenes: Overview address*. In: Rodricks, J.W., Hesseltine, C.W. & Mehlman, M.A., eds, *Mycotoxins in Human and Animal Health*, Park Forest South, IL, Pathotox Publishers, Inc., pp. 189-207

Ueno, Y. & Kubota, K. (1976) DNA-attacking ability of carcinogenic mycotoxins in recombination-deficient mutant cells of *Bacillus subtilis*. *Cancer Res.*, *36*, 445-451

Ueno, Y. & Matsumoto, H. (1975) Inactivation of some thiol-enzymes by trichothecene mycotoxins from *Fusarium* species. *Chem. pharm. Bull.*, *23*, 2439-2442

Ueno, Y., Ueno, I., Tatsuno, T., Ohokubo, K. & Tsunoda, H. (1969) Fusarenon-X, a toxic principle of *Fusarium nivale* - Culture filtrate. *Experientia*, *25*, 1062

Ueno, Y., Ishikawa, Y., Amakai, K., Nakajima, M., Saito, M., Enomoto, M. & Ohtsubo, M. (1970) Comparative study on skin-necrotizing effect of scirpene metabolites of *Fusaria*. *Jpn. J. exp. Med.*, *40*, 33-38

Ueno, Y., Ueno, I., Iitoi, Y., Tsunoda, H., Enomoto, M. & Ohtsubo, K. (1971) Toxicological approaches to the metabolites of *Fusaria*. III. Acute toxicity of fusarenon-X. *Jpn. J. exp. Med.*, *41*, 521-539

Ueno, Y., Sato, N., Ishii, K., Sakai, K. & Enomoto, M. (1972a) Toxicological approaches to the metabolites of *Fusaria*. V. Neosolaniol, T-2 toxin and butenolide, toxic metabolites of *Fusarium sporotrichioides* NRRL 3510 and *Fusarium poae* 3287. *Jpn. J. exp. Med.*, *42*, 461-472

Ueno, Y., Ishii, K., Sakai, K., Kanaeda, S., Tsunoda, H., Tanaka, T. & Enomoto, M. (1972b) Toxicological approaches to the metabolites of *Fusaria*. IV. Microbial survey on 'bean-hulls poisoning of horses' with the isolation of toxic trichothecenes, neosolaniol and T-2 toxin of *Fusarium solani* M-1-1. *Jpn. J. exp. Med.*, *42*, 187-203

Ueno, Y., Sato, N., Ishii, K., Sakai, K., Tsunoda, H. & Enomoto, M. (1973) Biological and chemical detection of trichothecene mycotoxins of *Fusarium* species. *Appl. Microbiol.*, *25*, 699-704

Ueno, Y., Kubota, K., Ito, T. & Nakamura, Y. (1978) Mutagenicity of carcinogenic mycotoxins in *Salmonella typhimurium*. *Cancer Res.*, *38*, 536-542

Umeda, M., Yamamoto, T. & Saito, M. (1972) DNA-strand breakage of HeLa cells induced by several mycotoxins. *Jpn. J. exp. Med.*, *42*, 527-535

Umeda, M., Tsutsui, T. & Saito, M. (1977) Mutagenicity and inducibility of DNA single-strand breaks and chromosome aberrations by various mycotoxins. *Gann*, *68*, 619-652

Wilson, B.J. (1973) 12,13-Epoxytricothecenes: Potential toxic contaminants of foods. *Nutr. Rev.*, *31*, 169-172

GYROMITRIN (ACETALDEHYDE FORMYLMETHYLHYDRAZONE)

1. Chemical and Physical Data

1.1 Synonyms and trade names

Chem. Abstr. Services Reg. No.: 16568-02-8

Chem. Abstr. Name: Hydrazinecarboxaldehyde, ethylidenemethyl-

IUPAC Systematic Name: Formic acid, ethylidenemethylhydrazide

Synonyms: Acetaldehyde-*N*-formyl-*N*-methylhydrazone;   acetaldehyde-*N*-methyl-*N*-formylhydrazone; acetaldehyde methylformylhydrazone; ethylidene gyromitrin

1.2 Structural and molecular formulae and molecular weight

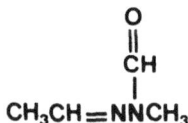

$$
\begin{array}{c}
O \\
\parallel \\
CH \\
\vert \\
CH_3CH \!\! = \!\! NNCH_3
\end{array}
$$

$C_4H_8N_2O$ Mol. wt: 100.1

1.3 Chemical and physical properties of the pure substance

From List & Luft (1968) and Pyysalo (1976)

(a) *Description*: Colourless liquid

(b) *Boiling-point*: 143°C

(c) *Melting-point:* 19.5°C (vacuum)

(d) *Density*: d_{20} 1.05

(e) *Spectroscopy data*: Infra-red, mass and nuclear magnetic resonance spectra have been determined.

(f) *Solubility*: Soluble in acetone, benzene, carbon tetrachloride, chloroform, diethyl ether, ethanol, ethyl acetate, methanol, dichloromethane and water

(g) *Stability*: Very sensitive to air oxidation (starts at -25°C); sensitive to hydrolysis by both acids and alkalis

1.4 Technical products and impurities

No technical product containing gyromitrin is available.

2. Production, Use, Occurrence and Analysis

2.1 Production and use

(a) *Production*

The first synthesis of gyromitrin was reported in 1968 (List & Luft, 1968) by the reaction of methylhydrazine and ethyl formate to produce N-methyl-N-formylhydrazine, which was condensed with acetaldehyde to give gyromitrin.

Gyromitrin is not produced commercially.

(b) *Use*

Gyromitrin is not used commercially.

2.2 Occurrence

The false morel, *Gyromitra esculenta*, is a mushroom which is widely eaten in northern Europe, both cooked and dried. It is estimated that 99.9% of gyromitrin in the mushroom is lost by boiling, and >99% by drying (Pyysalo, 1976). The gyromitrin content of dried false morels is reported to be between 0.05-0.3%; N-methyl-N-formylhydrazine, a hydro-lysis product of gyromitrin, is also present, at a concentration of 0.06% (Schmidlin-Mészáros, 1974).

Nine volatile N-methyl-N-formylhydrazones have been found in fresh false-morel mushrooms, *Gyromitra esculenta*, at an average combined level of 57 mg/kg; gyromitrin constituted about 85% of the total (Pyysalo & Niskanen, 1977). In earlier studies, a level of about 1.6 g/kg had been reported (List & Luft, 1969).

2.3 Analysis

Determination of the content of gyromitrin in fresh, dried or treated mushrooms has been performed by gas chromatography with flame ionization detection and identification by mass spectroscopy (Pyysalo & Niskanen, 1977; Raudaskoski & Pyysalo, 1978).

3. Biological Data Relevant to the Evaluation of Carcinogenic Risk to Humans

3.1 Carcinogenicity studies in animals

(a) *Oral administration*

Mouse: Groups of 50 male and 50 female Swiss mice, six weeks of age, were given gyromitrin (purity, >99%) by intragastric intubation weekly for 52 weeks at a concentration of 100 mg/kg bw in propylene glycol. Control groups of 50 male and 50 female Swiss mice of similar age received 10 ml/kg bw solvent intragastrically weekly for 52 weeks. The survival time of treated male mice was significantly shortened. In females, lung tumours were found in 35/50 (70%), *versus* 13/50 (26%) in controls (p <0.0002); forestomach tumours in 8/50 (16%), *versus* 0/50 in controls (p <0.01); and clitoral gland tumours in 6/50 (12%), *versus* 0/50 in controls (p < 0.04). In males, lung tumours were found in 20/50 (40%), *versus* 11/50 (22%) in controls (p >0.05); and preputial gland tumours in 45/50 (90%), *versus* 0/50 in controls (p <0.00001) (Toth *et al.*, 1981).

(b) *Carcinogenicity of metabolites*

Mouse: N-Methyl-N-formylhydrazine [purity unspecified], a metabolite of gyromitrin, was administered in the drinking-water at a dose level of 78 mg/l, daily for life, to groups of 50 male and 50 female Swiss mice. A group of 100 mice of each sex served as untreated controls. Hepatocellular tumours, benign and malignant, were found in 22/50 (44%) and 11/50 (22%) treated female and male mice, respectively (compared with 0/100 and 2/100 in female and male controls). Lung tumours, benign and malignant, were found in 30/50 (60%) females (71 tumours) and in 20/50 (40%) males (39 tumours) (compared with 15/100 and 22/100 in female and male controls, respectively). An increased incidence of gall-bladder tumours was observed in five treated males and four treated females; bile-duct tumours were seen in two treated females and five treated males (Toth, 1979). [The Working Group noted that no data on survival were given.]

Groups of 50 random-bred Swiss mice of each sex, six weeks old, were given 0.01% (100 mg/l) N-methylhydrazine [purity unspecified], a metabolite of gyromitrin, in the drinking-water for life. A group of 110 females and 110 males served as untreated controls. Female and male treated animals had died by 70 and 80 weeks of age, respectively, and control survivors were killed at 120 weeks of age. N-Methylhydrazine had a marked effect on the survival rates when compared with the respective controls: the numbers of survivors at 50 weeks of age were 13/50 and 6/50 in female and male treated mice, compared with 96/110 and 67/110 in female and male. controls, respectively. Lung adenomas were found in 12/50 (24%) (17 tumours) and in 11/50 (22%) (12 tumours) female and male treated animals (Toth, 1972). [The Working Group noted the lack of information on the lung tumour incidence in the untreated controls.]

Hamster: A group of 50 male and 50 female random-bred Syrian golden hamsters, six weeks old, were given 0.01% (100 mg/l) N-methylhydrazine [purity unspecified] in the drinking-water for life. An untreated group of 100 males and 100 females served as controls. All control survivors were killed at 120 weeks of age, and by 110 weeks all treated animals had died. The N-methylhydrazine treatment substantially reduced the survival when compared with the respective controls: 18/50 and 4/50 of the treated males and females were alive at 80 weeks of age (compared with 42/100 and 31/100 in male and female controls). Malignant histiocytomas (Kupffer-cell sarcomas) of the liver were found in 27/50 (54%) treated males and in 16/49 (32%) treated females. The first tumour was observed when the animals were 46 weeks of age. No such tumour was observed in the controls. Tumours of the caecum were observed in 7/50 (14%) treated males and in 9/49 (18%) treated females (compared with 1/97 and 1/99 in male and female controls) (Toth & Shimizu, 1973).

3.2 Other relevant biological data

(a) Experimental systems

Toxic effects

The acute oral LD$_{50}$s of gyromitrin are 344 mg/kg bw in NMRI mice (von Wright et al., 1978a), 320 mg/kg bw in Sprague-Dawley rats and 70 mg/kg bw in New Zealand white rabbits (Mäkinen et al., 1977).

Gyromitrin administered intragastrically to Wistar rats at levels of 50, 100 or 200 mg/kg bw caused a dose-dependent diuresis together with an increased excretion of sodium (five-fold) and potassium (two-fold). Administration of N-methyl-N-formylhydrazine, a metabolite of gyromitrin, had no effect on renal function (Braun et al., 1979a).

Gyromitrin was administered in the drinking-water to a group of ten New Zealand white rabbits at estimated doses of 0.05-5.0 mg/kg bw per day for 90 days. The most marked effect was degenerative changes in the tubular cells of the kidneys. The no-effect level was estimated to be 0.5 mg/kg bw per day (Niskanen et al., 1976).

After oral administration of 200 mg/kg bw gyromitrin to rats (80% of the LD$_{50}$), there was a transient time- and dose-dependent decrease in cytochrome P-450 and an inhibition of cytochrome P-450-mediated metabolism of aminopyrine and para-nitroanisole in liver microsomes. Comparable results were obtained after administration of N-methyl-N-formylhydrazine (Braun et al., 1979b).

Effects on reproduction and prenatal toxicity

No data were available to the Working Group.

Absorption, distribution, excretion and metabolism

Gyromitrin is rapidly hydrolysed, non-enzymatically, both in vitro and in vivo, to acetaldehyde and N-methyl-N-formylhydrazine; the latter is hydrolysed under physiological conditions at a much slower rate to form N-methylhydrazine and formic acid. At 37°C, 1 mM gyromitrin was hydrolysed to N-methylhydrazine, with a half-life of 122 min at pH 2; whereas at pH 3 only 9% appeared as N-methylhydrazine after 72 hours (Nagel et al., 1976, 1977; von Wright et al., 1978b).

N-Methylhydrazine was also found in the mouse stomach after oral administration of 4 mg per animal gyromitrin (Nagel et al., 1977). Gyromitrin, N-methylhydrazine and N-methyl-N-formylhydrazine were found in the peritoneal fluid of mice three hours after oral administration of 9 mg gyromitrin (von Wright et al., 1978c).

After an oral dose of 9 mg [³H-methyl]-gyromitrin to rats, [³H]-7-methylguanine was detected in the DNA of liver but not that of kidney or lung (Meier-Bratschi et al., 1983).

There is spectral evidence that rat liver cytochrome P-450 mediates oxidation of N-methyl-N-formylhydrazine to a hydroxylamine derivative (Braun et al., 1980).

Mutagenicity and other short-term tests

Gyromitrin was not mutagenic to *Salmonella typhimurium* TA100 (von Wright et al., 1978c) or to *Escherichia coli* WP2 hcr (von Wright et al., 1977) when tested in the presence or absence of a 9000 x g liver supernatant mix from phenobarbital-induced male NMRI mice. It was also negative in a host-mediated assay using S. typhimurium TA1950 (von Wright et al., 1978c).

N-Methylhydrazine, a metabolite of gyromitrin, was positive in the E. coli pol A assay and was weakly mutagenic in E. coli WP2 hcr (von Wright et al., 1977) and in a spot test with S. typhimurium TA100 (von Wright et al., 1978c). However, no mutagenic effect was observed in the plate test, with or without an exogenous metabolic activation system, or in the host-mediated assay (von Wright et al., 1978c). N-Methylhydrazine is highly bactericidal (von Wright et al., 1977), and the discrepancy between the results of the plate test and the spot test with S. typhimurium has been attributed to the fact that the mutagenic concentration of N-methylhydrazine is close to its lethal dose (von Wright et al., 1978c).

(b) Humans

Toxic effects

While no data were available on the toxicity of pure gyromitrin to man, poisoning by consumption of fresh *Gyromitra esculenta*, which contains gyromitrin, is relatively frequent in eastern Europe and in the Federal Republic of Germany. Reviews on the toxicity of these mushrooms are available (Franke et al., 1967). At least two fatal cases have been reported in North America (Dearness, 1924; Hendricks, 1940). Of 513 cases of intoxication described in the medical literature between 1782 and 1965, 74 proved to be fatal; 40 other fatal cases have been reported among an unspecified number of intoxications (Franke et al., 1967). Since then, further cases have occasionally been reported (Breuer & Stahler, 1966; Giusti & Carnevale, 1974; Garnier et al., 1978). Poisoning is characterized initially by nausea, vomiting and sometimes diarrhoea. About 38-48 hours after consuming the fresh mushroom, a variable degree of jaundice may develop, with enlargement of the liver and often also of the spleen. In the most severe cases, there is progressive liver necrosis with ensuing hepatic coma and death four or five days after ingestion (Garnier et al., 1978).

Effects on reproduction and prenatal toxicity

No data were available to the Working Group.

Absorption, distribution, excretion and metabolism

No data were available to the Working Group.

Mutagenicity and chromosomal effects

No data were available to the Working Group.

3.3 Case reports and epidemiological studies of carcinogenicity in humans

No data were available to the Working Group.

4. Summary of Data Reported and Evaluation

4.1 Experimental data

Gyromitrin was tested for carcinogenicity in one experiment in mice by gavage, producing increased incidences of lung, forestomach and clitoral gland tumours in females and of preputial tumours in males. N-Methyl-N-formylhydrazine, a metabolite, was tested in mice by administration in the drinking-water, increasing the incidence of tumours of the liver, lung, gall bladder and bile duct. N-Methylhydrazine, another metabolite, was tested in mice and hamsters by administration in the drinking-water; it produced increased incidences of histiocytomas and caecal tumours in hamsters.

Gyromitrin was not mutagenic in bacteria, but the metabolite N-methylhydrazine gave positive results. The data were *inadequate* to evaluate the activity of gyromitrin in short-term tests.

No data were available to evaluate the teratogenicity of this compound to experimental animals.

4.2 Human data

Gyromitrin is a natural substance found in the false morel. Although most of the compound is destroyed by proper preparation before eating, there is still a possibility for human exposure.

No data were available to assess the teratogenicity or chromosomal effects of this compound in humans.

No case report or epidemiological study of the carcinogenicity of gyromitrin was available to the Working Group.

4.3 Evaluation

Results of studies on gyromitrin itself, supported by studies on two of its metabolites, provide *sufficient evidence*[1] for the carcinogenicity of gyromitrin in experimental animals. No data on humans were available.

---

[1]In the absence of adequate data on humans, it is reasonable, for practical purposes, to regard chemicals for which there is sufficient evidence of carcinogenicity in animals as if they presented a carcinogenic risk to humans.

5. References

Braun, R., Kremer, J. & Rau, H. (1979a) Renal functional response to the mushroom poison gyromitrin. *Toxicology*, *13*, 187-196

Braun, R., Greeff, U. & Netter, K.J. (1979b) Liver injury by the false morel poison gyromitrin. *Toxicology*, *12*, 155-163

Braun, R., Greeff, U. & Netter, K.J. (1980) Indications for nitrosamide formation from the mushroom poison gyromitrin by rat liver microsomes. *Xenobiotica*, *10*, 557-564

Breuer, E.D. & Stahler, O. (1966) Haemolytic icterus due to *Gyromitra (Helvella) esculenta* poisoning (Ger.). *Med. Welt*, *18*, 1013-1018

Dearness, J. (1924) *Gyromitra* poisoning. *Mycologia*, *16*, 199

Franke, S., Freimuth, U. & List, P.H. (1967) On the virulence of the mushroom *Gyromitra (Helvella) esculenta* Fr. (Ger.). *Arch. Toxikol.*, *22*, 293-332

Garnier, R., Conso, F., Efthymiou, M.L., Riboulet, G. & Gaultier, M. (1978) Poisoning by *Gyromitra esculenta* (Fr.). *Toxicol. Eur. Res.*, *1*, 359-364

Giusti, G.V. & Carnevale, A. (1974) A case of fatal poisoning by *Gyromitra esculenta*. *Arch. Toxicol.*, *33*, 49-54

Hendricks, H.V. (1940) Poisoning by false morel (*Gyromitra esculenta*). Report of a fatal case. *J. Am. med. Assoc.*, *114*, 1625

List, P.H. & Luft, P. (1968) Components of mushrooms. 16. Gyromitrin, the poison of spring morels (Ger.). *Arch. Pharm.*, *301*, 294-305

List, P.H. & Luft, P. (1969) Components of mushrooms. 19. Detection and determination of gyromitrin in fresh *Gyromitra esculenta* (Ger.). *Arch. Pharm.*, *302*, 143-146

Mäkinen, S.M., Kreula, M. & Kauppi, M. (1977) Acute oral toxicity of ethylidene gyromitrin in rabbits, rats and chickens. *Food Cosmet. Toxicol.*, *15*, 575-578

Meier-Bratschi, A., Carden, B.M., Lutz, W.K. & Schlatter, C. (1983) Methylation by gyromitrin of DNA in the rat. *Food chem. Toxicol.* (in press)

Nagel, D., Toth, B. & Kupper, R. (1976) Formation of methylhydrazine from acetaldehyde N-methyl-N-formylhydrazone of *Gyromitra esculenta* (Abstract no. 36). *Proc. Am. Assoc. Cancer Res.*, *17*, 76

Nagel, D., Wallcave, L., Toth, B. & Kupper, R. (1977) Formation of methylhydrazine from acetaldehyde N-methyl-N-formylhydrazone, a component of *Gyromitra esculenta*. *Cancer Res.*, *37*, 3458-3460

Niskanen, A., Pyysalo, H., Rimaila-Pärnänen, E. & Hartikka, P. (1976) Short-term peroral toxicity of ethylidene gyromitrin in rabbits and chickens. *Food Cosmet. Toxicol.*, *14*, 409-415

Pyysalo, H. (1976) Test for gyromitrin, a poisonous compound in false morel *Gyromitra esculenta. Z. Lebensmittel. Untersuch.-Forsch.*, *160*, 325-330

Pyysalo, H. & Niskanen, A. (1977) On the occurrence of *N*-methyl-*N*-formylhydrazones in fresh and processed false morel, *Gyromitra esculenta. J. agric. Food Chem.*, *25*, 644-647

Raudaskoski, M. & Pyysalo, H. (1978) Occurrence of *N*-methyl-*N*-formylhydrazones in mycelia of *Gyromitra esculenta. Z. Naturforsch.*, *33c*, 472-474

Schmidlin-Mészáros, J. (1974) Gyromitrin in dried false morels (*Gyromitra esculenta* sicc.) (Ger.). *Mitt. Gebiete Lebensmittel. Hyg.*, *65*, 453-465

Toth, B. (1972) Hydrazine, methylhydrazine and methylhydrazine sulfate carcinogenesis in Swiss mice. Failure of ammonium hydroxide to interfere in the development of tumors. *Int. J. Cancer*, *9*, 109-118

Toth, B. (1979) Hepatocarcinogenesis by hydrazine mycotoxins of edible mushrooms. *J. Toxicol. environ. Health*, *5*, 193-202

Toth, B. & Shimizu, H. (1973) Methylhydrazine tumorigenesis in Syrian golden hamsters and the morphology of malignant histiocytomas. *Cancer Res.*, *33*, 2744-2753

Toth, B., Smith, J.W. & Patil, K.D. (1981) Cancer induction in mice with acetaldehyde methylformylhydrazone of the false morel mushroom. *J. natl Cancer Inst.*, *67*, 881-887

von Wright, A., Niskanen, A. & Pyysalo, H. (1977) The toxicities and mutagenic properties of ethylidene gyromitrin and *N*-methylhydrazine with *Escherichia coli* as test organism. *Mutat. Res.*, *56*, 105-110

von Wright, A., Niskanen, A., Pyysalo, H. & Korpela H. (1978a) The toxicity of some *N*-methyl-*N*-formylhydrazones from *Gyromitra esculenta* and related compounds in mouse and microbial tests. *Toxicol. appl. Pharmacol.*, *45*, 429-434

von Wright, A., Pyysalo, H. & Niskanen, A. (1978b) Qualitative evaluation of the metabolic formation of methylhydrazine from acetaldehyde-*N*-methyl-*N*-formylhydrazone, the main poisonous compound of *Gyromitra esculenta. Toxicol. Lett.*, *2*, 261-265

von Wright, A., Niskanen, A. & Pyysalo, H. (1978c) Mutagenic properties of ethylidene gyromitrin and its metabolites in microsomal activation tests and in the host-mediated assay. *Mutat. Res.*, *54*, 167-173

KAEMPFEROL

1. Chemical and Physical Data

1.1 Synonyms and trade names

Chem. Abstr. Services Reg. No.: 520-18-3

Chem. Abstr. Name: 4H-1-Benzopyran-4-one, 3,5,7-trihydroxy-2-(4-hydroxyphenyl)-

IUPAC Systematic Name: 3,4',5,7-Tetrahydroxyflavone

Synonyms: Campherol; C.I. 75640; indigo yellow; kaempherol; kampherol; kempferol; nimbecetin; pelargidenolon 1497; populnetin; rhamnolutein; rhamnolutin; robigenin; swartziol; trifolitin; 5,7,4'-trihydroxyflavonol

1.2 Structural and molecular formulae and molecular weight

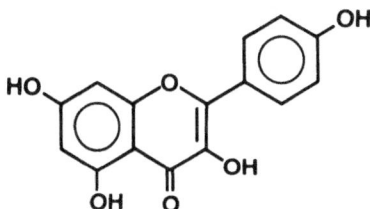

$C_{15}H_{10}O_6$ Mol. wt: 286.2

1.3 Chemical and physical properties of the pure substance

From Windholz (1976), unless otherwise specified

(a) *Description*: Yellow needles

(b) *Melting-point*: 276-278°C

(c) *Spectroscopy data*: λ_{max} 265 nm and 365 nm; mass spectral data have been tabulated (NIH/EPA Chemical Information System, 1981).

(d) *Identity and purity test*: Addition of sulphuric acid produces a blue fluorescent solution. Addition of alcoholic ferric chloride produces a green colour. Addition of iron alum produces a purple colour. Reduces ammoniacal silver nitrate and Fehling's solution (Anon., 1965)

(e) *Solubility*: Slightly soluble in water; soluble in diethyl ether, hot ethanol and alkaline solutions

(f) *Other properties*: Promotes the formation of nitrosamines (Walker *et al.*, 1982)

1.4 Technical products and impurities

No data were available to the Working Group.

2. Production, Use, Occurrence and Analysis

2.1 Production and use

(a) *Production*

Kaempferol is the aglycone of several glycosides which were described in the literature as early as 1900 (Anon., 1965). It has been obtained for use as a natural colouring agent (Natural Yellow 13) by extraction of the dried, unripe berries of various shrubs in the buckthorn family with hot water and evaporation of the extract under reduced pressure (The Society of Dyers & Colourists, 1971a). Kaempferol can be obtained from *para*-hydroxybenzoic acid in an overall yield of 35% in a four-step reaction (Ichikawa *et al.*, 1982).

No specific data on the commercial production of kaempferol in the US, Japan or western Europe are available. It is offered for sale in laboratory quantities.

(b) *Use*

Kaempferol has been reported to be useful as an analytical reagent for the determination of several metal ions, because the complexes which it forms can be determined spectrophotometrically. No evidence was found that it is being used in common practice for this purpose, however. Kaempferol or its glycosides are components of three natural dyes (C.I. Natural Yellow 13, C.I. Natural Yellow 10, and C.I. Natural Blue 1), which apparently have found some industrial use as textile dyes (The Society of Dyers & Colourists, 1971a,b).

2.2 Occurrence

Kaempferol is widely distributed in the plant kingdom, where it occurs as condensation products (glycosides) with various sugars. Several of these glycosides (afzelin, astragalin, equisetrin, kaempferitrin, multiflorin, populnin, robinin and trifolin) (Anon., 1965) have been found in the berries, flowers, fruits, leaves and roots of plants of the Ranunculaceae, Leguminosae and other families. Kaempferol has been isolated from *Pteridium aquilinum* (bracken fern) (Pamukcu *et al.*, 1980), *Allium porrum* (leek), *Brassica chinensis*, *Brassica napus*, *Brassica oleraceae var. botrytis*, *Brassica oleraceae var. botrytis subvar. cymosa*, *Brassica oleraceae var. buttata*, *Brassica oleraceae var. gemmifera* (plants of cabbage and mustard), *Capsicum anuum* (ornamental pepper), *Cichorium endivia* (endive), *Citrus paradisi Macf.* (grapefruit), *Delphinium consolida L.*, *Fragaria ananassa*, *Lactuca sativa* (lettuce), *Malus pumila* (apple), *Mangifera indica* (mango), *Prunus armeniaca*, *Prunus avium*, *Prunus domestica* (European plum), *Prunus persica*, *Pyrus communis*, *Raphanus sativus* (radish), *Ribes rubrum* (red currant), *Ribes ideaus*, *Solanum tuberosum* (potato), *Spinacea oleraceae* (spinach), *Vicia faba* (broad bean) (Ku"hnau, 1976; Vos-Stevenson, 1979), and from the stems and seeds of *Cuscuta reflexa* Roxb. (Windholz, 1976). China tea, *Camellia sinensis*, has been reported to contain relatively large amounts of triglycosides of kaempferol (Hainsworth, 1969). The total concentration of kaempferol and quercetin glycosides in tea [unspecified variety] was >10 000 mg/kg (Herrmann, 1976).

Kaempferol is the main colouring matter in C.I. Natural Yellow 13, an extract of Hungarian berries, and in dyer's knotgrass. Its glycosides are present in natural indigo, *Indigofera arrecta* (C.I. Natural Blue 1) and in red clover, *Trifolium pratense* L. (The Society of Dyers & Colourists, 1971b).

For concentrations of kaempferol in vegetables and fruits see Tables 1 and 2.

Table 1. Concentrations of kaempferol as its glycoside in tissues of edible plants[a]

Plant	Outer parts of tissues (skin, peel) (mg/kg)	Remaining tissues (mg/kg)
Apple	<1-7	0.0-<0.1
Pear	12	0.0
Quince	210	<0.01
Kohlrabi	6	<1.0
Small radish	27	0.6
Horse-radish	76	1.5
Scorzonera	<1	<1.0
Potato	*c.* 0.2-57	*c.* 0.1-9.0
Asparagus (white tips)	<0.1	0.0
Tomato	Contains nearly the total flavonol content in the outer parts of the tissues, which were 4-5% of the fruit	
Cucumber	Contains traces of flavon(ol) glycosides only in the peel	

[a]From Herrmann (1976)

Table 2. Concentrations of kaempferol as its glycoside in leaves and other parts of edible plants[a]

Plant	Location	Leaves (mg/kg)	Other parts of same plant (mg/kg)
Brussel sprouts		75	sprouts: 40
Cauliflower		270	curd: 2
Kohlrabi	open air	80	peel: 6 flesh: <1.0
	greenhouse	5	flesh: <0.1
Kale	open air	250	--
	greenhouse	70	--
Small radish		150-825	root: 1.3-8
	greenhouse	16	root: 1.0
Radish		130	root: c. 0.3
Rutabaga		400	root: c. 0.3
Horseradish		1600	root: 20
Scorzonera (salsify)		25	root: <1.0
Potato		50-60	tuber: 1.0
Tomato	open air	20	fruit: 0.2
	greenhouse	4	fruit: 0.2
Pea		140-150	pod without seeds: 3.0-5.0
			seed: <1.0
Broad bean		800	pod without seeds: 28
			pod: 5

[a]From Herrmann (1976)

2.3 Analysis

Kaempferol has been determined in plant material and food by thin-layer chromatography (Wildanger & Herrmann, 1973) and high-performance liquid chromatography (Charpentier & Cowles, 1981).

3. Biological Data Relevant to the Evaluation of Carcinogenic Risk to Humans

3.1 Carcinogenicity studies in animals

Oral administration

Rat: Six male and 6 female ACI rats, 1-1.5 months old, were fed a diet containing 400 mg/kg kaempferol (purity, 99%) for 540 days, at which time the experiment was terminated. A control group of 30 males and 22 females were fed basal diet only. There was no significant difference in the incidence of tumours between the experimental and control groups [$p > 0.05$] (Takanashi *et al.*, 1982). [The Working Group noted the small number of animals and the low dosage of kaempferol used.]

3.2 Other relevant biological data

(a) *Experimental systems*

Toxic effects

No data were available to the Working Group.

Effects on reproduction and prenatal toxicity

No data were available to the Working Group.

Absorption, distribution, excretion and metabolism

No data were available on kaempferol itself. Concentrations of 0.01-1mM kaempferol inhibit hydroxylation of benzo[a]pyrene by human liver microsomes (Buening *et al.*, 1981).

Mutagenicity and other short-term tests

The genetic effects of kaempferol and related flavonoids have been reviewed (Brown, 1980).

Kaempferol gave negative results in the *Bacillus subtilis rec* assay for DNA damage, when tested without exogenous metabolic activation (Brown, 1980). It is mutagenic to *Salmonella typhimurium* strains TA1537, TA98 and TA100, but not TA1535 or TA1538 (Sugimura *et al.*, 1977; Hardigree & Epler, 1978; MacGregor & Jurd, 1978; Brown & Dietrich, 1979). It requires activation by a mammalian microsomal fraction, and the mutagenicity is increased by prior induction with Aroclor or methylcholanthrene, but not phenobarbital (Hardigree & Epler, 1978).

Kaempferol, as well as other flavonoids, occurs in plants as various glycosides, which are not mutagenic to *S. typhimurium*. These are, however, hydrolysed to mutagenic aglycones by *beta*-glycosidases, such as those present in the mammalian intestinal flora (Brown, 1980).

Kaempferol was mutagenic in the sex-linked recessive lethal test in *Drosophila melanogaster* after feeding to adult males (Watson, 1982).

Kaempferol induces mutations to 8-azaguanine resistance in V79 Chinese hamster cells; activity was increased by the addition of a rat liver 15 000 x *g* supernatant fraction (Maruta *et al.*, 1979). [The Working Group noted the large variation in spontaneous mutation rates in the control series.]

No morphological transformation was observed in cryopreserved hamster embryo cells *in vitro* (Umezawa *et al.*, 1977).

There was an increase in the number of micronuclei in polychromatic erythrocytes in the bone marrow of male mice that had received i.p. injections of 200 and 400 mg/kg bw (Sahu *et al.*, 1981).

(*b*) *Humans*

No data were available to the Working Group.

3.3 Case reports and epidemiological studies of carcinogenicity in humans

No data were available to the Working Group.

4. Summary of Data Reported and Evaluation

4.1 Experimental data

Kaempferol was tested for carcinogenicity in one experiment in rats by administration in the diet. The data are inadequate to make an evaluation.

Kaempferol was mutagenic in bacteria and insects and in mammalian cells *in vitro*; it induced micronuclei in mice. There is *limited evidence* that kaempferol is active in short-term tests.

No data were available to evaluate the teratogenicity of kaempferol to experimental animals.

4.2 Human data

The natural occurrence of kaempferol, an aglycone widely distributed in fruit and other edible plants, results in wide human exposure to this compound.

No data were available to evaluate the teratogenicity or chromosomal effects of this compound in humans.

No case report or epidemiological study of the carcinogenicity of kaempferol was available to the Working Group.

4.3 Evaluation

The available data were inadequate to evaluate the carcinogenicity of kaempferol to experimental animals. In the absence of epidemiological data, no evaluation of the carcinogenicity of kaempferol to humans could be made.

5. References

Anon. (1965) *Dictionary of Organic Compounds*, Vol. 4, New York, Oxford University Press, p. 1981

Brown, J.P. (1980) A review of the genetic effects of naturally occurring flavonoids, anthraquinones and related compounds. *Mutat. Res.*, *75*, 243-277

Brown, J.P. & Dietrich, P.S. (1979) Mutagenicity of plant flavonols in the *Salmonella*/mammalian microsome test. Activation of flavonol glycosides by mixed glycosidases from rat cecal bacteria and other sources. *Mutat. Res.*, *66*, 223-240

Buening, M.K., Chang, R.L., Huang, M.-T., Fortner, J.G., Wood, A.W. & Conney, A.H. (1981) Activation and inhibition of benzo(a)pyrene and aflatoxin B_1 metabolism in human liver microsomes by naturally occurring flavonoids. *Cancer Res.*, *41*, 67-72

Charpentier, B. A. & Cowles, J.R. (1981) Rapid method of analysing phenolic compounds in *Pinus elliotti* using high-performance liquid chromatography. *J. Chromatogr.*, *208*, 132-136

Hainsworth, E. (1969) *Tea*. In: Kirk, R.E. & Othmer, D.F., eds, *Encyclopedia of Chemical Technology*, 2nd ed., Vol. 19, New York, John Wiley & Sons, pp. 743, 755

Hardigree, A.A. & Epler, J.L. (1978) Comparative mutagenesis of plant flavonoids in microbial systems. *Mutat. Res.*, *58*, 231-239

Herrmann, K. (1976) Flavonols and flavones in food plants: A review. *J. Food Technol.*, *11*, 433-448

Ichikawa, M., Pamukcu, A.M. & Byran, G.T. (1982) A convenient method for the synthesis of kaempferol. *Org. Prep. Proced. int.*, *14*, 183-187

Kühnau, J. (1976) The flavonoids. *A class of semi-essential food components: Their role in human nutrition*. In: Bourne, G.H., ed., *World Review of Nutrition and Dietetics*, Vol. 24, Basel/New York, Karger, pp. 117-191

MacGregor, J.T. & Jurd, L. (1978) Mutagenicity of plant flavonoids: Structural requirements for mutagenic activity in *Salmonella typhimurium*. *Mutat. Res.*, *54*, 297-309

Maruta, A., Enaka, K. & Umeda, M. (1979) Mutagenicity of quercetin and kaempferol on cultured mammalian cells. *Gann*, *70*, 273-276

NIH/EPA Chemical Information System (1981) *Mass Spectral Search System*, Washington DC, CIS Project, Information Sciences Corporation

Pamukcu, A.M., Yalciner, S., Hatcher, J.F. & Bryan, G.T. (1980) Quercetin, a rat intestinal and bladder carcinogen present in bracken fern (*Pteridium aquilinum*). *Cancer Res.*, *40*, 3468-3472

Sahu, R.K., Basu, R. & Sharma, A. (1981) Genetic toxicological testing of some plant flavonoids by the micronucleus test. *Mutat. Res.*, *89*, 69-74

The Society of Dyers & Colourists (1971a) *Colour Index*, 3rd ed., Vol. 3, Bradford, Yorkshire, Lund Humphries, pp. 3229, 3230

The Society of Dyers & Colourists (1971b) *Colour Index*, 3rd ed., Vol. 4, Bradford, Yorkshire, Lund Humphries, p. 4635

Sugimura, T., Nagao, M., Matsushima, T., Yahaghi, T., Seino, Y., Shirai, A., Sawamura, M., Natori, S., Yoshihira, K., Fukuoka, M. & Kuroyanagi, M. (1977) Mutagenicity of flavone derivatives. *Proc. Jpn. Acad.*, *53*, Ser. B, 194-197

Takanashi, H., Aiso, S., Hirono, I., Matsushima, T. & Sugimura, T. (1982) Carcinogenicity test of quercetin and kaempferol in rats by oral administration. *J. Food Saf.* (in press)

Umezawa, K., Matsushima, T., Sugimura, T., Hirakawa, T., Tanaka, M., Katoh, Y. & Takayama, S. (1977) *In vitro* transformation of hamster embryo cells by quercetin. *Toxicol. Lett.*, *1*, 175-178

Vos-Stevenson, H. (1979) *Mutagene Plantenmetabolieten; van Nature in Plantaardige Voedingsmiddelen Voorkomende Mutagenen* [*Mutagenic Plant Metabolites; Naturally Occurring Mutagens in Foods of Plant Origin*], Thesis

Walker, E.A., Pignatelli, B. & Friesen, M. (1982) The role of phenols in catalysis of nitrosamine formation. *J. Sci. Food. Agric.*, *33*, 81-88

Watson, W.A.F. (1982) The mutagenic activity of quercetin and kaempferol in *Drosophila melanogaster*. *Mutat. Res.*, *103*, 145-147

Wildanger, W. & Herrmann, K. (1973) Qualitative identification and quantitative determination of flavonols and flavones (Ger.). *J. Chromatogr.*, *76*, 433-440

Windholz, M., ed. (1976) *The Merck Index*, 9th ed., Rahway, NJ, Merck & Co., Inc., p. 692

NITHIAZIDE

1. Chemical and Physical Data

1.1 Synonyms and trade names

Chem. Abstr. Services Reg. No.: 139-94-6

Chem. Abstr. Name: Urea, N-ethyl-N'-(5-nitro-2-thiazolyl)-

IUPAC Systematic Name: 1-Ethyl-3-(5-nitro-2-thiazolyl)urea

Synonym: Nithiazid

Trade Names: Hepzide; Hepzide 30

1.2 Structural and molecular formulae and molecular weight

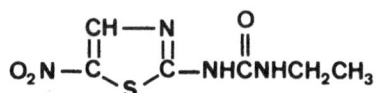

$$\begin{array}{c} CH \!-\! N \qquad O \\ \parallel \qquad \parallel \qquad \parallel \\ O_2N \!-\! C_{\diagdown S \diagup} C \!-\! NHCNHCH_2CH_3 \end{array}$$

$C_6H_8N_4O_3S$ Mol. wt: 216.2

1.3 Chemical and physical properties of the pure substance

From Windholz (1976), unless otherwise specified

(a) *Description:* Crystals

(b) *Melting-point*: 228°C (dec.)

(c) *Spectroscopy data*: λ_{max} 233 nm, A_1^1 = 341; 352 nm, A_1^1 = 601; 429 nm, A_1^1 = 92 (National Cancer Institute, 1979)

(d) *Solubility*: Practically insoluble in water (30 mg/l); the sodium and potassium salts are soluble in water.

1.4 Technical products and impurities

No technical product containing nithiazide is available.

2. Production, Use, Occurrence and Analysis

2.1 Production and use

(a) Production

Nithiazide was first prepared in 1956 by the condensation of ethyl isocyanate with 2-amino-5-nitrothiazole (see p. 71) in toluene (Cuckler et al., 1956).

Nithiazide was first produced commercially in the US in 1961 (US Tariff Commission, 1962). Because only one company reported production, separate production data were not published (see preamble, p. 21), and the company has not reported production of nithiazide since 1972 (US Tariff Commission, 1974). Separate data on US imports and exports of this compound are not published.

Nithiazide is not produced in commercial quantities in Japan or western Europe.

(b) Use

Nithiazide was used in veterinary medicine as an antiprotozoal agent. It was most commonly used against *Histomonas meleagridis*, the organism which causes blackhead in fowl (Shor & Magee, 1973).

2.2 Occurrence

Nithiazide is not known to occur as a natural product. No data were available to the Working Group on its persistence in the edible tissues of food-producing animals.

2.3 Analysis

No information on analytical methods for nithiazide was available to the Working Group.

3. Biological Data Relevant to the Evaluation of Carcinogenic Risk to Humans

3.1 Carcinogenicity studies in animals

Oral administration

Mouse: Groups of 50 male and 50 female B6C3F1 mice, six weeks of age, were fed diets containing 2500 or 5000 mg/kg nithiazide [purity unspecified] for 61 weeks, then control diet for nine weeks (due to a shortage of nithiazide), then nithiazide diets for 33 weeks, then control diet for one week - providing a total observation period of 104 weeks. The doses were selected on the basis of a range-finding study. A group of 20 mice of each sex served as matched controls. Mean body weight gain of treated male and female mice was distinctly reduced. No significant dose-related trend in mortality was seen for either sex: by the end of the study, 75, 72 and 78% of males and 85, 78 and 78% of females were still alive in the control, low-dose and high-dose groups, respectively. Statistically significant ($p = 0.002$), dose-related increased incidences of hepatocellular carcinomas or adenomas were observed in male mice: controls, 4/20 (2 carcinomas); low-dose, 15/46 (6 carcinomas); high-dose, 25/43 (12 carcinomas) ($p = 0.005$). A non-statistically significant increase in the incidence of pooled hepatocellular carcinomas or adenomas was observed in female mice: controls, 3/18 (1 carcinoma); low-dose, 4/41; high-dose, 12/43 (4 carcinomas). In historical controls in this laboratory, 9/207 (4%) untreated female B6C3F1 mice had hepatocellular carcinomas or adenomas; the incidence of these tumours in the control group of this bioassay was the highest of 11 female historical control groups (National Cancer Institute, 1979).

Rat: Groups of 50 male and 50 female Fischer 344 rats, six weeks of age, were fed diets containing 625 or 1250 mg/kg nithiazide [purity unspecified] for 38 weeks, then control diet for nine weeks (due to a shortage of nithiazide), then nithiazide diets for 56 weeks, then control diet for one week - providing a total observation period of 104 weeks. The doses were selected on the basis of a range-finding study. A group of 20 rats of each sex served as matched controls. Mean body weight gain of treated male and female rats was slightly reduced. No significant dose-related trend in mortality was seen for either sex: by the end of the study, 80, 64 and 66% of males and 85, 66 and 84% of females were still alive in the control, low-dose and high-dose groups, respectively. Statistically significant ($p = 0.003$) dose-related increased incidences of fibroadenomas or cystade-nomas of skin, subcutaneous tissue and mammary gland were observed in female rats: controls, 1/20; low-dose, 5/50; high-dose 15/50 ($p = 0.020$); and statistically significant dose-related increased incidences of chromophobe adenomas or acidophil adenomas of the pituitary ($p = 0.034$): controls, 5/18; low-dose, 13/39; high-dose, 24/47; and of endometrial stromal polyps of the uterus ($p = 0.039$): controls, 1/19; low-dose, 4/50; high-dose, 10/50, were also observed. No statistically significantly increased incidence of tumours was seen in treated male rats when compared with controls (National Cancer Institute, 1979). [The Working Group noted that historical control groups of female Fischer rats show an average incidence of pituitary gland tumours of 40% (Tarone *et al.*, 1981).]

3.2 Other relevant biological data

No data were available to the Working Group.

3.3 Case reports and epidemiological studies of carcinogenicity in humans

No data were available to the Working Group.

4. Summary of Data Reported and Evaluation

4.1 Experimental data

Nithiazide was tested for carcinogenicity in one experiment in mice and in one experiment in rats by administration in the diet. It increased the incidence of hepatocellular carcinomas and adenomas in male mice. In female rats, it increased the incidences of fibroadenomas and cystadenomas of the skin, subcutaneous tissue and mammary gland (significant only if individual incidences for each site were combined) and the incidence of endometrial stromal polyps of the uterus.

No data were available to assess the mutagenic or teratogenic effects of nithiazide in experimental systems.

4.2 Human data

Nithiazide, a synthetic antiprotozoal agent, was first produced in 1961. Humans may be exposed as a result of its manufacture and use in veterinary medicine.

No data were available to assess the teratogenicity or chromosomal effects of this compound in humans.

No case report or epidemiological study of the carcinogenicity of nithiazide was available to the Working Group.

4.3 Evaluation

There is *limited evidence*[1] for the carcinogenicity of nithiazide in experimental animals. In the absence of epidemiological data no evaluation of the carcinogenicity of nithiazide to humans could be made.

---

[1]See preamble, p. 18.

5. References

Cuckler, A.C., Malanga, C.M., Basso, A.J., O'Neill, R.C. & Pfister, K., III (1956) Nithiazide. I. Chemical and biologial studies on 1-ethyl-3-(5-nitro-2-thiazolyl)urea and related compounds. *Proc. Soc. exp. Biol. Med.*, *92*, 483-485

National Cancer Institute (1979) *Bioassay of Nithiazide for Possible Carcinogenicity (Tech. Rep. Ser. No. 146; DHEW Publication No. (NIH) 79-1702)*, Washington DC, US Government Printing Office

Shor, A.L. & Magee, R.J. (1973) *Veterinary drugs*. In: Kirk, R.E. & Othmer, D.F., eds, *Encyclopedia of Chemical Technology*, 2nd ed., Vol. 21, New York, John Wiley & Sons, pp. 248, 253, 254

Tarone, R.E., Chu, K.C. & Ward, J.M. (1981) Variability in the rates of some common naturally occurring tumors in Fischer 344 rats and (C57BL/6N x C3H/HeN)F_1 (B6C3F$_1$) mice. *J. natl Cancer Inst.*, *66*, 1175-1181

US Tariff Commission (1962) *Synthetic Organic Chemicals, US Production and Sales, 1961 (TC Publication 72)*, Washington DC, US Government Printing Office, p. 127

US Tariff Commission (1974) *Synthetic Organic Chemicals, US Production and Sales, 1972 (TC Publication 681)*, Washington DC, US Government Printing Office, p. 109

Windholz, M., ed. (1976) *The Merck Index*, 9th ed., Rahway, NJ, Merck & Co., Inc., p. 853

NITROVIN

1. Chemical and Physical Data

1.1 Synonyms and trade names

Chem. Abstr. Services Reg. No.: 804-36-4

Chem. Abstr. Name: Hydrazinecarboximidamide, 2-[3-(5-nitro-2-furanyl)-1-[2-(5-nitro-2-furanyl)ethenyl]-2-propenylidene]-

IUPAC Systematic Name: [[3-(5-Nitro-2-furyl)-1-[2-(5-nitro-2-furyl)vinyl]allylidene]amino] guanidine

Synonyms: 1,5-Bis(5-nitro-2-furanyl)-1,4-pentadien-3-one, (aminoiminomethyl)hydrazone; sym-bis(5-nitro-2-furfurylidene) acetone guanylhydrazone; 1,5-bis(5-nitro-2-furyl)-3-pentadienone guanylhydrazone; 1,5-bis(5-nitro-2-furyl)-3-pentadienone amidinohydrazone; bis(5-nitrofurfurylidene)acetone guanylhydrazone

Trade Names: Difuran; Difurazone; Panazon; Payzone

1.2 Structural and molecular formulae and molecular weight

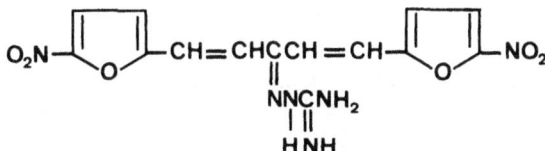

$$O_2N-\overset{\displaystyle\bigcirc}{}-CH=CHCCH=CH-\overset{\displaystyle\bigcirc}{}-NO_2$$

$$\underset{\overset{\displaystyle|}{H}\ \overset{\displaystyle|}{NH}}{NNCNH_2}$$

$C_{14}H_{12}N_6O_6$ Mol. wt: 360.3

1.3 Chemical and physical properties of the pure substance

(a) *Description:* Blackish-violet crystals recrystallized from ethanol (Windholz, 1976)

(b) *Melting-point*: 217°C (dec.) (Windholz, 1976)

(c) *Solubility*: Soluble in dimethyl formamide (Sestáková & Skarka, 1976)

1.4 Technical products and impurities

No data were available to the Working Group.

2. Production, Use, Occurrence and Analysis

2.1 Production and use

(a) Production

The synthesis of nitrovin was first described in 1952. It was prepared by treatment of bis(5-nitrofurfurylidene) acetone with aminoguanidine hydrochloride to give nitrovin hydrochloride, and conversion to the free base was effected by treatment with alkali (Uota et al., 1952).

Nitrovin is produced in Japan by one company, the production of which in recent years is estimated to have been about 25 thousand kg per year.

It is also believed to be produced by one company in Italy and two companies in Spain.

Nitrovin has not been produced in commercial quantities in the US, and no evidence was found that it has ever been imported into that country.

(b) Use

Nitrovin is used in Japan and other countries as a growth promoter in chickens because of its bacteriostatic and bactericidal action (Windholz, 1976; Ebetino, 1978). It is given in feed at a concentration of 10-30 mg/kg (Kodama et al., 1964).

2.2 Occurrence

Nitrovin is not known to occur as a natural product. No data were available to the Working Group on its persistence in the edible tissues of food-producing animals.

2.3 Analysis

A non-specific method for the determination of nitrovin in animal tissues has been reported, based on pulse polarography, which can detect levels down to 10 µg/kg (Sestáková & Skarka, 1976; Skarka & Sestáková, 1978).

3. Biological Data Relevant to the Evaluation of Carcinogenic Risk to Humans

3.1 Carcinogenicity studies in animals

Oral administration

Rat: A group of 28 female Sprague-Dawley rats, three weeks of age, was fed a diet containing 1000 mg/kg nitrovin hydrochloride [purity unspecified] for 46 weeks, followed by control diet for an additional 22 weeks until study termination at the 68th week (total cumulative dose, 5 g/rat). A group of 40 weanling female rats served as controls. No significant difference in survival or weight was seen between treated and control rats. No statistically significantly increase in the incidence of tumours was seen in treated female rats when compared with controls: controls, 6/37, treated, 3/26 solitary mammary fibroadenoma (Ertürk *et al.*, 1980, 1983). [The Working Group noted that a single test dose was used, the duration of treatment was short, the observation period was short and the fact that only female rats were used.]

3.2 Other relevant biological data

(*a*) *Experimental systems*

Toxic effects

No toxic effect was reported after oral administration of 9 g/kg bw nitrovin to mice or after long-term administration of 0.001-0.004% in the diet to rats (Plísek *et al.*, 1975).

Effects on reproduction and prenatal toxicity

No data were available to the Working Group.

Absorption, distribution, excretion and metabolism

Following oral administration of ^{14}C-nitrovin to rats, 0.6% of the radioactivity was absorbed through the intestine, the highest amount being found in the liver and kidneys. Activity was excreted rapidly in the faeces, with approximately 90% recovery within 48 hours. Only 1% of the radioactivity was found in the urine, and traces of radioactivity were detected in exhaled carbon dioxide. A small amount of radioactivity was still detected in animal bodies 12 days after its administration (Struck *et al.*, 1980a).

It has been demonstrated that some nitrovin metabolites, but not nitrovin *per se*, undergo enterohepatic circulation (Struck *et al.*, 1980b).

Mutagenicity and other short-term tests

Nitrovin was positive in the *Bacillus subtilis rec* assay measuring DNA damage (Ohta *et al.*, 1980).

Nitrovin and its hydrochloride were mutagenic to *Salmonella typhimurium* TA98 and TA100 (Joner *et al.*, 1977; Klemencic & Wang, 1978; Ohta *et al.*, 1980; Ertürk *et al.*, 1983). [In the studies by Ertürk *et al.*, the sample tested was the same as that used in the carcinogenicity assay described in section 3.1.] Mutagenic activity is abolished if the chemical is incubated previously with rat liver 9000 x *g* supernatant mix (Ohta *et al.*, 1980). Nitrovin was also mutagenic to *Escherichia coli* WP2 *hcr* repair-deficient strains (McCalla & Voutsinos, 1974; Ohta *et al.*, 1980), and (as reported in an abstract) in a fluctuation test using *Klebsiella pneumoniae* (Knapp *et al.*, 1983). It was reported in another abstract that nitrovin did not cause gene conversion in *Saccharomyces cerevisiae* strain D4 (Knapp *et al.*, 1983).

Nitrovin induced sex-linked recessive lethals in *Drosophila melanogaster* (Kramers, 1978, 1982; Knapp *et al.*, 1983, Abstract).

(*b*) *Humans*

No data were available to the Working Group.

3.3 Case reports and epidemiological studies of carcinogenicity in humans

No data were available to the Working Group.

4. Summary of Data Reported and Evaluation

4.1 Experimental data

Nitrovin was tested for carcinogenicity in one experiment in female rats by administration in the diet. The experiment was inadequate for evaluation.

Nitrovin induces DNA damage and mutations in bacteria and mutations in insects. There is *limited evidence* that nitrovin is active in short-term tests.

No data were available to evaluate the teratogenicity of this compound to experimental animals.

4.2 Human data

Nitrovin, a veterinary bacteriostatic and bactericidal compound, has been used since 1952 as a growth promotor in chickens. Humans may be exposed as a result of its manufacture and use in veterinary medicine.

No data were available to assess the teratogenicity or chromosomal effects of this compound in humans.

No case report or epidemiological study of the carcinogenicity of nitrovin was available to the Working Group.

4.3 Evaluation

No evaluation of the carcinogenicity of nitrovin to experimental animals could be made. In the absence of epidemiological data, no evaluation of the carcinogenicity of nitrovin to humans could be made.

5. References

Ebetino, F.F. (1978) *Antibacterial agents, nitrofurans.* In: Kirk, R.E. & Othmer, D.F., eds, *Encyclopedia of Chemical Technology*, 3rd ed., Vol. 2, New York, John Wiley & Sons, pp. 792, 794

Ertürk, E., Headley, D.B., Matsushima, M., Hatcher, J.F., Ichikawa, M. & Bryan, G.T. (1980) Comparisons between carcinogenicity, mutagenicity, antibacterial activity and induction of vesical ornithine decarboxylase (ODC) of some 5-nitrofuran analogs (Abstract no. 3975). *Fed. Proc.*, *39*, 1022

Ertürk, E., Headley, D.B., Matsushima, M., Hatcher, J.F., Ichikawa, M. & Bryan, G.T. (1983) Relationship between mutagenic, antibacterial, and induced murine vesical ornithine decarboxylase activity, and carcinogenicity of some 5-nitro- and nornitro-furyl analogues in rats. *Cancer Res.* (in press)

Joner, P.E., Dahle, H.K., Aune, T. & Dybing, E. (1977) Mutagenicity of nitrovin-A nitrofuran feed additive. *Mutat. Res.*, *48*, 313-318

Klemencic, J.M. & Wang, C.Y. (1978) *Mutagenicity of nitrofurans.* In: Bryan, G.T., ed., *Carcinogenesis - A Comprehensive Survey*, Vol. 4, *Nitrofurans: Chemistry, Metabolism, Mutagenesis and Carcinogenesis*, New York, Raven Press, pp. 99-130

Knaap, A.G.A.C., Voogd, C.E., Kramers, P.G.N., van Went, G.F. & Ond, J.H. (1983) *Mutagenicity of feed additives.* In: *Proceedings of the European Environmental Mutation Society, June 1982, Helsinki* (in press)

Kodama, H., Fujiwara, T. & Inagaki, T. (1964) Domestic-animal growth regulator. *Japanese Patent No. 6986* (to Toyama Chemical Industries Co.) [*Chem. Abstr.*, *62*, 5151f]

Kramers, P.G. (1978) Mutagenicity of nitro compounds in *Drosophila melanogaster* (Abstract no. 116). *Mutat. Res.*, *53*, 213

Kramers, P.G.N. (1982) Studies on the induction of sex-linked recessive lethal mutations in *Drosophila melanogaster* by nitroheterocyclic compounds. *Mutat. Res.*, *101*, 209-236

McCalla, D.R. & Voutsinos, D. (1974) On the mutagenicity of nitrofurans. *Mutat. Res.*, *26*, 3-16

Ohta, T., Moriya, M., Kaneda, Y., Watanabe, K., Miyazawa, T., Sugiyama, F. & Shirasu, Y. (1980) Mutagenicity screening of feed additives in the microbial system. *Mutat. Res.*, *77*, 21-30

Plísek, K., Malhocká, A. & Billová, V. (1975) Acute and long term toxicity of nitrovin (Lachema) (Czech.). *Biol. Chem. Vyz. Zvirat.*, *11*, 243-251

Sestáková, I. & Skarka, P. (1976) Polarographic determination of the [growth] stimulator nitrovin in biofactor supplements of premixes and in food mixtures (Czech.). *Biol. Chem. Vyz. Zvirat*, *12*, 321-328 [*Chem. Abstr.*, *86*, 104533t]

Skarka, P. & Sestáková, I. (1978) A new procedure for estimation of nitrovin and carbadox residues and their metabolites in food of animal origin. *Arch. Toxicol.*, *Suppl. 1*, 207-210

Struck, S., ter Meulen, U., Hillemeir, H. & Gunther, K.D. (1980a) Studies on the metabolic effects of growth promoters using nitrovin as a model. 1. Trace studies on the absorption, distribution, and excretion of ¹⁴C-nitrovin and its metabolites in young rats, chicks and piglets (Ger.). *Z. Tierphysiol. Tierernähr. Futtermittelkd.*, *43*, 173-190

Struck, S., Günther, K.D., Hillemeir, H. & ter Meulen, U. (1980b) Studies on the metabolic effect of growth promoters, using nitrovin as a model. 2. Studies on the enterohepatic circulation of ¹⁴C-labelled in the rat (Ger.). *Z. Tierphysiol. Tierernähr. Futtermittelkd.*, *43*, 191-197

Uota, H. *et al.* (1952) Bis(5-nitrofurfurylidene) acetone guanylhydrazone hydrochloride. *Japanese Patent No. 2673* (to Toyama Chemical Industries Co.) [*Chem. Abstr.*, *48*, 2115h]

Windholz, M., ed. (1976) *The Merck Index*, 9th ed., Rahway, NJ, Merck & Co., Inc., p. 864

OCHRATOXIN A

This substance was considered by a previous working group in October 1975 (IARC, 1976). Since that time, new data have become available, and these have been incorporated and taken into consideration in the present evaluation.

1. Chemical and Physical Data

1.1 Synonyms and trade names

Chem. Abstr. Services Reg. No.: 303-47-9

Chem. Abstr. Name: L-Phenylalanine, *N*-[(5-chloro-3,4-dihydro-8-hydroxy-3-methyl-1-oxo-1*H*-2-benzopyran-7-yl)carbonyl]-, (*R*)-

IUPAC Systematic Name: *N*-[[(3*R*)-5-Chloro-8-hydroxy-3-methyl-1-oxo-7-isochroma-nyl]carbonyl]-3-phenyl-*L*-alanine

Synonym:
(-)-*N*-[(5-Chloro-8-hydroxy-3-methyl-l-oxo-7-isochromanyl)carbonyl]-3-phenylalanine

1.2 Structural and molecular formulae and molecular weight

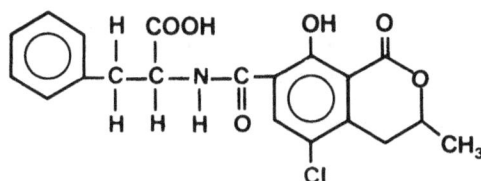

$C_{20}H_{18}ClNO_6$ Mol. wt: 403.8

1.3 Chemical and physical properties of the pure substance

From van der Merwe *et al.* (1965a,b) and Windholz (1976), unless otherwise specified

(*a*) *Description*: Crystals (recrystallized from xylene); intensely fluorescent in utra-violet light, emitting green and blue fluorescence in acid and alkaline solutions, respectively

(b) *Melting-point*: 169°C (recrystallized from xylene)

(c) *Optical rotation*: $[\alpha]_D^{20}$ -118° (c 1.1, in chloroform)

(d) *Spectroscopy data*: λ_{max} 215 nm, A_1^1 = 911; 333 nm, A_1^1 = 59 in ethanol; mass spectrometry data have been reported (NIH/EPA Chemical Information System, 1982).

(e) *Solubility*: The free acid is moderately soluble in organic solvents (e.g., chloroform, ethanol and methanol).

(f) *Stability*: Stable in the solid state

(g) *Reactivity*: The lactone group is saponified by alkalis

1.4 Technical products and impurities

No technical product containing ochratoxin A is available.

2. Production, Use, Occurrence and Analysis

2.1 Production and use

(a) *Production*

Ochratoxin A was first isolated in 1965 (van der Merwe *et al.*, 1965a) from a culture of *Aspergillus ochraceus* Wilh. grown on sterile, moistened maize meal. The structure was subsequently established by synthesis (Steyn & Holzapfel, 1967; Roberts & Woollven, 1970). An efficient method for obtaining small amounts of ochratoxin A from fermented wheat has been reported (Peterson & Ciegler, 1978).

Ochratoxin A is not produced commercially.

(b) *Use*

Ochratoxin A is not used commercially.

2.2 Occurrence

Ochratoxin A is produced naturally, primarily by members of the *Aspergillus ochraceus* group and by some species of the *Penicillium* group. *Penicillium viridicatum* Westling seems to be the major producer within the *Penicillium* group, but some other species have been found to form detectable amounts of ochratoxin A (van Walbeek *et al.*, 1969; Ciegler *et al.*, 1972).

An overview of the occurrence of ochratoxin A by foodstuff and geographical area has been published (FAO, 1979; Krogh & Nesheim, 1983) (see Table 1).

Table 1. Natural occurrence of ochratoxin A in foods and feeds of plant origin

Commodity	Country	Number of samples analysed	Percent contaminated	Ochratoxin A level (range, µg/kg)	Reference
Foods					
Maize	USA	293	1.0	83-166	Shotwell et al. (1971)
Maize (1973)	France	463	2.6	15-200	Galtier et al. (1977)
Maize (1974)	France	461	1.3	20-200	Galtier et al. (1977)
Wheat (red winter)	USA	291	1.0	15-35	Shotwell et al. (1976)
Wheat (red spring)	USA	286	2.8	15-115	Shotwell et al. (1976)
Barley (malt)	Denmark	50	6.0	9-189	Krogh (1978)
Barley	USA	182	12.6	10-29	Krogh & Nesheim (1983)
Coffee beans	USA	267	7.1	20-360	Levi et al. (1974)
Maize	Yugoslavia[a]	542	8.3[b]	<19-140	Pavlović et al. (1979)
Wheat	Yugoslavia[a]	130	8.5[b]	<19->100	Pavlović et al. (1979)
Wheat bread	Yugoslavia[a]	32	18.8[b]	--	Pavlović et al. (1979)
Barley	Yugoslavia[a]	64	12.5[b]	14-26	Pavlović et al. (1979)
Barley	Czechoslovakia	48	2.1	3800	Vesela et al. (1978)
Bread	UK[c]	50	2	210	Osborne (1980)
Flour	UK	7	28.5	490-2900	Osborne (1980)
Rice	Japan[c]	2	not given	230-430	Sugimoto et al. (1977)
Beans	Sweden	71	8.5	10-442	Akerstrand & Josefsson (1979)
Peas	Sweden	72	2.8	10	Akerstrand & Josefsson (1979)

Commodity	Country	Number of samples analysed	Percent contaminated	Ochratoxin A level (range, μg/kg)	Reference
Feeds					
Barley, wheat, oats, rye, maize	Poland	150	5.3	50-200	Juszkiewicz & Piskorska-Pliszczynska (1976)
Mixed feed	Poland	203	4.9	10-50	Juszkiewicz & Piskorska-Pliszczynska (1977)
Maize	Yugoslavia	191	2	45-5125	Balzer et al. (1977)
Barley, oats	Sweden	84	8	16-409	Krogh et al. (1974a)
Wheat, hay	Canada	95	7.4	30-6000	Prior (1976)
Wheat, oats, barley, rye	Canada[c]	29	62	30-27 000	Scott et al. (1972)
Barley, oats	Denmark[c]	33	57.6	28-27 500	Krogh et al. (1973)

[a] From an area of endemic human nephropathy
[b] Average values for a period of two to five years
[c] All samples suspected of containing mycotoxins

Ochratoxin A has been detected in cereals (wheat, rye, barley and oats), beans and peanuts; the range of levels was 9-27 500 μg/kg (Scott et al., 1970, 1972; Krogh et al., 1973). In a study conducted in Canada between 1975 and 1979, ochratoxin A was detected in four of 148 specimens of grain and two of 19 specimens of corn, at levels up to 500 μg/kg (Prior, 1981). In a study conducted in Poland between 1975 and 1981, ochratoxin A was found in about 8% of cereal samples, at a maximum level of 1200 μg/kg (Chelkowski & Golinéskia, 1982).

Ochratoxin A has been detected in barley intended for beer production. The malting process seems to completely degrade the ochratoxin A present in moderately contamina-ted barley lots, but in heavily contaminated lots a 2-7% carryover of the toxin was found, corresponding to 6-20 μg/l (Krogh et al., 1974b).

When food animals (pigs) are exposed to ochratoxin A-contaminated feed immediately prior to slaughter, a small fraction (less than 1%) of the ingested toxin is retained as residues in the tissues. Thus, surveys of meat plants in Denmark and Sweden have revealed that the kidneys of 25-35% of pigs suffering from nephropathy contain residues of ochratoxin A (Krogh, 1977; Rutqvist et al., 1978).

In an area of endemic nephropathy, ochratoxin A was found in 28.9% of ham samples at levels of 40-70 μg/kg, 18.9% of bacon samples at levels of 37-200 μg/kg, 13.3% of kulen (specially prepared sausage) samples at levels of 10-460 μg/kg and 12% of sausage samples at levels of 10-920 μg/kg (Pepeljnjak & Blazevicé, 1982).

2.3 Analysis

A manual of methods for the analysis of mycotoxins has been published (Egan et al, 1983) and includes two validated methods for ochratoxin A.

Typical methods for the analysis of ochratoxin A are summarized in Table 2.

Table 2. Methods for the analysis of ochratoxin A

Sample matrix	Sample preparation	Assay procedure[a]	Limit of detection	Reference
Cereals	Extract (phosphoric acid-chloroform); clean up (silica gel column)	HPLC/UV	1-5 μg/kg	Josefsson & Möl-ler (1979)
Cereals and coffee	Extract (chloroform); purify (diatomaceous earth column)	TLC	12 μg/kg	Nesheim et al. (1973); Levi (1975)
Food and feedstuffs	Extract (chloroform-methanol); clean up by a series of extractions	HPLC/FL	5 μg/kg	Schweighardt et al. (1980)

Sample matrix	Sample preparation	Assay procedure[a]	Limit of detection	Reference
	Extract (10:1 chloro-form:water for feedstuffs or 10:1 chloroform:0.1 M phosphoric acid for foods); add hexane; transfer to silica gel cartridge; elute aflatoxins first, then ochra-toxin A, using 19:1 metha-nol:90% formic acid	TLC	20 μg/kg	Roberts et al. (1981)
Feedstuffs	Extract (chloroform-water); add standard solution; clean up (chromatographic column)	TLC or HPLC/FL	TLC: 10 μg/kg HPLC: 1 μg/kg	Howell & Taylor (1981)

[a]Abbreviations: TLC, thin-layer chromatography; HPLC/FL, high-performance liquid chromatography with fluorescence detection; HPLC/UV, high-performance liquid chromatography with ultra-violet spectrometry

3. Biological Data Relevant to the Evaluation of Carcinogenic Risk to Humans

3.1 Carcinogenicity studies in animals[1]

(a) Oral administration

Mouse: A group of ten male ddy mice (average weight, 26 g) received a diet containing 40 mg/kg ochratoxin A (crystalline) [purity unspecified] for 44 weeks. A group of 10 untreated controls were fed the basal diet. All survivors were killed 49 weeks after the start of treatment. Hepatic-cell tumours (well-differentiated trabecular adenomas) were found in 5/9 treated mice and in 0/10 of the controls; hyperplastic liver nodules were found in 1/9 treated mice and in 2/10 controls. Solid renal-cell tumours were found in 2/9 treated mice and in 0/10 of the controls; cystic adenomas of the kidney were found in 9/9 treated mice and in 0/10 controls (Kanisawa & Suzuki, 1978). [The Working Group noted the small size of the experimental groups.]

---

[1]The Working Group was aware of a study in progress in which rats were being administered ochratoxin A by oral gavage (National Toxicology Program, 1982)

Rat: Groups of five Wistar-derived weanling rats of each sex (average weight, 50 g) received 100 or 300 μg ochratoxin A (crystalline, chromatographically pure) dissolved in 0.5 ml sodium bicarbonate orally on five days/week for 50 weeks. Controls consisted of five females and five males that received 0.5 ml sodium bicarbonate only and five females and five males that received no treatment. All survivors were killed at week 110. One rat in the high-dose group developed a hamartoma of the kidney. No tumour was observed in the control groups (Purchase & van der Watt, 1971). [The Working Group noted the incomplete reporting of the experiment, in that no data were available on the survival of treated rats or on the tumour incidence in untreated controls, and the small size of the experimental groups.]

(b) *Subcutaneous administration*

Mouse: A group of 10 male and 10 female mice received s.c. injections of 10 μg ochratoxin A suspended in 0.1 ml arachis oil twice weekly for 36 weeks; no tumour was observed in treated or control animals after 81 weeks (Dickens & Waynforth, 1968). [The Working Group noted the incomplete reporting of the experimental results.]

Rat: A group of 10 female Wistar-derived rats (average body weight, 85 g) received s.c. doses of 2.5 mg/kg bw ochratoxin A in sunflower seed oil twice weekly for a total of 35 doses. Solvent controls consisted of 10 female rats. All survivors were killed at week 87. Two treated rats and two controls developed fibrosarcomas at the injection site (Purchase & van der Watt, 1971). [The Working Group noted the incomplete reporting of the experiment, in that data on survival and tumour incidence were not available, and the small size of the experimental groups.]

3.2 Other relevant biological data

(a) *Experimental systems*

Toxic effects

The oral, i.p. and i.v. LD_{50} values of ochratoxin A in mice are about 60, 40 and 30 mg/kg bw, respectively (Galtier *et al.*, 1974). Oral LD_{50} values in rats range from 20-28 mg/kg bw (Purchase & Theron, 1968; Chu, 1974; Kanisawa *et al.*, 1977); i.p. and i.v. LD_{50} values in rats were about 13 mg/kg bw (Galtier *et al.*, 1974).

In mice, rats, dogs and pigs, both the acute and chronic effects of ochratoxin A are localized in the kidney, in which it causes necrosis of proximal tubular epithelium (reviewed by Krogh, 1976). Ochratoxin A in feed is believed to be the most important agent in the causation of mycotoxic porcine nephropathy (Krogh, 1978). In beagle dogs, treatment with oral doses of 0.1 or 0.2 mg/kg bw ochratoxin A for 14 days caused necrosis of the lymphoid tissues, of the lymph nodules of the ileum, colon and rectum (Kitchen *et al.*, 1977) and of the mucosa of the colon (Szczech *et al.*, 1973).

In isolated hepatoma cells, ochratoxin A inhibited nucleic acid and protein synthesis by competing with phenylalanine at the phenylalanyl-t-RNA-synthetase active site (Creppy *et al.*, 1980). Cells entering mitosis after exposure to ochratoxin A show abnormal metaphases and formation of polynucleated cells (Steyn *et al.*, 1975). Ochratoxin A, incubated in the presence of fresh renal cortex slices from rats, caused an inhibition of *para*-aminohippurate uptake, thus altering renal function (Berndt & Hayes, 1979a,b).

Effects on reproduction and prenatal toxicity

The effects of prenatal exposure to mycotoxins have been reviewed (Hayes & Hood, 1976; Hayes, 1978).

A single i.p. dose of 5 mg/kg bw ochratoxin A given to pregnant SAF/ICR mice on one of days 7-12 of gestation caused increases in prenatal mortality and in foetal malformations and a decrease in foetal weight. The highest number of malformations was seen in foetuses of animals treated on day 8 of gestation (35% dead or absorbed; 58% grossly malformed; 84% with skeletal malformations) (Hayes *et al.*, 1974).

A single i.p. injection of 2 mg/kg bw to CD-1 mice induced craniofacial malformations when given on day 8 but not when given on day 10 (Hood *et al.*, 1978). Cerebral necrosis occurred in most foetuses of CD-1 or ICR mice treated orally or intraperitoneally with 3-5 mg/kg bw on days 15-17 of gestation (Szczech & Hood, 1979 (abstract), 1981).

In several studies, pregnant Wistar or Sprague-Dawley rats were treated with ochratoxin A on various days during the period of organogenesis. Single oral doses of 6.25, 12.5 and 25 mg/kg bw on day 10 of gestation induced high resorption rates (25, 82 and 78%, respectively). At the highest dose, there was 100% resorption in 6/7 animals (Still *et al.*, 1971). An abnormal proportion of haemorrhagic foetuses and a significant decrease in foetal body weight, an increase in the resorption rate and a decrease in litter size were noted after total i.p. or oral doses of 4 or 5 mg/kg bw (Moré & Galtier, 1974, 1975, 1978). Furthermore, multiple oral doses of 0.75 mg/kg bw on days 6-15 were embryotoxic and teratogenic: various gross, visceral and skeletal anomalies were induced (Brown *et al.*, 1976). The effects of single s.c. injections of 0.5-5 mg/kg bw on one of days 4-10 of gestation were studied. The minimum teratogenic dose in rats was 1.75 mg/kg, which caused decreased foetal weight and various foetal malformations. Higher doses caused foetal resorption. Ochratoxin A was most effective when given on day 5 or day 6 of gestation (Mayura *et al.*, 1982).

Similar results were obtained in pregnant golden hamsters after single i.p. injections of 2.5-20 mg/kg bw on one of days 7-10 of gestation; days 8 and 9 were the most critical with regard to malformations. The foetal mortality rate was significantly increased in litters exposed to the highest dose level on days 7, 8 or 9 (Hood *et al.*, 1975, 1976).

Absorption, distribution, excretion and metabolism

In rats, ochratoxin A is absorbed through the stomach wall (Galtier, 1974a) and the jejunum (Kumagai & Aibara, 1982). It is distributed to most tissues, but mainly to liver, kidneys and muscle (Galtier, 1974a; Chang & Chu, 1977; Lillehoj *et al.*, 1979). In rats, it is excreted *via* the faeces and urine; the plasma half-life of ochratoxin A is about 60 hours (Galtier, 1974b).

Ochratoxin A is cleaved into phenylalanine and a less toxic iso-coumarin derivative (ochratoxin α) by the microbial flora of the colon (Galtier, 1974a; Galtier & Alvinerie, 1976) and by carboxypeptidase A and α-chymotrypsin (Pitout, 1969).

When ochratoxin A was incubated with pig, rat or human liver microsomes, (4R)- and (4S)-4-hydroxyochratoxin A were formed, the (4R):(4S) ratios varying with the species (Størmer et al., 1981). When 6.6 mg/kg ochratoxin A were administered intraperitoneally or orally to Wistar rats, 27% ochratoxin α, 12% parent compound and 1-2% (4R)-4-hydroxyochratoxin A were recovered in the urine after 8 days. Traces of ochratoxin A and ochratoxin α were detected in the faeces (Støren et al., 1982).

Mutagenicity and other short-term tests

The genetic effects of mycotoxins, including ochratoxin A, have been reviewed (Stark, 1980).

Ochratoxin A had no effect in a *Bacillus subtilis rec* assay, measuring DNA damage, when tested at 20 and 100 μg/plate (Ueno & Kubota, 1976).

Ochratoxin A was not mutagenic to *Salmonella typhimurium* TA1535, TA1537, TA1538, TA98 or TA100 at doses of up to 500 μg/plate, with or without exogenous metabolic activation (Kuczuk et al., 1978; Wehner et al., 1978). No increase in genetic changes at the *ade 2* locus of *Saccharomyces cerevisiae* was observed after treatment with 50 and 100 μg/plate ochratoxin A, with or without exogenous metabolic activation (Kuczuk et al., 1978). Ochratoxin A did not induce mutations to 8-azaguanine resistance in C3H mouse mammary carcinoma cells (FM3A) treated with doses of 5 and 10 μg/ml (Umeda et al., 1977).

(*b*) *Humans*

Toxic effects

The human disease, Balkan endemic nephropathy, has been suggested to be the result of fungal poisoning (Anon., 1973), and similarities in the changes of renal function and structure seen in this disease and in mycotoxin A-induced porcine nephropathy have been noted (Krogh, 1974). In a survey of 768 samples of cereals and bread produced locally in an area of Yugoslavia where Balkan nephropathy is prevalent, ochratoxin A was found at a higher frequency than that reported in cereals for human consumption elsewhere (Pavlovicé et al., 1979). In an endemic area for Balkan nephropathy, 7% of the population had ochratoxin A in the blood compared with none in a control group from another area (Krogh & Nesheim, 1983).

Effects on reproduction and prenatal toxicity

No data were available to the Working Group.

Absorption, distribution, excretion and metabolism

No data were available to the Working Group.

Mutagenicity and chromosomal effects

No data were available to the Working Group.

3.3 Case reports and epidemiological studies of carcinogenicity in humans

The geographical distribution of Balkan endemic nephropathy in Bulgaria and Yugoslavia correlates with the incidence and mortality of urothelial urinary-tract tumours (Chernozemsky et al., 1977; Stojanov et al., 1977; Radovanovicé & Krajinovicé, 1979). No biological explanation exists for this association. The evidence for a role of ochratoxin A in causation of Balkan endemic nephropathy was reviewed (3.2.b), but no report of a direct association in human studies between ochratoxin A and urinary tract or other tumours was available to the Working Group.

4. Summary of Data Reported and Evaluation

4.1 Experimental data

Ochratoxin A has been tested for carcinogenicity in mice and rats by oral administration and by subcutaneous injection. In one limited feeding study in mice, hepatic-cell adenomas, solid renal-cell tumours and cystic adenomas of the kidney were observed. The other experiments were considered inadequate for evaluation.

Ochratoxin A was not mutagenic in bacteria or yeast or in mammalian cells *in vitro*; it was also negative in a bacterial repair test. There is no evidence that ochratoxin A is active in short-term tests; however, no data on tests measuring chromosomal anomalies were available for evaluation.

Ochratoxin A is embryolethal and teratogenic to mice, rats and hamsters.

4.2 Human data

Ochratoxin A, a naturally occurring mycotoxin, was first isolated in 1965. Its occurrence in a wide variety of human and animal foodstuffs results in human exposure.

No data were available to evaluate the teratogenicity or chromosomal effects of this compound in humans.

The only epidemiological evidence available of an association between ochratoxin A and cancer occurrence was considered inadequate for evaluation.

4.3 Evaluation

The results of one study in mice provide *limited evidence*[1] for the carcinogenicity of ochratoxin A in experimental animals. In the absence of adequate epidemiological data, no evaluation of the carcinogenicity of ochratoxin A to humans could be made.

---

[1]See preamble, p. 18.

5. References

Akerstrand, K., & Josefsson, E. (1979) Fungi and mycotoxins in beans and peas. *Var Foeda*, *31*, 405-414

Anon. (1973) Endemic nephropathy. *Lancet*, *i*, 472

Balzer, I., Bogdanic, C. & Muzic, S. (1977) Natural contamination of corn (*Zea mays*) with mycotoxins in Yugoslavia. *Ann. Nutr. Alim.*, *31*, 425-430 [*Chem. Abstr.*, *89*, 58454e]

Berndt, W.O. & Hayes, A.W. (1979a) *Factors related to the nephrotoxicity produced by certain mycotoxins* (Abstract no. 35). In: *18th Annual Meeting of the Society of Toxicology, New Orleans*, p. A18

Berndt, W.O. & Hayes, A.W. (1979b) *In vivo* and *in vitro* changes in renal function caused by ochratoxin A in the rat. *Toxicology*, *12*, 5-17

Brown, M.H., Szczech, G.M. & Purmalis, B.P. (1976) Teratogenic and toxic effects of ochratoxin A in rats. *Toxicol. appl. Pharmacol.*, *37*, 331-338

Chang, F.C. & Chu, F.S. (1977) The fate of ochratoxin A in rats. *Food Cosmet. Toxicol.*, *15*, 199-204

Chelkowski, J. & Golinéski, P. (1982) *Mycotoxins and toxinogenic fungi in mixed feeds and their cereal components*. In: *Fifth International IUPAC Symposium on Mycotoxins and Phycotoxins*, Vienna, Austrian Chemical Society, pp. 68-71

Chernozemsky, I.N., Stoyanov, I.S., Petkova-Bocharova, T.K., Nocolov, I.G., Draganov, I.V., Stoichev, I.I., Tanchev, Y., Naidenov, D. & Kalcheva, N.D. (1977) Geographic correlation between the occurrence of endemic nephropathy and urinary tract tumours in Vratza district, Bulgaria. *Int. J. Cancer*, *19*, 1-11

Chu, F.S. (1974) Studies on ochratoxins. *CRC crit. Rev. Toxicol.*, *2*, 499-524

Ciegler, A., Fennell, D.J., Mintzlaff, H.-J. & Leistner, L. (1972) Ochratoxin synthesis by *Penicillium* species. *Naturwissenschaften*, *59*, 365-366

Creppy, E.-E., Lorkowski, G., Beck, G., Röschenthaler, R. & Dirheimer, G. (1980) Combined action of citrinin and ochratoxin A on hepatoma tissue culture cells. *Toxicol. Lett.*, *5*, 375-380

Dickens, F. & Waynforth, H.B. (1968) Studies on carcinogenesis by lactones and related substances. *Rep. Br. Emp. Cancer Campaign*, *46*, 108

Egan, H., Stoloff, L., Castegnaro, M., Scott, P., O'Neill, I.K. & Bartsch, H., eds (1983) *Environmental Carcinogens. Selected Methods of Analysis*, Vol. 5, *Mycotoxins* (*IARC Scientific Publications No. 44*), Lyon, International Agency for Research on Cancer

FAO (1979) *Perspective on Mycotoxins* (*Food and Nutrition Paper No. 13*), Rome, pp. 15-120

Galtier, P. (1974a) Fate of ochratoxin A in the animal organism. II. Distribution in the tissues and excretion in the rat (Fr.). *Ann. Rech. vét.*, *5*, 319-328

Galtier, P. (1974b) Fate of ochratoxin A in the animal organism. I. Transport of the toxin in the blood of the rat (Fr.). *Ann. Rech. vét.*, *5*, 311-318

Galtier, P. & Alvinerie, M. (1976) *In vitro* transformation of ochratoxin A by animal microbial floras. *Ann. Rech. vét.*, *7*, 91-98

Galtier, P., Moré, J. & Bodin, G. (1974) Toxins of *Aspergillus ochraceus* Wilheim. III. Acute toxicity of ochratoxin A in adult rats and mice (Fr.). *Ann. Rech. vét.*, *5*, 233-247

Galtier, P., Jemmali, M. & Larrieu, G. (1977) Investigation on the possible occurrence of aflatoxin and ochratoxin A in maize harvested in France in 1973 and 1974 (Fr.). *Ann. Nutr. Alim.*, *31*, 381-389

Hayes, A.W. (1978) *Mycotoxin teratogenicity.* In: Rosenberg, P., ed., *Toxins: Animal, Plant and Microbial*, New York, Pergamon Press, pp. 739-758

Hayes, A.W. & Hood, R.D. (1976) Effects of prenatal exposure to mycotoxins. *Proc. Eur. Soc. Toxicol.*, *17*, 209-219

Hayes, A.W., Hood, R.D. & Lee, H.L. (1974) Teratogenic effects of ochratoxin A in mice. *Teratology*, *9*, 93-98

Hood, R.D., Naughton, M.J. & Hayes, A.W. (1975) Teratogenic effects of ochratoxin A in hamsters (Abstract). *Teratology*, *11*, 23A

Hood, R.D., Naughton, M.J. & Hayes, A.W. (1976) Prenatal effects of ochratoxin A in hamsters. *Teratology*, *13*, 11-14

Hood, R.D., Kuczuk, M.H. & Szczech, G.M. (1978) Effects in mice of simultaneous prenatal exposure to ochratoxin A and T-2 toxin. *Teratology*, *17*, 25-29

Howell, M.V. & Taylor, P.W. (1981) Determination of aflatoxins, ochratoxin A, and zearalenone in mixed feeds, with detection by thin layer chromatography or high performance liquid chromatography. *J. Assoc. off. anal. Chem.*, *64*, 1356-1363

IARC (1976) *IARC Monographs on the Evaluation of Carcinogenic Risk of Chemicals to Man*, Vol. 10, *Some Naturally Occurring Substances*, Lyon, France, pp. 191-197

Josefsson, E. & Möller, T. (1979) High pressure liquid chromatographic determination of ochratoxin A and zearalenone in cereals. *J. Assoc. off. anal. Chem.*, *62*, 1165-1168

Juszkiewicz, T. & Piskorksa-Pliszczynska, J. (1976) Occurrence of aflatoxins B_1, B_2, G_1 and G_2, ochratoxins A and B, sterigmatocystin, and zearalenone in cereals (Pol.). *Med. Weter.*, *32*, 617-619 [*Chem. Abstr.*, *86*, 54044m]

Juszkiewicz, T. & Piskorska-Pliszczynska, J. (1977) Occurrence of mycotoxins in mixed feeds and concentrates. *Med. Weter.*, *33*, 193-196

Kanisawa, M. & Suzuki, S. (1978) Induction of renal and hepatic tumors in mice by ochratoxin A, a mycotoxin. *Gann*, *69*, 599-600

Kanisawa, M., Suzuki, S., Kozuka, Y. & Yamazaki, M. (1977) Histopathological studies on the toxicity of ochratoxin A in rats. I. Acute oral toxicity. *Toxicol. appl. Pharmacol.*, *42*, 55-64

Kitchen, D.N., Carlton, W.W. & Tuite, J. (1977) Ochratoxin A and citrinin induced nephrosis in beagle dogs. II. Pathology. *Vet. Pathol.*, *14*, 261-272

Krogh, P. (1974) *Mycotoxin porcine nephropathy: A possible model for Balkan endemic nephropathy*. In: Puchlev, A., Dinev, I.V., Milev, B. & Doichinov, D., eds, *Endemic Nephropathy*, Sofia, Bulgarian Academy of Sciences, pp. 266-270

Krogh, P. (1976) Mycotoxic nephropathy. *Adv. vet. Sci. comp. Med.*, *20*, 147-170

Krogh, P. (1977) Ochratoxin A residues in tissues of slaughter pigs with nephropathy. *Nord. Vet. Med.*, *29*, 402-405

Krogh, P. (1978) Causal associations of mycotoxic nephropathy. *Acta pathol. microbiol. scand. A, Suppl. 269*

Krogh, P. & Nesheim, S. (1983) *Ochratoxin A*. In: Egan, H., Stoloff, L., Castegnaro, M., Scott, P., O'Neill, I.K. & Bartsch, H., eds, *Environmental Carcinogens. Selected methods of Analysis*, Vol. 5, *Mycotoxins (IARC Scientific Publications No. 44)*, Lyon, International Agency for Research on Cancer, pp. 247-253

Krogh, P., Hald, B. & Pedersen, E.J. (1973) Occurrence of ochratoxin A and citrinin in cereals associated with mycotoxic porcine nephropathy. *Acta pathol. microbiol. scand. sect. B.*, *81*, 689-695

Krogh, P., Hald, B., Englund, P., Rutqvist, L. & Swahn, O. (1974a) Contamination of Swedish cereals with ochratoxin A. *Acta pathol. microbiol. scand. sect. B.*, *82*, 301-302

Krogh, P., Hald, B., Gjertsen, P. & Myken, F., (1974b) Fate of ochratoxin A and citrinin during malting and brewing experiments. *Appl. Microbiol.*, *28*, 31-34

Kuczuk, M.H., Benson, P.M., Heath, H. & Hayes, A.W. (1978) Evaluation of the mutagenic potential of mycotoxins using *Salmonella typhimurium* and *Saccharomyces cerevisiae*. *Mutat. Res.*, *53*, 11-20

Kumagai, S. & Aibara, K. (1982) Intestinal absorption and secretion of ochratoxin A in the rat. *Toxicol. appl. Pharmacol.*, *64*, 94-102

Levi, C.P. (1975) Collaborative study of a method for the determination of ochratoxin A in green coffee. *J. Assoc. off. anal. Chem.*, *58*, 258-262

Levi, C.P., Trenk, H.L. & Mohr, H.K. (1974) Study of the occurrence of ochratoxin A in green coffee beans. *J. Assoc. off. anal. Chem.*, *57*, 866-870

Lillehoj, E.B., Kwolek, W.F., Elling, F. & Krogh, P. (1979) Tissue distribution of radioactivity from ochratoxin A-^{14}C in rats. *Mycopathologia*, *68*, 175-177

Mayura, K., Hayes, A.W. & Berndt, W.O. (1982) Teratogenicity of Ochratoxin A in rats (Abstract no. 263). *Toxicologist*, *2*, 74 van der Merwe, K.J., Steyn, P.S., Fourie, L., Scott, De B. & Theron, J.J. (1965a) Ochratoxin A, a toxic metabolite produced by *Aspergillus ochraceus* Wilh. *Nature, 205*, 1112-1113

van der Merwe, K.J., Steyn, P.S. & Fourie, L. (1965b) Mycotoxins. Part II. The constitution of ochratoxins A, B, and C, metabolites of *Aspergillus ochraceus* Wilh. *J. chem. Soc.*, 7083-7088

Moré, J. & Galtier, P. (1974) Toxicity of ochratoxin A. I. Embryotoxic and teratogenic effect in the rat (Fr.). *Ann. Rech. vét., 5*, 167-178

Moré, J. & Galtier, P. (1975) Toxicity of ochratoxin A. II. Effects of treatment on the progeny (F_1 and F_2) of poisoned rats (Fr.). *Ann. Rech. vét., 6*, 379-389

Moré, J. & Galtier, P. (1978) *Embryotoxic and teratogenic effects of ochratoxin A in rats.* In: *XIXth Morphological Congress Symposia*, Prague, Charles University, pp. 321-326

National Toxicology Program (1982) *Status of Ochratoxin A. Tox-TIPS*, February, Bethesda, MD, Toxicology Information Program, 69-5 - 69-6

Nesheim, S., Hardin, N.F., Francis, O.J. Jr & Langham, W.S. (1973) Analysis of ochratoxins A and B and their esters in barley using partition and thin layer chromatography. I. Development of the method. *J. Assoc. off. anal. Chem., 56*, 817-821

NIH/EPA Chemical Information System (1982) *Mass Spectral Search System*, Washington DC, CIS Project, Information Sciences Corporation

Osborne, B.G. (1980) The occurrence of ochratoxin in moldy bread and flour. *Food Cosmet. Toxicol., 18*, 615-617

Pavlovicé, M., Plestina, R. & Krogh, P. (1979) Ochratoxin A contamination of foodstuffs in an area with Balkan (endemic) nephropathy. *Acta pathol. microbiol. scand. sect. B., 87*, 243-246

Pepeljnjak, S. & Blazevicé, N. (1982) *Contamination with moulds and occurrence of ochratoxin A in smoked meat products from endemic nephropathy region of Yugoslavia.* In: *Fifth International IUPAC Symposium on Mycotoxins and Phycotoxins*, Vienna, Austrian Chemical Society, pp. 102-105

Peterson, R.E. & Ciegler, A. (1978) Ochratoxin A: Isolation and subsequent purification by high-pressure liquid chromatography. *Appl. environ. Microbiol., 36*, 613-614

Pitout, M.J. (1969) The hydrolysis of ochratoxin A by some proteolytic enzymes. *Biochem. Pharmacol., 18*, 485-491

Prior, M.G. (1976) Mycotoxin determinations on animal feedstuffs and tissues in Western Canada. *Can. J. comp. Med., 40*, 75-79

Prior, M.G. (1981) Mycotoxins in animal feedstuffs and tissues in Western Canada 1975 to 1979. *Can. J. comp. Med., 45*, 116-119

Purchase. I.F.H. & Theron, J.J. (1968) The acute toxicity of ochratoxin A to rats. *Food Cosmet. Toxicol.*, *6*, 479-483

Purchase, I.F.H. & van der Watt, J.J. (1971) The long-term toxicity of ochratoxin A to rats. *Food Cosmet. Toxicol.*, *9*, 681-682

Radovanovicé, Z. & Krajinovicé, S. (1979) The Balkan endemic nephropathy and urinary tract tumors. *Arch. Geschwultstforsch.*, *49*, 444-447

Roberts, J.C. & Woollven, P. (1970) Studies in mycological chemistry. Part XXIV. Synthesis of ochratoxin A, a metabolite of *Aspergillus ochraceus* Wilh. *J. chem. Soc. (C)*, 278-281

Roberts, B.A., Glancy, E.M. & Patterson, D.S.P. (1981) Rapid, economical method for determination of aflatoxin and ochratoxin in animal feedstuffs. *J. Assoc. off. anal. Chem.*, *64*, 961-963

Rutqvist, L., Björklund, N.-E., Hult, K., Hökby, E. & Carlsson, B. (1978) Ochratoxin A as the cause of spontaneous nephropathy in fattening pigs. *Appl. environ. Microbiol.*, *36*, 920-925

Schweighardt, H., Schuh, M., Abdelhamid, A.M., Böhm, J. & Leibetseder, J. (1980) Method for quantitative determination of ochratoxin A in foods and feeds by high-pressure liquid chromatography (HPLC) (Ger.). *Z. Lebensmittel. Untersuch. Forsch.*, *170*, 355-359

Scott, P.M., van Walbeek, W., Harwig, J. & Fennell, D.I. (1970) Occurrence of a mycotoxin, ochratoxin A, in wheat and isolation of ochratoxin A and citrinin producing strains of *Penicillium viridicatum. Can. J. Plant Sci.*, *50*, 583-585

Scott, P.M., van Walbeek, W., Kennedy, B. & Anyeti, D. (1972) Mycotoxins (ochratoxin A, citrinin, and sterigmatocystin) and toxigenic fungi in grains and agricultural products. *J. agric. Food Chem.*, *20*, 1103-1109

Shotwell, O.L., Hesseltine, C.W., Vandegraft, E.E. & Goulden, M.L. (1971) Survey of corn from different regions for aflatoxin, ochratoxin and zearalenone. *Cereal Sci. Today*, *16*, 266-273

Shotwell, O.L., Goulden, M.L. & Hesseltine, C.W. (1976) Survey of US wheat for ochratoxin and aflatoxin. *J. Assoc. off. anal. Chem.*, *59*, 122-124

Stark, A.-A. (1980) Mutagenicity and carcinogenicity of mycotoxins: DNA binding as a possible mode of action. *Ann. Rev. Microbiol.*, *34*, 235-262

Steyn, P.S. & Holzapfel, C.W. (1967) The synthesis of ochratoxins A and B, metabolites of *Aspergillus ochraceus* Wilh. *Tetratredron*, *23*, 4449-4461

Steyn, P.S., Vleggaar, R., Du Preez, N.P., Blyth, A.A. & Seegers, J.C. (1975) The *in vitro* toxicity of analogs of ochratoxin A in monkey kidney epithelial cells. *Toxicol. appl. pharmacol.*, *32*, 198-203

Still, P.E., Macklin, A.W., Ribelin, W.E. & Smalley, E.B. (1971) Relationship of ochratoxin A to foetal death in laboratory and domestic animals. *Nature*, *234*, 563-564

Stojanov, I.S., Stojchev, I.I., Nicolov, I.G., Draganov, I.V., Petkova-Bocharova, T.K. & Chernozemsky, I.N. (1977) Cancer mortality in a region with endemic nephropathy. *Neoplasma, 24,* 625-632

Støren, O., Helgerud, P., Holm, H. & Størmer, F.C. (1982) *Formation of (4R)-hydroxyochratoxin A and ochratoxin α from ochratoxin A by rats.* In: *Fifth International IUPAC Symposium on Mycotoxins and Phycotoxins,* Vienna, Austrian Chemical Society, pp. 321-324

Størmer, F.C., Hansen, C.E., Pedersen, J.I., Hvistendahl, G. & Aasen, A.J. (1981) Formation of (4R)- and (4S)-4-hydroxyochratoxin A from ochratoxin A by liver microsomes from various species. *Appl. environ. Microbiol., 42,* 1051-1056

Sugimoto, T., Minamisawa, M., Takano, K., Sasamura, Y. & Tsuruta, O. (1977) Detection of ochratoxin A, citrinin and sterigmatocystin from stored rice contaminated by a natural occurrence of *Penicillium viricatum* and *Aspergillus versicolor* (Jpn.). *Shokuhin Eiseigaku Zasshi, 18,* 176-181 [*Chem. Abstr., 87,* 166168g]

Szczech, G.M. & Hood, R.D. (1979) Necrosis produced in fetal mouse brain by transplacental exposure to the mycotoxin, ochratoxin A (Abstract no. 104). *Toxicol. appl. Pharmacol., 48,* A52

Szczech, G.M. & Hood, R.D. (1981) Brain necrosis in mouse fetuses tranplacentally exposed to the mycotoxin ochratoxin A. *Toxicol. appl. Pharmacol., 57,* 127-137

Szczech, G.M., Carlton, W.W. & Tuite, J. (1973) Ochratoxicosis in beagle dogs. II. Pathology. *Vet. Pathol., 10,* 219-231

Ueno, Y. & Kubota, K. (1976) DNA-attacking ability of carcinogenic micotoxins in recombination-deficient mutant cells of *Bacillus subtilis. Cancer Res., 36,* 445-451

Umeda, M., Tsutsui, T. & Saito, M. (1977) Mutagenicity and inducibility of DNA single-strand breaks and chromosome aberrations by various mycotoxins. *Gann, 68,* 619-625

Vesela, D., Vesely, D., Jelinek, S. & Kusak, V. (1978) Detection of ochratoxin in feed barley. *Vet. Med. (Prague), 23,* 431-436

van Walbeek, W., Scott, P.M., Harwig, J. & Lawrence, J.W. (1969) *Penicillium viridicatum* Westling: a new source of ochratoxin A. *Can. J. Microbiol., 15,* 1281-1285

Wehner, F.C., Thiel, P.G., van Rensburg, S.J. & Demasius, I.P.C. (1978) Mutagenicity to *Salmonella typhimurium* of some *Aspergillus* amd *Penicillium* mycotoxins. *Mutat. Res., 58,* 193-203

Windholz, M., ed. (1976) *The Merck Index,* 9th ed., Rahway, NJ, Merck & Co., Inc., p. 877

PETASITENINE

1. Chemical and Physical Data

1.1 Synonyms and trade names

Chem. Abstr. Services Reg. No.: 60102-37-6

Chem. Abstr. Name: 4,8-Secosenecionan-8,11,16-trione, 15,20-epoxy-15,20-dihydro-12-hydroxy-4-methyl-,(15β,20R)-

IUPAC Systematic Name: Petasitenine (neutral) or (1R,3'R,4R,6R,7R,11Z)-7-hydroxy-3',6,7,14-tetramethylspiro(2,9-dioxa-14-azabicyclo[9.5.1]heptadec-11-ene-4,2'-oxirane)-3,8,17-trione

Synonym: Fukinotoxin

1.2 Structural and molecular formulae and molecular weight

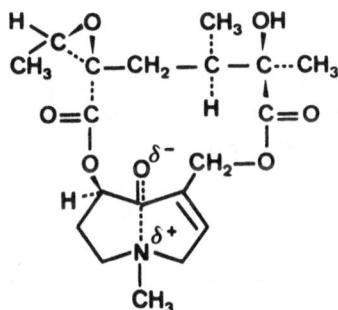

$C_{19}H_{27}NO_7$ Mol. wt: 380.4

1.3 Chemical and physical properties of the pure substance

From Furuya *et al.* (1976) and Yamada *et al.* (1976)

 (*a*) *Description:* Colourless crystals (recrystallized from acetone)

 (*b*) *Melting-point:* 129.0-131.0°C (recrystallisation from acetone)

 (*c*) *Optical rotation:* $[\alpha]_D^{19}$ + 44° (c 1.08 in ethanol)

 (*d*) *Spectroscopy data:* Infra-red, mass, nuclear magnetic resonance and X-ray spectral data have been determined.

 (*e*) *Solubility:* Soluble in methanol and water

 (*f*) *Stability:* Sensitive to hydrolysis by alkalis and to oxidation

1.4 Technical products and impurities

No technical product containing petasitenine is available.

2. Production, Use, Occurrence and Analysis

2.1 Production and use

 (*a*) *Production*

Petasitenine is not produced commercially. It can be isolated by extraction from *Petasites japonicus* Maxim. for use in biological evaluations (Yamada *et al.*, 1976). Preparations of *Petasites japonicus* Maxim. are commercially available in Japan and in the Federal Republic of Germany.

 (*b*) *Use*

The young flower stalks of *Petasites japonicus* Maxim., a kind of coltsfoot, have long been used in Japan as a food and as a herbal remedy, e.g., as a cough remedy, expectorant or stomachic (Hirono *et al.*, 1973).

2.2 Occurrence

Petasitenine is a naturally occurring pyrrolizidine alkaloid found in the herb *Petasites japonicus* Maxim. (*fukinotoh* in Japanese) of the tribe Senecioneae in the family Compositae [at a maximum concentration of 0.01%] (Hirono *et al.*, 1979).

2.3 Analysis

No data were available to the Working Group.

3. Biological Data Relevant to the Evaluation of Carcinogenic Risk to Humans

3.1 Carcinogenicity studies in animals

(a) Oral administration

Rat: A group of five male and six female ACI rats, one month old, were given drinking-water containing a 0.01% solution of petasitenine [purity unspecified], which was isolated from wild flower stalks of *Petasites japonicus* Maxim., dissolved in ethanol and diluted with distilled water. A group of 10 male and nine female controls were administered tap-water. The experiment was terminated 480 days after start of treatment, when all survivors were killed. Haemangioendothelial sarcomas of the liver developed in 5/10 treated rats, the first appearing 300-330 days after initiation of the experiment; four were in females. Liver-cell adenomas were observed in 5/10 animals, after latent periods of 150-180 days. No such tumour was observed in the matched control group or in a group of 266 historical controls (Hirono *et al.*, 1977).

(b) Carcinogenicity of plants containing petasitenine

Mouse: Groups of 20-24 male and 20-21 female ddN, Swiss and C57BL/6 mice, six weeks old, were fed a diet containing 4% of young flower stalks (dried and milled) of *Petasites japonicus* Maxim. for 480 days. Appropriate controls were also available. The experiment was terminated 480 days after the start of feeding, when all the survivors were killed. Lung adenomas and adenocarcinomas were found in 30/45 male and female ddN mice combined (compared with 1/50 in the respective controls.) No significant difference in tumour incidence was observed between treated Swiss and C57BL/6 mice and the corresponding controls (Fushimi *et al.*, 1978). [The Working Group noted that no data were given on the tumour incidence, separated by sex, in treated and control animals or on survival of controls.]

Rat: Groups of 11-12 male and 8-15 female ACI rats, one month old, received diets containing freshly dried, young flower stalks of wild *Petasites japonicus* Maxim. according to the following schedules: the first group received 4% in the diet until the termination of the study; a second group received the 4% diet for six months then, alternately, 8% for one week and a control diet for one week, until the end of the experiment; a third group received 1% in the diet until the end of the experiment. A group of 14 rats served as untreated controls. All survivors were killed 480 days after the start of treatment. Of the first group, 13/19 rats survived until the end of the experiment; 8 (6 males and 2 females) had haemangioendothelial sarcomas, 4 developed hepatocellular adenomas and 1 a hepatocellular carcinoma. Of the second group, 24/27 were still alive at the end of the experiment; 3 males developed haemangioendothelial sarcomas, 6 had hepatocellular adenomas and 2 had hepatocellular carcinomas. No liver tumour was observed in animals of the third group. No such tumour was observed in the untreated concurrent controls nor in another group of about 50 controls (Hirono *et al.*, 1973, 1975).

One group of 16 ACI rats [sex unspecified], one month old, received a diet containing 8% of flower stalks of cultivated *Petasites japonicus* Maxim. for 120 days. Another group of 30 rats received, alternately, the 8% diet for one week and a control diet for one week.

All experiments were terminated at 480 days. The flower stalks of cultivated *Petasites* induced much less hepatotoxicity than those of the wild type. However, 1/16 animals that received the 8% diet had a haemangioendothelial sarcoma of the liver. The same control groups as were used in the study above served as controls (Hirono *et al.*, 1975).

Hamster: A group of 13 male and 17 female Syrian golden hamsters, six weeks old, received a diet containing 4% of young flower stalks (dried and milled) of *Petasites japonicus* Maxim. for 480 days. All survivors were killed 480 days after the start of feeding. No significant difference in tumour incidence was observed between treated and control hamsters (Fushimi *et al.*, 1978).

3.2 Other relevant biological data

Reviews of the toxicology and pharmacology of pyrrolizidine alkaloids are available (McClean, 1970; Hirono, 1981; Culvenor, 1983); a general discussion of their metabolism and hepatotoxicity was published previously in the *IARC Monographs* series (IARC, 1976).

(a) *Experimental systems*

Toxic effects

A group of 3 ACI rats receiving 0.05% petasitenine in the drinking-water died or were moribund within 72 days after beginning treatment; all showed liver-cell necrosis, haemorrhage and proliferation of the bile duct (Hirono *et al.*, 1977). The flower stalks of cultivated *Petasites* induced much less hepatotoxicity than those of the wild type (Hirono *et al.*, 1975).

Effects on reproduction and prenatal toxicity

No data were available to the Working Group.

Absorption, distribution, excretion and metabolism

No data were available to the Working Group.

Mutagenicity and other short-term tests

Petasitenine induced mutations in *Salmonella typhimurium* TA100 when tested in the presence of polychlorinated biphenyl-induced rat or hamster liver 9000 x *g* supernatant mix, using a preincubation assay (Yamanaka *et al.*, 1979).

Petasitenine caused a significant increase in unscheduled DNA synthesis in rat hepatocytes (Williams *et al.*, 1980). It induced chromosomal aberrations and forward mutations to 8-azaguanine resistance in V79 Chinese hamster cells, the mutagenic effect being increased by the addition of phenobarbital-induced rat liver 9000 x *g* supernatant fraction (Takanashi *et al.*, 1980).

It was reported that petasitenine transforms cryopreserved hamster embryo cells (Hirono *et al.*, 1979). [No detail was provided.]

(b) *Humans*

No data specific to petasitenine were available to the Working Group.

3.3 Case reports and epidemiological studies of carcinogenicity in humans

No data were available to the Working Group.

4. Summary of Data Reported and Evaluation

4.1 Experimental data

Petasitenine isolated from young flower stalks of wild *Petasites japonicus* Maxim. was tested for carcinogenicity in rats by administration in the drinking-water; haemangioendothelial sarcomas of the liver and liver-cell adenomas were observed. Flower stalks of *Petasites japonicus* Maxim. were tested in mice, rats and hamsters by administration in the diet. They increased the incidence of lung adenomas and adenocarcinomas in mice of one strain and of haemangioendothelial sarcomas of the liver and of hepatocellular adenomas and hepatocellular carcinomas in rats. No increase in tumour incidence was observed in hamsters.

Petasitenine is mutagenic in bacteria and in mammalian cells *in vitro*. It also induced chromosomal aberrations, unscheduled DNA synthesis and transformation in mammalian cells *in vitro*. There is *sufficient evidence* that petasitenine is active in short-term tests.

No data were available to evaluate the teratogenicity of this compound to experimental animals.

4.2 Human data

Petasitenine is found in a plant species to which limited human exposure occurs from its use as a herbal remedy and as a food.

No data were available to evaluate the teratogenicity or chromosomal effects of this compound in humans.

No case report or epidemiological study of the carcinogenicity of petasitenine was available to the Working Group.

4.3 Evaluation

There is *limited evidence*[1] for the carcinogenicity of both petasitenine and flower stalks of *Petasites japonicus* Maxim. in experimental animals. In the absence of epidemiological data, no evaluation of the carcinogenicity of petasitenine to humans could be made.

---

[1]See preamble, p. 18.

5. References

Culvenor, C. (1983) Estimated intakes of pyrrolizidine alkaloids by humans. A comparison with dose rates causing tumours in rats. *J. Toxicol. environ. Health* (in press)

Furuya, T., Hikichi, M. & Iitaka, Y. (1976) Fukinotoxin, a new pyrrolizidine alkaloid from *Petasites japonicus. Chem. pharm. Bull.*, *24*, 1120-1122

Fushimi, K., Kato, K., Kato, T., Matsubara, N. & Hirono, I. (1978) Carcinogenicity of flower stalks of *Petasites japonicus* Maxim. in mice and Syrian golden hamsters. *Toxicol. Lett.*, *1*, 291-294

Hirono, I. (1981) Natural carcinogenic products of plant origin. *CRC crit. Rev. Toxicol.*, *8*, 235-277

Hirono, I., Shimizu, M., Fushimi, K., Mori, H. & Kato, K. (1973) Carcinogenic activity of *Petasites japonicus* Maxim., a kind of coltsfoot. *Gann*, *64*, 527-528

Hirono, I., Sasaoka, I., Shibuya, C., Shimizu, M., Fushimi, K., Mori, H., Kato, K. & Haga, M. (1975) Natural carcinogenic products of plant origin. *Gann Monogr.*, *17*, 205-217

Hirono, I., Mori, H., Yamada, K., Hirata, Y., Haga, M., Tatematsu, H. & Kanie, S. (1977) Brief communication: Carcinogenic activity of petasitenine, a new pyrrolizidine alkaloid isolated from *Petasites japonicus* Maxim. *J. natl Cancer Inst.*, *58*, 1155-1157

Hirono, I., Mori, H., Haga, J., Fujii, M., Yamada, K., Hirata, Y., Takanashi, H., Uchida, E., Hosaka, S., Ueno, I., Matsushima, T., Umezawa, K. & Shirai, A. (1979) *Edible plants containing carcinogenic pyrrolizidine alkaloids in Japan.* In: Miller, E.C., Miller, J.A., Hirono, I., Sugimura, T. & Takayama, S., eds, *Naturally Occurring Carcinogens-Mutagens and Modulators of Carcinogenesis*, Tokyo/Baltimore, Japan Scientific Societies Press/University Park Press, pp. 79-87

IARC (1976) *IARC Monographs on the Evaluation of Carcinogenic Risk of Chemicals to Man*, Vol. 10, *Some Naturally Occurring Substances*, Lyon, pp. 263-342

McLean, E.K. (1970) The toxic actions of pyrrolizidine (*Senecio*) alkaloids. *Pharmacol. Rev.*, *22*, 429-483

Takanashi, H., Umeda, M. & Hirono, I. (1980) Chromosomal aberrations and mutation in cultured mammalian cells induced by pyrrolizidine alkaloids. *Mutat. Res.*, *78*, 67-77

Williams, G.M., Mori, H., Hirono, I. & Nagao, M. (1980) Genotoxicity of pyrrolizidine alkaloids in the hepatocyte primary culture/DNA-repair test. *Mutat. Res.*, *79*, 1-5

Yamada, K., Tatematsu, H., Suzuki, M., Hirata, Y., Haga, M. & Hirono, I. (1976) Isolation and the structures of two new alkaloids, petasitenine and neopetasitenine from *Petasites japonicus* Maxim. *Chem. Lett.*, *5*, 461-464

Yamanaka, H., Nagao, M., Sugimura, T., Furuya, T., Shirai, A. & Matsushima, T. (1979) Mutagenicity of pyrrolizidine alkaloids in the *Salmonella*/mammalian-microsome test. *Mutat. Res.*, *68*, 211-216

QUERCETIN

1. Chemical and Physical Data

1.1 Synonyms and trade names

Chem. Abstr. Services Reg. No.: 117-39-5

Chem. Abstr. Name: 4H-1-Benzopyran-4-one, 2-(3,4-dihydroxyphenyl)-3,5,7-trihydroxy-

IUPAC Systematic Name: 3,3',4',5,7-Pentahydroxyflavone

Synonyms: C.I. 75670; C.I. Natural Red 1; C.I. Natural Yellow 10 & 13; cyanidenolon 1522; meletin; 3,5,7,3',4'-pentahydroxyflavone; quercetine; quercetol; quercitin; quertine; sophoretin; xanthaurine

1.2 Structural and molecular formulae and molecular weight

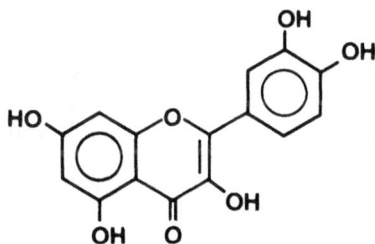

$C_{15}H_{10}O_7$

Mol. wt: 302.2

1.3 Chemical and physical properties of the pure substance

From Windholz (1976), unless otherwise specified

  (a) *Description*: Yellow needles recrystallized from dilute ethanol (dihydrate)

  (b) *Melting-point*: 314°C (dec.); dihydrate changes to anhydrous form at 95-97°C

  (c) *Spectroscopy data*: λ_{max} 258 nm, A_1^1 = 186; 375 nm, A_1^1 = 186

  (d) *Identiity and purity test*: Addition of sulphuric acid produces a yellow solution with a faint green fluorescence. Reduces ammoniacal silver nitrate in the cold, and Fehling's solution on heating (Anon., 1965).

  (e) *Solubility*: Practically insoluble in water; soluble in ethanol (3.4 g/l), boiling ethanol (43.5 g/l), acetic acid and aqueous alkaline solutions

  (f) *Reactivity*: A strong antioxidant and a metal chelator (Kühnau, 1976)

  (g) *Other properties*: Promotes the formation of nitrosamines (Walker *et al.*, 1982)

1.4 Technical products and impurities

No data were available to the Working Group.

2. Production, Use, Occurrence and Analysis

2.1 Production and use

  (a) *Production*

Quercetin is the aglycone of quercitrin, rutin and other glycosides, which were described in the literature as early as 1888 (Anon., 1965). It has been obtained for use as a natural colouring agent (Natural Yellow 10) by the rapid extraction of powdered quercitron bark with dilute ammonia and boiling of the extract with sulphuric acid (The Society of Dyers & Colourists, 1971a). It is apparently still made from such natural sources, although it can be made by chemical synthesis.

The first successful synthesis of quercetin was reported in 1962 (Shakhova *et al.*, 1962), in which treatment of 2-methoxyacetyl phloroglucinol with *O*-benzylvanillic acid anhydride in triethylamine and then with potassium hydroxide produced 5,7-dihydroxy-4'-benzyloxy-3,3'-dimethoxyflavone. The benzyl ether was cleaved with acetic acid-hydrochloric acid, and the methyl ethers were then cleaved with hydriodic acid to produce quercetin.

No data were available on the method or extent of US production, imports or exports.

Quercetin is produced from natural sources by two Japanese companies with an estimated annual production in recent years of about 20 kg.

Quercetin is believed to be produced by two companies in France and one company each in Spain and Switzerland. No information was available on whether the product is isolated from natural sources or synthesized.

(b) *Use*

No information was found on the present uses, if any, of quercetin, although Hawley (1981) reported that reaction of quercetin with epichlorohydrin could be used to produce epoxy resins, and Windholz (1975) reported that quercetin and its pentabenzyl ether were used in human medicine to decrease capillary fragility.

Quercetin and its glucosides are components of three natural dyes - C.I. Natural Red 1, C.I. Natural Yellow 10 and C.I. Natural Yellow 13 - which have apparently had some industrial use as textile dyes (The Society of Dyers & Colourists, 1971b).

In 1970, the US Food and Drug Administration withdrew its approval of drugs containing rutin, quercetin, hesperidin and any other bioflavonoid on the grounds that there was no substantial evidence that they had the effect that they were purported to have (US Food & Drug Administration, 1970).

2.2 Occurrence

Quercetin is widely distributed in the plant kingdom, where it occurs as a condensation product (a glycoside) with sugars (e.g., one of these, called rutin, is the 3-rhamnogluco-side of quercetin). Many fruits and other parts (e.g., seeds, bark, leaves, and wood) of plants contain these glycosides: *Allium ascalonicum, Allium cepa* (onion), *Allium porrum* (leek), *Anethum graveolens, Apium graveolens, Asperagus officinalis* (asparagus), *Brassica chinensis, Brassica napus, Brassica oleracae var. butrytis subvar. cymosa, Brassica oleraceae var. buttata, Brassica oleraceae var. captata, Brassica oleraceae var. gemmifera* (plants of cabbage and mustrard), *Capsicum annuum* (ornamental pepper), *Cichorium endivia* (endive), *Citrus paradisi* (grapefruit), *Fragaria ananassa, Humulus lupulus, Latuca sativa* (lettuce), *Malus pumila* (apple), *Malus silvestris, Mangifera indica* (mango), *Petroselinum crispum, Prunus armeniaca, Prunus avium, Prunus domestica* (European plum), *Raphanus sativus* (radish), *Rheum* spp, *Ribes* L., *Ribes nigrum* (blackcurrant), *Ribes grossularia, Rubus* L., *Rubus ideaus, Rumex acetosa, Sambuccus nigra* (elder), *Solanum tuberosum* (potato), *Solanum lycopersicum, Spinacea oleraceae* (spinach), *Vaccinium macrocarpum* (Vos-Stevenson, 1979). A chief source of rutin is the buckwheat plant *Fagopyrum esculentum* (Gennaro, 1975). Quercetin has been isolated from grapes, *Vitis vinifera* (1.4 mg/kg, fresh fruit), from leaves of the 'huckleberry', *Vaccinium myrtillus* (11 g/kg, dry weight, for quercetin and its glucosides), and from the leaves of *Rhododendron cinnabarinum* Hook (Williams & Wender, 1952; Ice & Wender, 1953; Rangaswami *et al.*, 1962). China tea, *Camellia sinensis*, has been reported to contain relatively large amounts of triglycosides of quercetin (Hainsworth, 1969). The total concentration of kaempferol and quercetin glycosides in tea [unspecified variety] is >10 000 mg/kg (Herrmann, 1976). This compound occurs in bracken fern (*Pteridium aquilinum*) (Pamukcu *et al.*, 1980).

Quercetin is a major component of C.I. Natural Yellow 10, an extract of powdered quercitron bark. It is also a minor component of Persian berries extract (C.I. Natural Yellow 13) and is found as a glucoside in gunar, the flowers of *Cedrela toona*, the toon or Indian mahogany tree (Natural Red 1) (The Society of Dyers & Colourists, 1971a).

Concentrations of quercetin in vegetables and fruit are given in Tables 1 and 2.

The concentration in onions varies widely depending on the type of onion. Those with coloured skins (*Allium cepa* L.) contain 25 000-65 000 mg/kg quercetin mainly as the aglycone; however, onions with white skins have only traces of flavonols, e.g., 10 mg/kg quercetin in dry skins. The quercetin concentration decreases from the outer to inner scales, with the highest levels in the outer epidermis (Herrmann, 1976).

Table 1. Concentration of quercetin as its glycoside in tissues of edible plants[a]

Plant	Concentration of quercetin (mg/kg)	
	Outer parts of tissues (skin, peel)	Remaining tissues
Apple	58-263	<1.0-2.0
Pear	28	<0.1
Quince	180	<0.01
Bell pepper (outer parts of tissues = 28% of fruit)	63	<1.0
Kohlrabi	7	<1.0
Scorzonera (salsify)	<1	<1.0
Potato (green)	47	~ 0.2
Asparagus (white tips)	0.3	<0.1
Tomato	Contains nearly the total flavonol content in the outer parts of the tissues, which were 4-5% of the fruit	
Cucumber	Contains traces of flavon(ol) glycosides only in the peel	

[a]From Herrmann (1976)

Table 2. Concentration of quercetin as its glycoside in leaves and other parts of edible plants[a]

Plant	Location	Concentration of quercetin (mg/kg)		
		Leaves	Other parts of the same plants	
Brussels sprout		50	Sprouts	25
Cauliflower		30	Curd	1
Kohlrabi	open air	25	Peel	7
			Flesh	<1
	greenhouse	<0.1	Flesh	<0.1
Kale	open air	50	--	
	greenhouse	35	--	
Small radish		0-30	Root	0-<0.1
Radish		35	Root	0
Rutabaga		40	Root	~ 0.1
Horseradish		50	Root	0
Scorzonera (salsify)		230	Root	<1
Potato		770-1000	Tuber	2
Tomato	open air	420	Fruit	7
	greenhouse	155	Fruit	2.5
Pea		1580-1590	Pods without seeds	125-130
			Seed	<1
Broad bean		1340	Pods without seeds	36
			Pod	19

[a]From Herrmann (1976)

2.3 Analysis

Quercetin has been separated from a crude plant extract by high-performance liquid chromatography (Becker *et al.*, 1979). The reaction of quercetin with vanadyl sulphate has been used as basis for a sensitive spectrophotometric method for estimation of quercetin, with a limit of detection of about 0.3 mg/l (Kaushal *et al.*, 1979). Gel filtration followed by ultra-violet spectroscopy is reported to offer another selective method for determination of quercetin at a level of 5 mg/l (Lattanzio & Marchesini, 1981).

3. Biological Data Relevant to the Evaluation of Carcinogenic Risk to Humans

3.1 Carcinogenicity studies in animals[1]

(a) Oral administration

Mouse: Thirty-eight male and 35 female ddY mice, six weeks old, were fed a diet containing 2% quercetin [purity unspecified] throughout their life span (842 days). A control group of 16 males and 15 females was fed a normal diet. Mortality was high: 44% of males and 47% of females in the control group and 58% of males and 37% of females in the experimental group. The incidence of tumours in experimental and control groups was not statistically different (Saito *et al.*, 1980).

Twenty-three male and 24 female strain A (A/JJms) mice, six to eight weeks old, were fed a diet containing 5% quercetin (purity, 99%) for 23 weeks, at which time the experiment was terminated. A control group of 21 males and 27 females was fed a basal diet only. No significant difference in the incidence or multiplicity of lung adenomas was seen in the two groups (Hosaka & Hirono, 1981). [The Working Group noted the short duration of the experiment.]

Rat: Three groups of non-inbred albino rats, bred from a local stock derived in 1930 from the Norwegian strain, 35 days old, were fed a basic grain diet (9 males and 10 females: controls) or a basal diet containing 0.1% quercetin (purity, > 99%) (7 males and 18 females), or a basal diet supplemented with 33% bracken fern as a positive control (8 males and 11 females), until termination of the experiment at 58 weeks. The incidences of intestinal and bladder tumours were as follows: controls - intestinal and bladder: 0/9 males, 0/10 females; quercetin-treated - intestinal: 6/7 males, 14/18 females [$p < 0.001$], bladder: 2/7 males, 3/18 females [$p > 0.05$]; bracken fern-treated - intestinal: 7/8 males, 10/11 females, bladder: 6/8 males, 8/11 females. The histopathology of intestinal and bladder tumours was identical for the two groups of treated rats. Multiple ileal tumours in quercetin-treated rats included 4 adenomas, 7 fibroadenomas and 9 adenocarcinomas (3 with mesenteric metastases). The 5 bladder tumours were transitional-cell carcinomas (Pamukcu *et al.*, 1980).

Three groups of ACI rats, 1-1.5 months old, were fed a diet containing 1% quercetin (purity, 99%) (10 males and 10 females; Group 1), or 5% quercetin (8 males and 9 females; Group 2) for 540 days, or 10% quercetin (20 males and 20 females; Group 3) for 850 days, at which time the experiment was terminated. Control groups (30 males and 22 females for Groups 1 and 2; 33 males and 33 females for Group 3) were fed a normal basal diet. In Group 1, 19/20 rats survived for more than 335 days, and 17 survived until the end of the experiment; all rats in Group 2 survived for more than 388 days, and 14 survived until the end of the experiment; and in Group 3, 37/40 rats survived for more than 349 days, and 27 for more than 600 days. There was no significant difference in the incidence of tumours between Groups 1 and 2 and controls; one caecal adenoma was observed in Group 2. No significant difference was observed in the incidence of any tumour in Group 3 and control animals; 3 male rats in Group 3 had 1 caecal adenoma and 2 caecal adenocarcinomas (Hirono *et al.*, 1981). [The Working Group noted that this strain of rats is sensitive to the carcinogenic effects of bracken fern (see Hirono *et al.*, 1970, 1972, 1973).]

---

[1]Several studies by oral or i.p. administration in mice and rats are in progress (IARC, 1981).

Fifteen male and 15 female Fischer 344 rats, 1.5 months old, were fed a diet containing 0.1% quercetin dihydrate (purity, 99%) for 540 days, at which time the experiment was terminated. A control group of 16 males and 16 females was fed a normal diet. All animals in the experimental group and all but two rats in the control group (1 male and 1 female) survived until the end of the experiment. There was no significant difference in the incidence of tumours between experimental and control groups; one treated rat had a jejunal adenocarcinoma (Takanashi et al., 1983).

Hamster: Twenty male and 20 female non-inbred golden hamsters, six weeks old, were fed a diet containing 10% quercetin dihydrate (purity, > 95%) for 735 days, at which time the experiment was terminated. A control group of 20 males and 20 females was fed the normal basal diet for the same period. By day 480, more than 70% of males and females in the experimental groups and of male controls, and 55% of females in the control group were still alive. There was no significant difference in the incidence of tumours between the experimental and control groups. A non-significant difference in tumour incidence was observed between hamsters fed a control diet and those fed a diet containing 4% quercetin for 709 days or a diet containing 1% quercetin for 351 days followed by basal diet for 350 days (Morino et al., 1982).

(b) Skin application

Mouse: Doses of 25 mg of a purified sample of quercetin in 0.1 ml dimethylsulphoxide were applied to the dorsal skin of 50 female ICR/Ha Swiss mice, six to eight weeks old, thrice weekly for 368 days, at which time the experiment was terminated. No skin tumour was induced (Van Duuren & Goldschmidt, 1976). [The Working Group noted the short period of observation.]

(c) Other experimental systems

Bladder implantation: A group of female albino Swiss mice weighing 40 g received purified cholesterol pellets weighing 20 mg and containing 4 mg purified quercetin by bladder implantation. A control group of female mice received similar sized pellets composed of cholesterol only. Mice surviving more than 175 days or up to one year, when the experiment was terminated, were evaluated for the presence of bladder tumours. Bladder carcinomas occurred in 10/46 (21.7%) of the quercetin-treated group and in 10/62 (16.1%) of the control group (p > 0.5) (Wang et al., 1976).

(d) Carcinogenicity of combinations containing quercetin

In skin painting experiments in mice, quercetin was shown to inhibit the carcinogenicity of various polycyclic aromatic hydrocarbons (Van Duuren & Goldschmidt, 1976; DiGiovanni et al., 1978; Slaga et al., 1978).

(e) Carcinogenicity of the 3-rhamnoglucoside of quercetin (rutin)

Rat: A group of 11 male and 10 female ACI rats, 1-1.5 months old, were fed a diet containing 5% rutin (a glycoside of quercetin; purity, 99.5%) for 540 days, at which time the experiment was terminated. A second group of 20 males and 20 females received a diet containing 10% rutin for 850 days. Groups of 30 males and 22 females and of 33 males and 33 females, respectively, were fed a normal diet and served as controls. Of the animals fed 5% rutin, 20/21 survived for more than 404 days and 15/21 until the end of the experiment; of those fed 10% rutin, 39/40 lived longer than 410 days and 26/40 more than 600 days. No significant difference in the incidence of tumours was observed between the two groups (p > 0.05) (Hirono et al., 1981).

Hamster: A group of 20 male and 20 female non-inbred golden hamsters, six weeks old, were fed a diet containing 10% rutin (>95% pure) for 735 days, at which time the experiment was terminated. A group of 20 males and 20 females fed a normal diet served as controls. Seventeen treated males survived for more than 480 days after the start of the experiment, and 14/20 females survived for more than 480 days. There was no significant difference between the incidence of tumours in the experimental and control groups (Morino et al., 1982).

3.2 Other relevant biological data

(a) Experimental systems

Toxic effects

The acute oral and s.c. $LD_{50}s$ of quercetin in the mouse are 160 and 100 mg/kg bw (Sullivan et al., 1951). Rabbits were unaffected by i.v. administration of 100 mg/kg bw or by the feeding of diets containing 1% quercetin for 410 days (Ambrose et al., 1952).

Quercetin is an inhibitor of Na^+-K^+ ATPase in both plasma and mitochondrial membranes (Lang & Racker, 1974; Suolinna et al., 1975). Inhibition of glucose oxidation in neutrophils via the hexosemonophosphate pathway and inhibition of uptake of 2-deoxyglucose were also reported (Long et al., 1981). Quercetin inhibited glycolysis in Erhlich ascites tumour cells. This effect is explained by a lowering of the intracellular pH through inhibition of lactate efflux (Belt et al., 1979). There was pronounced inhibition of growth of several cell lines by 5-20 μg/ml quercetin (Suolinna et al., 1975). Liposome-encapsulated quercetin inhibited DNA synthesis in Ehrlich ascites tumour cells (Podhajcer et al., 1980).

Concentrations of 0.005-1 mM quercetin inhibit hydroxylation of benzo[a]pyrene by human liver microsomes (Buening et al., 1981).

Effects on reproduction and prenatal toxicity

Pregnant Sprague-Dawley rats received oral doses of 0 (control), 2, 20, 200 or 2000 mg/kg bw quercetin on days 6-15 of gestation. There were no teratogenic effects attributable to the treatment (Willhite, 1982).

Absorption, distribution, excretion and metabolism

Autoradiographic analysis of a rat three hours after receiving a single oral dose of 2.3 mg/kg bw [4-^{14}C]-quercetin showed that, although most of the radioactivity remained in the digestive tract, it also occurred in blood, liver, kidney, lung and ribs. Following oral administration of 630 mg/kg bw of the labelled compound to rats, the radioactivity was excreted within 24 h, in expired carbon dioxide (34%), in bile (12%) and in urine (9%), and within 48 h in faeces (45%). Aproximately 60% of the radioactivity in the faeces was identified as unmetabolized quercetin. Sulphate and glycuronide conjugates of quercetin and of an unidentified flavonoid were found in bile and urine (Ueno *et al.*, 1983).

Following oral administration of 0.5 g/kg bw quercetin to rabbits, the main urinary metabolites were: 3,4-dihydroxyphenylacetic acid, 3-methoxy-4-hydroxyphenylacetic acid and 3-hydroxyphenylacetic acid (Booth *et al.*, 1956).

Incubation of [4-^{14}C]-quercetin with rat caecal and colon contents *in vitro* resulted in the release of 6% of the radioactivity as $^{14}CO_2$ (Ueno *et al.*, 1983).

Mutagenicity and other short-term tests

The genetic effects of quercetin and related flavonoids have been reviewed (Brown, 1980). (See also 'General Remarks on the Substances Considered', p. 34.) Quercetin was reported to give positive results in the *Escherichia coli* pol A$^-$/A$^+$ assay in the presence of a 9000 x *g* supernatant mix (details not given), but gave negative results in a *Bacillus subtilis rec* assay when tested without activation (Brown, 1980).

The mutagenicity of quercetin in the *Salmonella*/microsomal system has been established in strains TA1537, TA1538, TA98 and TA100, but no effect has been shown in TA1535 (Wang *et al.*, 1976; Bjeldanes & Chang, 1977; Brown *et al.*, 1977; Sugimura *et al.*, 1977; Hardigree & Epler, 1978; MacGregor & Jurd, 1978; Brown & Dietrich, 1979). It is a direct mutagen; however, the addition of a liver activation system increases the mutagenic effect (Brown, 1980)

Quercetin as well as most other flavonoids occur in plants as various glycosides, which are not mutagenic to *Salmonella*. The glycosides can be converted into the mutagenic aglycone by β-glycosidases, including those present in the intestinal flora (Brown, 1980). Hydrolysis of quercetin glycoside has been performed in the *Salmonella* test system by the addition of extract from rat caecal bacteria (Brown & Dietrich, 1979), hesperidinase, a crude extract from *Aspergillus niger* (Nagao *et al.*, 1979) and extracts from human faeces (Tamura *et al.*, 1980). The urine from rats treated orally or intraperitoneally with 1 g/kg bw quercetin was mutagenic to *S. typhimurium* strains TA98 and TA100 (MacGregor, 1979).

Following metabolic activation, quercetin increased reversion in *E. coli* of the frameshift *nad* allele; but no effect was observed on forward mutations at the *gal* locus or on reverse mutations at the *arg* locus (Hardigree & Epler, 1978). Quercetin also gave negative results in a forward mutation system measuring sporulation mutations in *B. subtilis* (MacGregor, 1979; MacGregor & Sacks, 1979).

Quercetin increased gene conversion at the tryptophan and adenine loci in *Saccharomyces cerevisiae*, strain D4. Tests on forward mutations to canavanine resistance and reverse mutations of *lys*, *his* and *hom* loci were negative with or without activation (Hardigree & Epler, 1978). Negative results with or without a 9000 x *g* supernatant have also been reported for strain D7, measuring mitotic crossing over, gene conversion and reverse mutations at the *ade*, *trp* and *ilv* loci (Brown, 1980; details not given).

Quercetin has been reported to cause a significant increase in the number of sex-linked recessive lethals in *Drosophila melanogaster* after feeding to adult males (Watson, 1982).

In V79 Chinese hamster cells, quercetin caused a dose-dependent increase in 8-azaguanine resistance, both with and without the addition of a rat liver 15 000 x g supernatant fraction (Maruta et al., 1979). However, van der Hoeven et al. (1982) reported in an abstract that they had found no increase in mutation induction at the HGPRT locus in V79 Chinese hamster cells, tested with or without rat liver 9000 x g supernatant mix, or in chick embryo hepatocytes. Quercetin induced forward mutations at the TK locus of L5178Y mouse lymphoma cells (Amacher et al., 1979; Meltz & MacGregor, 1981). Meltz and MacGregor (1981) reported that the addition of rat liver 9000 x g supernatant decreases the mutagenic effect; they also observed a dose-related increase in single-strand breaks in DNA. van der Hoeven et al. (1982), in an abstract, confirmed these results at the TK locus of L5178Y mouse lymphoma cells, but found no effect at the HGPRT locus.

Quercetin induced chromosomal aberrations in Chinese hamster fibroblasts, Chinese hamster ovary cells, human fibroblasts and polycyclic aromatic hydrocarbon-stimulated human lymphocytes (MacGregor et al., 1980; Yoshida et al., 1980; Stich et al., 1981). Sister chromatid exchanges were reported to be induced by quercetin in Chinese hamster fibroblasts, human fibroblasts, polycyclic aromatic hydrocarbon-stimulated human lymphocytes and human lymphoblastoid cells (Brown, 1980; Yoshida et al., 1980). It was reported in two abstracts that no sister chromatid exchange was induced in Chinese hamster ovary cells or in V79 Chinese hamster cells (Carver et al., 1981; van der Hoeven et al., 1982).

In-vitro morphological transformation occurs in exposed cryopreserved Syrian golden hamster embryo cells (Umezawa et al., 1977). Morphological transformation by quercetin was also suggested by results in Balb/c 3T3 cells (Meltz & MacGregor, 1981).

Quercetin given intraperitoneally to male Swiss mice at doses of 200 and 400 mg/kg bw caused a significant dose-related increase in micronuclei in bone-marrow erythrocytes (Sahu et al., 1981). [The Working Group noted the unexpectedly high frequency of micronuclei in monochromatic as compared to polychromatic erythrocytes in the treated series.] However, both MacGregor (1979) and Aeschbacher (1982) have reported that oral or i.p. administration of up to 1 g/kg bw gave negative results in the micronucleus test in mice.

The glycoside of quercetin, rutin (quercetin-3-rhamnoglucoside) gave negative results in the B. subtilis rec assay and in E. coli Sd-4-73 (Brown, 1980). After treatment with glycosidases, rutin was mutagenic in S. typhimurium TA100, TA1537 and TA98 (Brown & Dietrich, 1979; Nagao et al., 1981). No increase in the incidence of micronuclei was observed in bone-marrow erythrocytes of Swiss mice given i.p. injections of 100 or 200 mg/kg bw rutin (Sahu et al., 1981).

(b) Humans

Toxic effects

No data were available to the Working Group.

Effects on reproduction and prenatal toxicity

No data were available to the Working Group.

Absorption, distribution, excretion and metabolism

Following oral administration of a single dose of 4 g quercetin to human volunteers, neither quercetin nor its conjugates was detected in the blood or urine; 53% of the dose was recovered in the faeces within 72 hours. After a single i.v. injection of 100 mg quercetin, blood plasma levels declined biphasically, with half-lives of 8.8 min and 2.4 hours; protein binding exceeded 98%. In the urine, 0.65% of the i.v. dose was excreted as unchanged quercetin and 7.4% as a conjugate within nine hours; no further excretion occurred up to 24 hours (Gugler et al., 1975).

Mutagenicity and chromosomal effects

No data were available to the Working Group.

3.3 Case reports and epidemiological studies of carcinogenicity in humans

No data were available to the Working Group.

4. Summary of Data Reported and Evaluation

4.1 Experimental data

Quercetin has been tested for carcinogenicity in mice, rats and hamsters in several experiments by administration in the diet and in mice by skin application and urinary bladder implantation. Increased incidences of ileal and urinary bladder carcinomas were observed in only one experiment in rats fed quercetin, whereas several other experiments, using the same or higher doses, do not provide evidence of a carcinogenic effect.

The 3-rhamnoglucoside of quercetin (rutin) was tested in rats and hamsters by administration in the diet. No evidence of carcinogenicity was found.

Quercetin is mutagenic in bacteria and insects and caused gene conversion in yeast. Equivocal results were obtained with respect to mutations in mammalian cells *in vitro*. It induced chromosomal anomalies in cultured cells, but equivocal results were obtained in the micronucleus test *in vivo*. Quercetin induced morphological transformation of hamster embryo cells *in vitro*. There is *sufficient evidence* that quercetin is active in short-term tests.

In one experiment with rats, no teratogenic effect was seen.

4.2 Human data

The natural occurrence of quercetin in fruit and other edible plants results in wide human exposure to this compound.

No data were available to evaluate the teratogenicity or chromosomal effects of this compound in humans.

No case report or epidemiological study of the carcinogenicity of quercetin was available to the Working Group.

4.3 Evaluation

Results from one experiment in rats provide *limited evidence*[1] for the carcinogenicity of quercetin in experimental animals. In the absence of epidemiological data, no evaluation of the carcinogenicity of quercetin to humans could be made.

5. References

Aeschbacher, H.U. (1982) *The significance of mutagens in food.* In: Sorsa, M. & Vainio, H., eds, *Mutagens in Our Environment*, New York, Alan R. Liss, Inc., pp. 349-362

Amacher, D.E., Paillet, S. & Ray, V.A. (1979) Point mutations at the thymidine kinase locus in L5178Y mouse lymphoma cells. I. Application to genetic toxicological testing. *Mutat. Res., 64*, 391-406

Ambrose, A.M., Robbins, D.J. & DeEds, F. (1952) Comparative toxicities of quercetin and quercitrin. *J. Am. pharm. Assoc., 41*, 119-122

Anon. (1965) *Dictionary of Organic Compounds*, Vol. 5, New York, Oxford University Press, pp. 2832, 2833

Becker, H., Exner, J. & Bingler, T. (1979) Comparative investigation of polyamides DC11- and RP-2-, RP-8- and RP-18-layers for separation of methylated quercetin derivatives (Ger.). *J. Chromatogr., 172*, 420-423

Belt, J.A., Thomas, J.A., Buchsbaum, R.N. & Racker, E. (1979) Inhibition of lactate transport and glycolysis in Ehrlich ascites tumor cells by bioflavonoids. *Biochemistry, 18*, 3506-3511

Bjeldanes, L.F. & Chang, G.W. (1977) Mutagenic activity of quercetin and related compounds. *Science, 197*, 577-578

Booth, A.N., Murray, C. W., Jones, F.T. & DeEds, F. (1956) The metabolic fate of rutin and quercetin in the animal body. *J. biol. Chem., 223*, 251-257

---

[1]See preamble, p. 18.

Brown, J.P. (1980) A review of the genetic effects of naturally occurring flavonoids, anthraquinones and related compounds. *Mutat. Res.*, *75*, 243-277

Brown, J.P. & Dietrich, P.S. (1979) Mutagenicity of plant flavonols in the *Salmonella*/mammalian microsome test. Activation of flavonol glycosides by mixed glycosidases from rat cecal bacteria and other sources. *Mutat. Res.*, *66*, 223-240

Brown, J.P., Dietrich, P.S. & Brown, R.J. (1977) Frameshift mutagenicity of certain naturally occurring phenolic compounds in the *Salmonella*/microsome test: Activation of anthraquinone and flavonol glycosides by gut bacterial enzymes. *Biochem. Soc. Trans.*, *5*, 1489-1492

Buening, M.K., Chang, R.L., Huang, M.-T., Fortner, J.G., Wood, A.W. & Conney, A.H. (1981) Activation and inhibition of benzo(a)pyrene and aflatoxin B_1 metabolism in human liver microsomes by naturally occurring flavonoids. *Cancer Res.*, *41*, 67-72

Carver, J.H., Carrano, A.V. & MacGregor, J.T. (1981) Genetic effects of galangin, kaempferol, and quercetin in Chinese hamster ovary cells *in vitro* (Abstract no. Eb-2). *Environ. Mutagenesis*, *3*, 383

DiGiovanni, J., Slaga, T.J., Viaje, A., Berry, D.L., Harvey, R.G. & Juchau, M.R. (1978) Effects of 7,8-benzoflavone on skin tumor-initiating activities of various 7- and 12-substituted derivatives of 7,12-dimethylbenz[a]anthracene in mice. *J. natl Cancer Inst.*, *61*, 135-140

Gennaro, A.R. (1975) *Natural products*. In: Osol, A., ed., *Remington's Pharmaceutical Sciences*, 15th ed., Easton, PA, Mack Publishing Co., pp. 416-422

Gugler, R., Leschik, M. & Dengler, H.J. (1975) Disposition of quercetin in man after single oral and intravenous doses. *Eur. J. clin. Pharmacol.*, *9*, 229-234

Hainsworth, E. (1969) *Tea*. In: Kirk, R.F. & Othmer, D.F., eds, *Encyclopedia of Chemical Technology*, 2nd ed., Vol. 19, New York, John Wiley & Sons, pp. 743, 755

Hardigree, A.A. & Epler, J.L. (1978) Comparative mutagenesis of plant flavonoids in microbial systems. *Mutat. Res.*, *58*, 231-239

Hawley, G.G. (1981) *The Condensed Chemical Dictionary*, New York, Van Nostrand Reinhold Company, p. 878

Herrmann, K. (1976) Flavonols and flavones in food plants; A review. *J. Food Technol.*, *11*, 433-448

Hirono, I., Shibuya, C., Fushimi, K. & Haga, M. (1970) Studies on carcinogenic properties of bracken, *Pteridium aquilinum*. *J. natl Cancer Inst.*, *45*, 179-188

Hirono, I., Shibuya, C., Shimizu, M. & Fushimi, K. (1972) Carcinogenic activity of processed bracken used as human food. *J. natl Cancer Inst.*, *48*, 1245-1250

Hirono, I., Fushimi, K., Mori, H., Miwa, T. & Haga, M. (1973) Comparative study of carcinogenic activity in each part of bracken. *J. natl Cancer Inst.*, *50*, 1367-1371

Hirono, I., Ueno, I., Hosaka, S., Takanashi, H., Matsushima, T., Sugimura, T. & Natori, S. (1981) Carcinogenicity examination of quercetin and rutin in ACI rats. *Cancer Lett.*, *13*, 15-21

van der Hoeven, J.C.M., Debets, F.M.H., Bruggeman, I.M., Van Erp, I.H.M., Rutgers, M. & Koeman, J.H. (1982) *Evaluation of the genotoxicity of some mutagenic compounds of plant origin in in vitro mammalian test systems (Abstract).* In: Donner, M. & Hytönen, S., eds, *Proceedings of the 12th Annual Meeting of European Environmental Mutagen Society, Espoo, Finland* (Abstracts), Helsinki, Institute of Occupational Health

Hosaka, S. & Hirono, I. (1981) Carcinogenicity test of quercetin by pulmonary-adenoma bioassay in strain A mice. *Gann, 72*, 327-328

IARC (1981) *Information Bulletin on the Survey of Chemicals Being Tested for Carcinogenicity*, No. 9, Lyon, pp. 77, 83, 123

Ice, C.H. & Wender, S.H. (1953) Quercetin and its glycosides in leaves of *Vaccinium myrtillus. J. Am. chem. Soc., 75*, 50-52

Kaushal, G.P., Sekhon, B.S. & Bhatia, I.S. (1979) Spectrophotometric determination of quercetin with VO^{2+}. *Mikrochim. Acta, 1*, 365-370

Kühnau, J. (1976) The flavonoids. A class of semi-essential food components: Their role in human nutrition. *World Rev. Nutr. Diet, 24*, 117-191

Lang, D.R. & Racker, E. (1974) Effects of quercetin and F_1 inhibitor on mitochondrial ATPase and energy-linked reactions in submitochondrial particles. *Biochim. biophys. Acta, 333*, 180-186

Lattanzio, V. & Marchesini, A. (1981) Determination of plant phenols by gel filtration. *J. Food Sci., 46*, 1907-1909, 1917

Long, G.D., DeChatelet, L.R., O'Flaherty, J.T., McCall, C.E., Bass, D.A., Shirley, P.S. & Parce, J.W. (1981) Effects of quercetin on magnesium-dependent adenosine triphosphatase and the metabolism of human polymorphonuclear leukocytes. *Blood, 57*, 561-566

MacGregor, J.T. (1979) Mutagenicity studies of flavonoids *in vivo* and *in vitro* (Abstract no. 94). *Toxicol. appl. Pharmacol., 48*, A47

MacGregor, J.T. & Jurd, L. (1978) Mutagenicity of plant flavonoids: Structural requirements for mutagenic activity in *Salmonella typhimurium. Mutat. Res., 54*, 297-309

MacGregor, J.T. & Sacks, L.E. (1979) The *Bacillus subtilis* multi-gene sporulation test: Sensitivity to known mutagens and carcinogens (Abstract no. 3). *Environ. Mutagenesis, 1*, 121

MacGregor, J.T., Carrano, A.V. & Carver, J.H. (1980) Genetic effects of flavonols in Chinese hamster ovary (CHO) cells *in vitro*, and in rabbit lymphocytes and mouse erythroblasts *in vivo* (Abstract no. 4). *Environ. Mutagenesis, 2*, 231

Maruta, A., Enaka, K. & Umeda, M. (1979) Mutagenicity of quercetin and kaempferol on cultured mammalian cells. *Gann, 70*, 273-276

Meltz, M.L. & MacGregor, J.T. (1981) Activity of the plant flavanol quercetin in the mouse lymphoma L5178Y TK$^{+/-}$ mutation, DNA single-strand break, and Balb/c 3T3 chemical transformation assays. *Mutat. Res., 88*, 317-324

Morino, K., Matsukura, N., Kawachi, T., Ohgaki, H., Sugimura, T. & Hirono, I. (1982) Carcinogenicity test of quercetin and rutin in golden hamsters by oral administration. *Carcinogenesis, 3*, 93-97

Nagao, M., Takahashi, Y., Yamanaka, H. & Sugimura, T. (1979) Mutagens in coffee and tea. *Mutat. Res., 68*, 101-106

Nagao, M., Morita, N., Yahagi, T., Shimizu, M., Kuroyanagi, M., Fukuoka, M., Yoshihira, K., Natori, S., Fugino, T. & Sugimura, T. (1981) Mutagenicity of 61 flavonoids and 11 related compounds. *Environ. Mutagenesis, 3*, 401-419

Pamukcu, A.M., Yalciner, S., Hatcher, J.F. & Bryan, G.T. (1980) Quercetin, a rat intestinal and bladder carcinogen present in bracken fern (*Pteridium aquilinum*). *Cancer. Res., 40*, 3468-3472

Podhajcer, O.L., Friedlander, M. & Graziani, Y. (1980) Effect of liposome-encapsulated quercetin on DNA synthesis, lactate production, and cyclic adenosine 3':5'-monophosphate level in Ehrlich ascites tumor cells. *Cancer Res., 40*, 1344-1350

Rangaswami, S., Sambamurthy, K. & Mallayga Sastry, K. (1962) Chemical examination of the leaves of *Rhododendron cinnabarinum*. *Proc. Indian Acad. Sci. Sect. A, 56*, 239-24I [*Chem. Abstr., 58*, 9413h]

Sahu, R.K., Basu, R. & Sharma, A. (1981) Genetic toxicological testing of some plant flavonoids by the micronucleus test. *Mutat. Res., 89*, 69-74

Saito, D., Shirai, A., Matsushima, T., Sugimura, T. & Hirono, I. (1980) Test of carcinogenicity of quercetin, a widely distributed mutagen in food. *Teratog. Carcinog. Mutagenesis, 1*, 213-221

Shakhova, M.K., Samokhvalov, G.I. & Preobrazhenskii, N.A. (1962) Synthetic studies of flavonoids. III. Total synthesis of quercetin 3β-rutinoside, rutin. *Zh. Obshch. Khim., 32*, 390-396 [*Chem. Abstr., 58*, 1426e]

Slaga, T.J., Bracken, W.M., Viaje, A., Berry, D.L., Fischer, S.M. & Miller, D.R. (1978) Lack of involvement of 6-hydroxymethylation in benzo[a]pyrene skin tumor initiation in mice. *J. natl Cancer Inst., 61*, 451-455

The Society of Dyers & Colourists (1971a) *Colour Index*, 3rd ed., Vol. 4, Bradford, Yorkshire, Lund Humphries, p. 4636

The Society of Dyers & Colourists (1971b) *Colour Index*, 3rd ed., Vol. 3, Bradford, Yorkshire, Lund Humphries, pp. 3229, 3230, 3235

Stich, H.F., Stich, W. & Lam, P.P.S. (1981) Potentiation of genotoxicity by concurrent application of compounds found in betel quid: arecoline, engenol, quercetin, chlorogenic acid and Mn^{2+}. *Mutat. Res.*, *90*, 355-363

Sugimura, T., Nagao, M., Matsushima, T., Yahagi, T., Seino, Y., Shirai, A., Sawamura, M., Natori, S., Yoshihira, K., Fukuoka, M. & Kuroyanagi, M. (1977) Mutagenicity of flavone derivatives. *Proc. Jpn. Acad. Ser. B*, *53*, 194-197

Sullivan, M., Follis, R.H., Jr & Hilgartner, M. (1951) Toxicology of podophyllin. *Proc. Soc. exp. Biol. Med.*, *77*, 269-272

Suolinna, E.-M., Buchsbaum, R.N. & Racker, E. (1975) The effect of flavonoids on aerobic glycolysis and growth of tumor cells. *Cancer Res.*, *35*, 1865-1872

Takanashi, H., Aiso, S., Hirono, I., Matsushima, T. & Sugimura, T. (1983) Carcinogenicity test of quercetin and kaempferol in rats by oral administration. *J. Food Saf.* (in press)

Tamura, G., Gold, C., Ferro-Luzzi, A. & Ames, B.N. (1980) Fecalase: A model for activation of dietary glycosides to mutagens by intestinal flora. *Proc. natl Acad. Sci. USA*, *77*, 4961-4965

Ueno, I., Nakano, N. & Hirono, I. (1983) Metabolic fate of [^{14}C]quercetin in the ACI rat. *Jpn. J. exp. Med.* (in press)

Umezawa, K., Matsushima, T., Sugimura, T., Hirakawa, T., Tanaka, M., Katoh, Y. & Takayama, S. (1977) *In vitro* transformation of hamster embryo cells by quercetin. *Toxicol. Lett.*, *1*, 175-178

US Food & Drug Administration (1970) Drugs containing rutin, quercetin, hesperidin, or any other bioflavonoids. *Fed. Regist.*, *35*, 10872, 10873, 16332

Van Duuren, B.L. & Goldschmidt, B.M. (1976) Cocarcinogenic and tumor-promoting agents in tobacco carcinogenesis. *J. natl Cancer Inst.*, *56*, 1237-1242

Vos-Stevenson, H. (1979) *Mutagene Plantenmetabolieten; van Nature in Plantaardige Voedingsmiddelen Voorkomende Mutagenen* [*Mutagenic Plant Metabolites; Naturally Occurring Mutagens in Foods of Plant Origin*], Thesis

Walker, E.A., Pignatelli, B. & Friesen, M. (1982) The role of phenols in catalysis of nitrosamine formation. *J. Sci. Food Agric.*, *33*, 81-88

Wang, C.Y., Chiu, C.W., Pamukcu, A.M. & Bryan, G.T. (1976) Identification of carcinogenic tannin isolated from bracken fern (*Pteridium aquilinum*). *J. natl Cancer Inst.*, *56*, 33-36

Wang, C.Y., Pamucku, A.M. & Bryan, G.T. (1976) *Bracken fern a naturally-occurring carcinogen*. In: Stock, C.C., Santamaria, L., Mariani, P. & Gorin, S., eds, *Ecological Perspectives on Carcinogens and Cancer Control* (*Médecine Biologie Environnement 4*), Basel, Karger, pp. 565-572

Watson, W.A.F. (1982) The mutagenic activity of quercetin and kaempferol in *Drosophila melanogaster*. *Mutat. Res.*, *103*, 145-147

Willhite, C.C. (1982) Teratogenic potential of quercetin in the rat. *Food Chem. Toxicol.*, *20*, 75-79

Williams, B.L. & Wender, S.H. (1952) The isolation and identification of quercetin and isoquercitrin from grapes (*Vitis vinifera*). *J. Am. chem. Soc.*, *74*, 4372-4373

Windholz, M., ed. (1975) *The Merck Index*, 9th ed., Rahway, NJ, Merck & Co., Inc., p. 1043

Yoshida, M.A., Sasaki, M., Sugimura, K. & Kawachi, T. (1980) Cytogenetic effects of quercetin on cultured mammalian cells. *Proc. Jpn. Acad. Ser. B*, *56*, 443-447

SENKIRKINE

This substance was considered by a previous Working Group, in October 1975 (IARC, 1976a). Since that time, new data have become available, and these have been incorporated into the monograph and taken into consideration in the present evaluation.

1. Chemical and Physical Data

1.1 Synonyms and trade names

Chem. Abstr. Services Reg. No.: 2318-18-5

Chem. Abstr. Name: 4,8-Secosenecionan-8,11,16-trione, 12-hydroxy-4-methyl-

IUPAC Systematic Name: Senkirkine (neutral); renardine (neutral) or (1R,4Z,6R,7R,11Z)-4-ethylidene-7-hydroxy-6,7,14-trimethyl-2,9-dioxa-14-azabicyclo[9.5.1]heptadec-11-ene-3,8,17-trione

Synonyms: *trans*-15-Ethylidene-12β-hydroxy-4,12α,13β-trimethyl 8-oxo-4,8 secosenec-1-enine; NSC-89945; renardin; renardine; senkirkin

1.2 Structural and molecular formulae and molecular weight

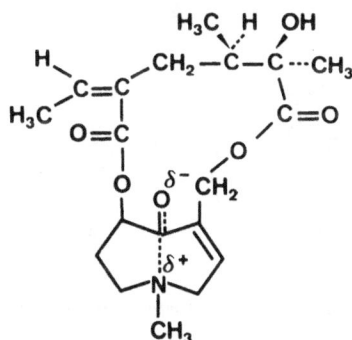

$C_{19}H_{27}NO_6$

Mol. wt: 365.4

1.3 Chemical and physical properties of the pure substance

From Briggs *et al.* (1965)

(a) *Description*: Colourless plates recrystallized from ethyl acetate or acetone

(b) *Melting-point*: 196.5-197.5°C

(c) *Optical rotation*: $[\alpha]_b^{25}$ -16° $\pm$ 1° (c = 1.89 in methanol); $[a]_b^{23}$ - 19° $\pm$ 1° (c = 1.33 in ethanol)

(d) *Spectroscopy data*: λ_{max} 219 nm (A_1^1 = 287)

(e) *Solubility*: Readily soluble in chloroform and ethyl acetate; less soluble in acetone, benzene, ethanol and water

(f) *Stability*: Stable at room temperature in closed containers; for lengthy periods, it is best stored under nitrogen at -15°C. Readily hydrolysed by alkali; sensitive to air oxidation

1.4 Technical products and impurities

No data were available to the Working Group.

2. Production, Use, Occurrence and Analysis

2.1 Production and use

(a) *Production*

Senkirkine, a macrocyclic pyrrolizidine alkaloid, was isolated from plant material under the name of 'renardine' (Danilova & Konovalova, 1950; Danilova *et al.*, 1961). The alkaloid was also investigated by Briggs *et al.* (1948, 1965), who gave it the name senkirkine. When the structure was elucidated in 1965, it was found that the structures of renardine and senkirkine were identical.

Senkirkine can be obtained by extraction from various parts of dried or fresh *Senecio kirkii*; the crude extract is subsequently purified by column chromatography and crystallization to give the pure alkaloid (Briggs *et al.*, 1965).

Senkirkine is not produced commercially.

(b) Use

Farfugium japonicum, in which senkirkine occurs, is used in Japanese folk medicine for treatment of suppuration and eczema (Furuya *et al.*, 1971). *Petasites japonicus*, in which senkirkine occurs, is used both as a food and herbal remedy.

The dried flowering shoots, leaves and roots of *Tussilago farfara* are used in Europe in anti-irritants for the relief of coughs and chest complaints (Wade, 1977; Borka & Onshuus, 1979); and the young flowers, which have been shown to contain senkirkine, are used medicinally in the People's Republic of China and Japan (Culvenor *et al.*, 1976). *Tussilago farfara* is also used in cleansing gels and shampoos.

2.2 Occurrence

Senkirkine occurs in several species of the tribe *Senecioneae* (family Compositae), including *Brachyglottis repanda* Forst. et Forst. F.; *Petasites laevigatis* (Willd.) Reichenb. [*Nardosmia laevigata* (Willd.) DC.]; *Senecio kirkii* Hook. f. ex Kirk; *S. kleinia* Sch. Bip.; *S. renardii* Winkl. (Smith & Culvenor, 1981); *S. antieuphorbium* (L.) Sch. Bip. (Rodrigues & Gonzáles, 1971); *S. procerus* L. (Jovceva *et al.*, 1978); *S. jacobaea* L. (Smith & Culvenor, 1981); *S. vernalis* (Röder *et al.*, 1979); *Farfugium japonicum* Kitam. (Furuya *et al.*, 1971); *Petasites japonicus* Maxim. (1 mg/kg based on the weight of the dried plant) (Yamada *et al.*, 1978); and *Tussilago farfara* (Culvenor *et al.*, 1976). It also occurs in *Crotalaria laburnifolia* L. subsp. *eldomae* (family *Leguminosae*) (Crout, 1972); and *Syneilesis palmata* Maxim. (Smith & Culvenor, 1981).

Senkirkine has been found to be the only pyrrolizidine alkaloid present in *Tussilago farfara* (0.15 g/kg) (Culvenor *et al.*, 1976).

2.3 Analysis

The analysis of pyrrolizidine alkaloids such as senkirkine in plant material can be accomplished by separation of the alkaloids and estimation of the amount by thin-layer, paper or gas chromatography (Chalmers *et al.*, 1965; Mattocks, 1967).

More recently described methods for analysing senkirkine make use of gas chromatography (Röder *et al.*, 1979; Wiedenfeld *et al.*, 1981) and high-performance liquid chromatography (Qualls & Segall, 1978; Tittel *et al.*, 1979). A method has been developed specifically for senkirkine in plant material, using a combination of gas chromatography and mass spectrometry (Borka & Onshuus, 1979). The limit of detection is approximately 5 mg/kg.

3. Biological Data Relevant to the Evaluation of Carcinogenic Risk to Humans

3.1 Carcinogenicity studies in animals

(a) Intraperitoneal administration

Rat: A group of 20 male inbred ACI rats, 1-1.5 months old, received i.p. injections of 22 mg/kg bw (10% of the LD_{50}) senkirkine [extracted from dried milled buds of coltsfoot (*Tussilago farfara* L.); purity unspecified] dissolved in physiological saline twice a week for four weeks and then once a week for 52 weeks. A control group of 20 male rats was given i.p. injections of physiological saline (0.1 ml/100 g bw) by the same injection schedule. The experiment was terminated 650 days after initiation of injections. All rats in the experimental group survived for more than 290 days after the start of injections; 9/20 rats developed liver-cell adenomas. No liver tumour was observed in the control group [p < 0.005] (Hirono *et al.*, 1979a,b).

(b) Carcinogenicity of plants containing senkirkine

Rat: A group of 6 male and 6 female ACI rats, 1.5 months old, were fed a diet containing 32% coltsfoot buds (*Tussilago farfara* L.) for four days and subsequently a diet containing 16% coltsfoot until the end of the experiment (Group 1). Groups of 5 male and 5 female rats (Group 2) and 6 males and 5 females (Group 3) were fed diets containing 8% and 4% coltsfoot, respectively, for 600 days, at which time the experiment was terminated. A group of 8 males and 8 females fed a normal diet served as controls. All the rats in Group 1 survived longer than 380 days after the start of feeding, and 8/12 rats developed haemangioendothelial sarcomas. In Group 2, all but one animal survived longer than 420 days, 1/10 rats developed a haemangioendothelial sarcoma. No liver tumour was observed in Group 3 or in control animals. The incidence of liver tumours in Group 1 was significantly higher than that in the control group [p < 0.001] (Hirono *et al.*, 1976).

3.2 Other relevant biological data

The toxicology and pharmacology of pyrrolizidine alkaloids have been reviewed (McClean, 1970; Hirono, 1981; Culvenor, 1983); a general discussion of their metabolism and hepatotoxicity was published previously in the *IARC Monographs* series (IARC, 1976b).

(a) Experimental systems

Toxic effects

The i.p. LD_{50} of senkirkine in rats has been reported to be 220 mg/kg bw (Hirono *et al.*, 1979a,b).

Weanling rats [numbers unspecified] given >300 mg/kg bw senkirkine by stomach tube died within a few days; those surviving had lesions in the liver typical of those induced by pyrrolizidine alkaloids (Schoental, 1970).

Effects on reproduction and prenatal toxicity

No data were available to the Working Group.

Absorption, distribution, excretion and metabolism

No data specific to senkirkine were available to the Working Group.

Mutagenicity and related short-term tests

Senkirkine induced mutations in *Salmonella typhimurium* strain TA100 in the presence of polychlorinated biphenyl-induced rat or hamster liver 9000 x *g* supernatant mix, in a preincubation assay (Yamanaka *et al.*, 1979).

Senkirkine caused a significant increase in unscheduled DNA synthesis in rat hepatocytes (Williams *et al.*, 1980).

It induced chromosomal aberrations and forward mutations to 8-azaguanine resistance in V79 Chinese hamster cells. The mutagenicity was increased by the addition of a phenobarbital-induced rat liver 9000 x *g* supernatant fraction (Takanashi *et al.*, 1980).

It was reported that senkirkine does not transform cryopreserved hamster embryo cells (Hirono *et al.*, 1979b) [details not given].

(*b*) Humans

No data specific to senkirkine were available to the Working Group.

3.3 Case reports and epidemiological studies of carcinogenicity in humans

No data were available to the Working Group.

4. Summary of Data Reported and Evaluation

4.1 Experimental data

Senkirkine was tested for carcinogenicity in male rats by intraperitoneal administration; it significantly increased the incidence of liver-cell adenomas. In rats fed the herb *Tussilago farfara* L., which has been shown to contain senkirkine as the only pyrrolizidine alkaloid, an increased incidence of liver haemangioendothelial sarcomas was observed.

Senkirkine is mutagenic in bacteria and in mammalian cells *in vitro*. It also induced chromosomal aberrations and unscheduled DNA synthesis in mammalian cells *in vitro*. There is *sufficient evidence* that senkirkine is active in short-term tests.

No data were available to evaluate the teratogenicity of this compound to experimental animals.

4.2 Human data

Senkirkine is found in a number of plant species which are used as foods, herbal remedies and toiletries, resulting in limited human exposure.

No data were available to evaluate the teratogenicity or chromosomal effects of this compound in humans.

No case report or epidemiological study of the carcinogenicity of senkirkine was available to the Working Group.

4.3 Evaluation

There is *limited evidence*[1] for the carcinogenicity of both senkirkine and *Tussilago farfara* L. in experimental animals. In the absence of epidemiological data, no evaluation of the carcinogenicity of senkirkine to humans could be made.

5. References

Borka, L. & Onshuus I. (1979) Senkirkine content in the leaves of *Tussilago farfara* L. *Medd. Norsk. Farm. Selsk.*, *41*, 165-168

Briggs, L.H., Mangan, J.L. & Russell, W.E. (1948) Alkaloids of New Zealand *Senecio* species. Part I. The alkaloid from *Senecio kirkii*. *J. chem. Soc.*, 1891-1892

Briggs, L.H., Cambie, R.C., Candy, B.J., O'Donovan, G.M., Russell, R.H. & Seelye, R.N. (1965) Alkaloids of New Zealand *Senecio* species. Part II. Senkirkine. *J. chem. Soc.*, April, 2492-2498

Chalmers, A.H., Culvenor, C.C.J. & Smith, L.W. (1965) Characterisation of pyrrolizidine alkaloids by gas, thin-layer and paper chromatography. *J. Chromatogr.*, *20*, 270-277

---

[1]See preamble, p. 18.

Crout, D.H.G. (1972) Pyrrolizidine and seco-pyrrolizidine alkaloids of *Crotalaria laburnifolia* L. subspecies *eldomae. J. chem. Soc. Perkin Trans. I*, 1602-1607

Culvenor, C.C.J. (1983) Estimated intakes of pyrrolizidine alkaloids by humans. A comparison with dose rates causing tumours in rats. *J. Toxicol. environ. Health* (in press)

Culvenor, C.C.J., Edgar, J.A., Smith, L.W. & Hirono, I. (1976) The occurrence of senkirkine in *Tussilago farfara. Aust. J. Chem., 29*, 229-230

Danilova, A.V. & Konovalova, R.A. (1950) Alkaloids of *Senecio* species. VII. Alkaloids from *Senecio renardi. Zh. Obshch. Khim., 20*, 1921-1926 [*Chem. Abstr., 45*, 2960a]

Danilova, A.V., Koretskaya, N.I. & Utkin, L.M. (1961) Structure of the alkaloid renardine II. *Zh. Obshch. Khim., 31*, 3815-3818 [*Chem. Abstr., 57*, 9901d]

Furuya, T., Murakami, K. & Hikichi, M. (1971) Senkirkine, a pyrrolizidine alkaloid from *Farfugium japonicum. Phytochemistry, 10*, 3306-3307

Hirono, I. (1981) Natural carcinogenic products of plant origin. *CRC crit. Rev. Toxicol., 8*, 235-277

Hirono, I., Mori, H. & Culvenor, C.C.J. (1976) Carcinogenic activity of coltsfoot, *Tussilago farfara* L.. *Gann, 67*, 125-129

Hirono, I., Haga, M., Fujii, M., Matsuura, S., Matsubara, N., Nakayama, M., Furuya, T., Hikichi, M., Takanashi, H., Uchida, E., Hosaka, S. & Ueno, I. (1979a) Induction of hepatic tumors in rats by senkirkine and symphytine. *J. natl Cancer Inst., 63*, 469-472

Hirono, I., Mori, H., Haga, M., Fujii, M., Yamada, K., Hirata, Y., Takanashi, H., Uchida, E., Hosaka, S., Ueno, I., Matsushima, T., Umezawa, K. & Shirai, A. (1979b) *Edible plants containing carcinogenic pyrrolizidine alkaloids in Japan.* In: Miller, E.C., Miller, J.A., Hirono, I., Sugimura, T. & Takayama, S., eds, *Naturally Occurring Carcinogens-Mutagens and Modulators of Carcinogenesis*, Tokyo/Baltimore, Japan Scientific Society Press/University Park Press, pp. 79-87

IARC (1976a) *IARC Monographs on the Evaluation of Carcinogenic Risk of Chemicals to Man*, Vol. 10, *Some Naturally Occurring Substances*, Lyon, pp. 327-331

IARC (1976b) *IARC Monographs on the Evaluation of Carcinogenic Risk of Chemicals to Man*, Vol. 10, *Some Naturally Occurring Substances*, Lyon, pp. 263-342

Jovceva, R.J., Boeva, A., Potesilová, H., Klásek, A. & Santavyé, F. (1978) Pyrrolizidine alkaloids. XXVI. Alkaloids from *Senecio procerus* L. var. *procerus Stoj. Stef. et Kit. Coll. Czech. chem. Commun., 43*, 2312-2314

Mattocks, A.R. (1967) Detection of pyrrolizidine alkaloids on thin-layer chromatograms. *J. Chromatogr., 27*, 505-508

McLean, E.K. (1970) The toxic actions of pyrrolizidine (*Senecio*) alkaloids. *Pharmacol. Rev., 22*, 429-483

Qualls, C.W., Jr & Segall, H.J. (1978) Rapid isolation and identification of pyrrolizidine alkaloids (*Senecio vulgaris*) by use of high-performance liquid chromatography. *J. Chromatogr.*, *150*, 202-206

Röder, E., Wiedenfeld, H. & Pastewka, U. (1979) Pyrrolizidine alkaloids from *Senecio vernalis* (Ger.). *Planta med.*, *37*, 131-136

Rodrigues, D.F. & Gonzáles, A.G. (1971) Canary plant alkaloids. XII. Alkaloids from *Senecio antieuphorbium* (L.) Sch. Bip. (Sp.). *Farm. nueva*, *36*, 810-811

Schoental, R. (1970) Hepatotoxic activity of retrorsine, senkirkine and hydroxysenkirkine in newborn rats, and the role of epoxides in carcinogenesis by pyrrolizidine alkaloids and aflatoxins. *Nature*, *227*, 401-402

Smith, L.W. & Culvenor, C.C.J. (1981) Plant sources of hepatotoxic pyrrolizidine alkaloids. *J. nat. Prod.*, *44*, 129-152

Takanashi, H., Umeda, M. & Hirono, I. (1980) Chromosomal aberrations and mutation in cultured mammalian cells induced by pyrrolizidine alkaloids. *Mutat. Res.*, *78*, 67-77

Tittel, G., Hinz, H. & Wagner, H. (1979) Quantitative estimation of the pyrrolizidine alkaloids of *Symphyti radix* by HPLC (Ger.). *Planta med.*, *37*, 1-8

Wade, A., ed. (1977) *Martindale, The Extra Pharmacopoeia*, 27th ed., London, The Pharmaceutical Press, p. 1248

Wiedenfeld, H., Pastewka, U., Stengl, P. & Röder, E. (1981) Gas-chromatographic determination of pyrrolizidine-alkaloids of some *Senecio* species (Ger.). *Planta med.*, *41*, 124-128

Williams, G.M., Mori, H., Hironi, I. & Nagao, M. (1980) Genotoxicity of pyrrolizidine alkaloids in the hepatocyte primary culture/DNA-repair test. *Mutat. Res.*, *79*, 1-5

Yamada, K., Tatematsu, H., Kyotani, Y., Hirata, Y., Haga, M. & Hirono, I. (1978) Senkirkine and a new sesquiterpene glycoside, isopetasoside, from *Petasites japonicus*. *Phytochemistry*, *17*, 1667-1668

Yamanaka, H., Nagao, M., Sugimura, T., Furuya, T., Shirai, A. & Matsushima, T. (1979) Mutagenicity of pyrrolizidine alkaloids in the *Salmonella*/mammalian-microsome test. *Mutat. Res.*, *68*, 211-216

SYMPHYTINE

1. Chemical and Physical Data

1.1 Synonyms and trade names

Chem. Abstr. Services Reg. No.: 22571-95-5

Chem. Abstr. Name: 2-Butenoic acid, 2-methyl-, 7-[[2,3-dihydroxy-2-(1-methylethyl)-1-oxobutoxy]methyl]-2,3,5,7a-tetrahydro-1*H*-pyrrolizin-1-yl ester, [1*R*-[1α(*E*), 7(2*S**, 3*S**),7aβ]]-

IUPAC Systematic Name: Symphytine or (1*R*,7a*R*)-2,3,5,7a-tetrahydro-1-hydroxy-1*H*-pyrrolizine-7-methanol 7-[(2*S*,3*S*)-2,3-dihydroxy-2-isopropylbutyrate]-1-[(*E*)-2- methyl-crotonate

Synonyms: 7-Tiglylretronecine viridiflorate; 7-tiglyl-9-viridiflorylretronecine

1.2 Structural and molecular formulae and molecular weight

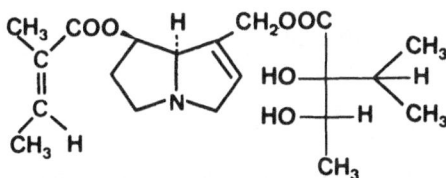

$C_{20}H_{31}NO_6$ Mol. wt: 381.5

1.3 Chemical and physical properties of the pure substance

From Furuya and Araki (1968) and Furuya and Hikichi (1971)

(a) *Description*: Almost colourless oil

(b) *Optical rotation*: $[\alpha]_D^{24}$ + 3.65° (c = 4.28 in ethanol)

(c) *Spectroscopy data*: Nuclear magnetic resonance and mass spectral data have been reported.

(d) *Stability*: Readily hydrolysed by alkalis; sensitive to oxidation

1.4 Technical products and impurities

No technical product containing symphytine is available.

2. Production, Use, Occurrence and Analysis

2.1 Production and use

(a) *Production*

Symphytine is a pyrrolizidine alkaloid which can be extracted from various parts of dried *Symphytum officinale* Linn. (comfrey); the alkaloid occurs mainly in the form of its *N*-oxide. Extraction of the dried roots with methanol produces a crude extract from which allantoin is removed. The residue is subsequently purified by reduction of the *N*-oxide with zinc dust and hydrochloric acid and column chromatography to give the pure alkaloid (Furuya & Araki, 1968).

Symphytine is not produced commercially.

(b) *Use*

The roots of the plant *Symphytum officinale* Linn. (comfrey), in which symphytine occurs, are reportedly used as a demulcent in chronic catarrh and certain mucous membrane affections of the gut in domestic medicine in Europe; it is also used as a tonic in Japan (Furuya & Araki, 1968). In the US, the herb comfrey is used commercially to make a common herbal tea. The hybrid *Symphytum* X *uplandicum* Nyman is is widely grown as a garden herb and is used as green feed for animals; the alkaloid content is variable but is usually low, and only 5% of the total alkaloid content is symphytine. It is reported to be widely consumed as a medicinal herb, salad plant or 'green drink' (Culvenor *et al.*, 1980a,b).

2.2 Occurrence

Symphytine occurs in the roots of the plant *Symphytum officinale* L. (a member of the family Boraginaceae), which occurs widely in Europe and is cultivated in Japan (Furuya & Araki, 1968). It also occurs in the roots of *Symphytum* X *uplandicum* Nyman, a hybrid of *Symphytum officinale* L. and *Symphytum asperum* Lepechin (Culvenor *et al.*, 1980b). It is found in the true forget-me-not, *Myosotis scorpioides* (Resch *et al.*, 1982). *Symphytum officinale* L. contains 1.7-2.5 g/kg symphytine (Tittel *et al.*, 1979).

2.3 Analysis

The isolation and analysis of symphytine are usually carried out by chromatographic methods. No direct quantitative method is available, but a few methods for its isolation and purification are described in Table 1.

Table 1. Methods for the analysis of symphytine

Sample matrix	Sample preparation	Assay procedure[a]	Limit of detection	Reference
Plant materials	Extract (methanol); reduct N-oxides (zinc dust and hydrochloric acid)	TLC/UV or HPLC/UV	not given	Tittel et al. (1979)
	Reduce N-oxides; purify (XAD-2 column using gradient elution with acidified methanol-water mixtures)	TLC	not given	Huizing & Malingré (1979)
	(chloranil spray)	TLC	0.15 μg	Huizing et al. (1980)
	Isolate alkaloids (ion-pair HPLC); derivatize (hexamethyldisilazane:trimethylchlorosilane [10:1])	GC/FID or GC/MS	not given	Huizing et al. (1981)

[a]Abbreviations: TLC/UV, thin-layer chromatography with ultra-violet spectrometry; HPLC/UV, high-performance liquid chromatography with ultra-violet spectrometry; TLC, thin-layer chromatography; GC/FID, gas chromatography with flame-ionization detection; GC/MS, gas chromatography with mass spectrometry

3. Biological Data Relevant to the Evaluation of Carcinogenic Risk to Humans

3.1 Carcinogenicity studies in animals

(a) Intraperitoneal administration

Rat: A group of 20 male inbred ACI rats, 1-1.5 months old, received i.p. injections of 13 mg/kg bw (10% of the LD_{50}) symphytine dissolved in physiological saline twice a week for four weeks and then once a week for 52 weeks. Symphytine was isolated from dried milled roots of comfrey (*Symphytum officinale* L.). A control group of 20 male rats was given i.p. injections of physiological saline (0.1 ml/100 g bw) by the same injection schedule. The experiment was terminated 650 days after initiation of injections. All rats in the experimental group survived for more than 330 days after the start of injections, and 4/20 had liver tumours (3 haemangioendothelial sarcomas and 1 liver-cell adenoma). No liver tumour was observed in the control group [p > 0.05] (Hirono et al., 1979a,b). [No liver tumour was observed in 359 rats serving as controls for another long-term experiment, suggesting a compound-related effect.]

(b) Carcinogenicity of plants containing symphytine

Rat: Four groups of 19-28 male and female ACI rats, 1-1.5 months old, were fed diets containing 8-33% comfrey leaves (Symphytum officinale L.) for 480-600 days. Five additional groups of 15-24 rats were fed diets containing 0.5-8% comfrey root for 245-480 days. A control group of 65 male and 64 female rats was fed a normal basal diet. Hepatocellular adenomas were induced in all experimental groups; no liver tumour was observed in control animals. Hepatocellular adenomas were induced in 7/21 rats [p < 0.001] and haemangioendothelial sarcomas of the liver in 1/21 rats fed 16% comfrey leaf diet for 600 days; hepatocellular adenomas were seen in 12/15 rats and haemangioendothelial sarcomas of the liver in 2/15 rats fed 1% comfrey root diet for 275 days and 0.5% weekly at 3-week intervals up to death [p < 0.001]. Despite the fact that the percentage of comfrey flour is higher in the leaf diet than in the root diet, the incidence of liver tumours tended to be higher in groups fed a diet containing comfrey root than that in those fed a diet containing comfrey leaf (Hirono et al ., 1978).

Fifteen male and 15 female rats were fed 0.5% comfrey root in the diet for 754 days, at which time the experiment was terminated. Of animals surviving longer than 590 days after the start of the experiment, 8/30 had hepatocellular adenomas, and 9/13 (69.2%) had haemangioendothelial sarcomas of the liver. No haemangioendothelial sarcoma occurred in an unspecified number of surviving controls (Hirono et al., 1979b).

3.2 Other relevant biological data

The toxicology and pharmacology of pyrrolizidine alkaloids have been reviewed (McLean, 1970; Hirono, 1981; Culvenor, 1983); a general discussion of their metabolism and hepatotoxicity was published previously in the IARC Monographs series (IARC, 1976).

(a) Experimental systems

Toxic effects

The i.p. LD_{50} of symphytine has been reported to be 130 mg/kg bw in rats (Hirono et al., 1979a,b).

Effects on reproduction and prenatal toxicity

No data were available to the Working Group.

Absorption, distribution, excretion and metabolism

No data specific to symphytine were available to the Working Group.

Mutagenicity and other short-term tests

Symphytine was reported to induce mutations in *Salmonella typhimurium* TA100 only in the presence of polychlorinated biphenyl-induced rat liver 9000 x *g* supernatant mix. It also induced forward mutations to 8-azaguanine resistance in V79 Chinese hamster cells; but it did not transform cryopreserved hamster embryo cells (Hirono *et al.*, 1979b) [details not given].

(*b*) *Humans*

No data specific to symphytine were available to the Working Group.

3.3 Case reports and epidemiological studies of carcinogenicity in humans

No data were available to the Working Group.

4. Summary of Data Reported and Evaluation

4.1 Experimental data

Symphytine was tested for carcinogenicity in male rats by intraperitoneal administration; a non-significant increase in the incidence of liver tumours was observed. When leaves and roots of *Symphytum officinale* L. were tested in rats by administration in the diet, the incidence of liver tumours was increased.

Symphytine was mutagenic in *Salmonella typhimurium* and in mammalian cells *in vitro*. The data were *inadequate* to evaluate the activity of symphytine in short-term tests.

No data were available to evaluate the teratogenicity of this compound to experimental animals.

4.2 Human data

Symphytine is found in several plant species which are used as foods and as herbal remedies, resulting in wide human exposure.

No data were available to evaluate the teratogenicity or chromosomal effects of this compound in humans.

No case report or epidemiological study of the carcinogenicity of symphytine was available to the Working Group.

4.3 Evaluation

No evaluation of the carcinogenicity of symphytine to experimental animals could be made. Results of experiments in rats provide *limited evidence*[1] that the leaves and roots of *Symphytum officinale* L. are carcinogenic to experimental animals. In the absence of epidemiological data, no evaluation of the carcinogenicity of symphytine to humans could be made.

5. References

Culvenor, C.C.J. (1983) Estimated intakes of pyrrolizidine alkaloids by humans. A comparison with dose rates causing tumours in rats. *J. Toxicol. environ. Health* (in press)

Culvenor, C.C.J., Clarke, M., Edgar, J.A., Frahn, J.L., Jago, M.V., Peterson, J.E. & Smith, L.W. (1980a) Structure and toxicity of the alkaloids of Russian comfrey (*Symphytum X uplandicum* Nyman), a medicinal herb and item of human diet. *Experientia, 36,* 377-379

Culvenor, C.C.J., Edgar, J.A., Frahn, J.L. & Smith, L.W. (1980b) The alkaloids of *Symphytum X uplandicum* (Russian comfrey). *Aust. J. Chem., 33,* 1105-1113

Furuya, T. & Araki, K. (1968) Studies on constituents of crude drugs. I. Alkaloids from *Symphytum officinale* Linn.. *Chem. pharm. Bull., 16,* 2512-2516

Furuya, T. & Hikichi, M. (1971) Alkaloids and triterpenoids of *Symphytum officinale*. *Phytochemistry, 10,* 2217-2220

Hirono, I. (1981) Natural carcinogenic products of plant origin. *CRC crit. Rev. Toxicol., 8,* 235-277

Hirono, I., Mori, H. & Haga, M. (1978) Carcinogenic activity of *Symphytum officinale*. *J. natl Cancer Inst., 61,* 865-869

Hirono, I., Haga, M., Fujii, M., Matsuura, S., Matsubara, N., Nakayama, M., Furuya, T., Hikichi, M., Takanashi, H., Uchida, E., Hosaka, S. & Ueno, I. (1979a) Induction of hepatic tumors in rats by senkirkine and symphytine. *J. natl Cancer Inst., 63,* 469-472

Hirono, I., Mori, H., Haga, M., Fujii, M., Yamada, K., Hirata, Y., Takanashi, H., Uchida, E., Hosaka, S., Ueno, I., Matsushima, T., Umezawa, K. & Shirai, A. (1979b) *Edible plants containing carcinogenic pyrrolizidine alkaloids in Japan.* In: Miller, E.C., Miller, J.A., Hirono, I., Sugimura, T. & Takayama, S., eds, *Naturally Occurring Carcinogens-Mutagens and Modulators of Carcinogenesis,* Tokyo/Baltimore, Japan Scientific Society Press/University Park Press, pp. 79-87

[1]See preamble, p. 18.

Huizing, H.J. & Malingré, T.M. (1979) Purification and separation of pyrrolizidine alkaloids from Boraginaceae on a polystyrene-divinylbenzene resin. *J. Chromatogr.*, *176*, 274-279

Huizing, H.J., De Boer, F. & Malingré, T.M. (1980) Chloranil, a sensitive reagent for pyrrolizidine alkaloids on thin-layer chromatograms. *J. Chromatogr.*, *195*, 407-411

Huizing, H.J., De Boer, F. & Malingré, T.M. (1981) Preparative ion-pair high-performance liquid chromatography and gas chromatography of pyrrolizidine alkaloids from comfrey. *J. Chromatogr.*, *214*, 257-262

IARC (1976) *IARC Monographs on the Evaluation of Carcinogenic Risk of Chemicals to Man*, Vol. 10, *Some Naturally Occurring Substances*, Lyon, pp. 263-342

McLean, E.K. (1970) The toxic actions of pyrrolizidine (*Senecio*) alkaloids. *Pharmacol. Rev.*, *22*, 429-483

Resch, J.F., Rosberger, D.F., Meinwald, J. & Appling, J.W. (1982) Biologically active pyrrolizidine alkaloids from the true forget-me-not, *Myosotis scorpioides*. *J. nat. Prod.*, *45*, 358-362

Tittel, G., Hinz, H. & Wagner, H. (1979) Quantitative estimation of the pyrrolizidine alkaloids of *Symphyti radix* by HPLC (Ger.). *Planta Med.*, *37*, 1-8

Trp-P-1 (3-AMINO-1,4-DIMETHYL-5*H*-PYRIDO[4,3-*b*]INDOLE) AND ITS ACETATE

A general review on this compound has been published (Sugimura *et al.* (1981).

1. Chemical and Physical Data

Trp-P-1

1.1 Synonyms and trade names

Chem. Abstr. Services Reg. No.: 62450-06-0

Chem. Abstr. Name: 5*H*-Pyrido[4,3-*b*]indol-3-amine, 1,4-dimethyl-

IUPAC Systematic Name: 3-Amino-1,4-dimethyl-5*H*-pyrido[4,3-*b*]indole

Synonyms: 3-Amino-1,4-dimethyl-γ-carboline; TRP-PI; Tryptophan P1

1.2 Structural and molecular formulae and molecular weight

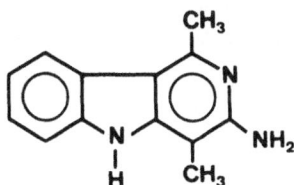

$C_{13}H_{13}N_3$ Mol. wt: 211.3

Trp-P-1 acetate

1.1 Synonyms and trade names

Chem. Abstr. Services Reg. No.: 75104-43-7 (acetate); 68808-54-8 (monoacetate)

Chem. Abstr. Name: 5*H*-Pyrido[4,3-*b*]indol-3-amine, 1,4-dimethyl-, acetate; 5*H*-pyrido[4,3-*b*]indol-3-amine, 1,4-dimethyl-, monoacetate

IUPAC Systematic Name: 3-Amino-1,4-dimethyl-5*H*-pyrido[4,3-*b*]indole acetate

1.2 Structural and molecular formulae and molecular weight

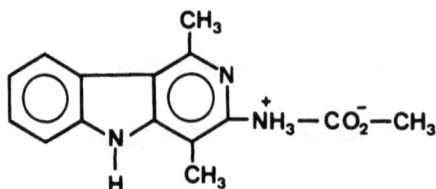

$$C_{13}H_{13}N_3.xC_2H_4O_2 \text{ (acetate)}$$
$$C_{13}H_{13}N_3.C_2H_4O_2 \text{ (monoacetate)}$$

Mol. wt: 271.3

1.3 Chemical and physical properties of the acetate salt

From Kosuge *et al.* (1978)

    (*a*) *Description*: Pale-brown needles or small prisms

    (*b*) *Melting-point*: 252-262°C (recrystallized from ethyl acetate)

    (*c*) *Spectroscopy data*: λ_{max} (methanol): 245, 265, 267, 292, 305 and 317 nm. Infra-red, nuclear magnetic resonance and mass spectral data have been determined.

    (*d*) *Solubility*: Soluble in methanol

1.4 Technical products and impurities

No technical product containing Trp-P-1 is available.

2. Production, Use, Occurrence and Analysis

2.1 Production and use

Trp-P-1 is not produced or used commercially.

2.2 Occurrence

Trp-P-1 has been detected in broiled sardines at a level of 13.3 µg/kg (Yamaizumi *et al.*, 1980) and in broiled beef at an unspecified level (Yamaguchi *et al.*, 1980). It has also been isolated by fractionation of the tar obtained from the pyrolysis of tryptophan (Kosuge *et al.*, 1978; Kasai *et al.*, 1979) and from the pyrolysis products of casein (0.54 mg/kg) and gluten (0.13 mg/kg) (Uyeta *et al.*, 1979).

2.3 Analysis

Trp-P-1 has been determined in broiled fish by gas chromatography-mass spectrometry (Yamaizumi *et al.*, 1980).

3. Biological Data Relevant to the Evaluation of Carcinogenic Risk to Humans

3.1 Carcinogenicity studies in animals[1]

(a) *Oral administration*

Mouse: Groups of 40 male and 40 female CDF$_1$ (BALB/cAnN x DBA/2N, Charles River Japan) mice, seven weeks old, were fed a pellet diet containing 200 mg/kg Trp-P-1 acetate (purity >99.5%) for 621 days, at which time the experiment was terminated. A group of 40 male and 40 female mice given the basal diet served as controls. By day 402, when the first hepatic tumour was found, the numbers of survivors were 24 males and 26 females in the experimental group and 25 males and 24 females in the control group. Hepatic tumours were found in 5/24 (21%) treated males and 16/26 (62%) treated females; female mice were more susceptible to Trp-P-1 carcinogenicity than males. In the control group, a hepatic tumour was found in 1/25 (4%) males but in 0/24 females; the increased incidence of hepatic tumours in Trp-P-1-treated females was statistically significant [p < 0.001]. Most of the hepatic tumours were hepatocellular carcinomas (14 in females and 4 in males); the hepatic tumour in the controls was a haemangioma (Matsukura *et al.*, 1981).

---

[1]The Working Group was aware of studies in progress in rats and hamster by oral administration (IARC, 1981).

(b) *Skin application*

Mouse: The interscapular region of the skin of 20 female ICR mice (Charles River Japan), eight weeks old, was painted with a 0.4% Trp-P-1 solution in acetone thrice weekly for six months. A control group of 20 animals was treated with acetone alone. Mice were necropsied 12 months after the start of the experiment, but no marked change was observed in either the control or test group (Ishikawa *et al.*, 1979a). [The Working Group noted the short duration of treatment and observation.]

(c) *Subcutaneous administration*

Rat: Ten male and 10 female Fischer rats, eight weeks old, received s.c. injections of 1.5 mg Trp-P-1 in 0.1 ml olive oil once a week for 20 weeks; an equal number of control rats were injected with olive oil alone. All animals survived until termination of the experiment at 10 months after the first injection, when they were killed. Tumours at the injection site developed only in 5/10 female [p = 0.02] Trp-P-1-treated rats; histologically these were fibrosarcomas, which were transplantable to other rats. No tumour occurred in treated males or in control animals of either sex (Ishikawa *et al.*, 1979a).

Hamster: Ten male and 10 female, eight-week-old Syrian golden hamsters received s.c. injections of 1.5 mg Trp-P-1 in 0.1 ml olive oil once a week for 20 weeks. The same number of hamsters injected with olive oil alone served as controls. All survivors were killed 10 months after the first injection. In most of the Trp-P-1-treated hamsters, subcutaneous nodules at the injection site became palpable within four to five months. Tumours were induced in 1/3 males and 2/5 females that survived for longer than five months; metastases to regional lymph nodes were found in two animals. Histologically, the tumours were classified as pleomorphic sarcomas, and two were successfully transplanted into other hamsters. No tumour was observed in controls (8 males and 9 females) (Ishikawa *et al.*, 1979a).

(d) *Other experimental systems*

Bladder implantation: A group of 33 female *mice* of ddy strain (18 g bw) received implantations of paraffin pellets containing 5% Trp-P-1 into the bladder. Another group of 55 female mice of the same strain were implanted with pellets of paraffin wax alone and served as a control group. The experiment was terminated 40 weeks after pellet implantation. Eleven of 23 treated mice that survived until termination of the experiment (47.8%) developed bladder carcinomas, whereas only one animal out of 36 surviving controls (2.7%) had a bladder carcinoma (p < 0.0001) (Hashida *et al.*, 1982).

3.2 Other relevant biological data

(a) *Experimental systems*

Toxic effects

The acute oral LD_{50} values of Trp-P-1 when given by intragastric intubation were 200 mg/kg bw in mice, 100 mg/kg bw in rats and 380 mg/kg bw in Syrian golden hamsters. Animals that received doses above the LD_{50} died in convulsions within one hour (Ishikawa et al., 1979a).

Trp-P-1 induced a local inflammatory reaction in mice, rats and hamsters when injected subcutaneously (Ishikawa *et al.*, 1979a).

Enzyme-altered foci, characterized by ATPase deficiency, were induced in the livers of male weanling Sprague-Dawley rats, 21 days old, treated daily with i.p. injections of 0.5 mg Trp-P-1 for six days and then fed a diet containing 0.05% phenobarbital for 16 weeks; they were also seen in similarly treated animals that had undergone a partial hepatectomy (Ishikawa *et al.*, 1979a,b).

Effects on reproduction and prenatal toxicity

No data were available to the Working Group.

Absorption, distribution, excretion and metabolism

No data were available on the absorption, distribution, excretion or metabolism of Trp-P-1.

Trp-P-1 binds non-covalently to DNA without prior metabolic activation and binds covalently to DNA in the presence of hepatic microsomes (Pezzuto *et al.*, 1980).

Mutagenicity and other short-term tests

Trp-P-1 was strongly mutagenic to *Salmonella typhimurium* TA98 and TA100 when tested in the presence of a liver 9000 x *g* supernatant preparation from polychlorinated biphenyl-induced rats (Nagao *et al.*, 1980).

In further experiments in *Salmonella*, Trp-P-1 was oxidized to a mutagenically inactive form by treatment with oxidizing agents such as beef liver catalase and horseradish peroxidase (Yagi, 1979; Yamada *et al.*, 1979).

Trp-P-1 was mutagenic in a forward-mutation assay to 8-azaguanine resistance in *S. typhimurium* strain TM677 in the presence of a liver microsomal preparation from 3-methylcholanthrene-induced rats (Pezzuto *et al.*, 1981).

Trp-P-1, in the absence of exogenous metabolic activation, induced chromosomal aberrations and sister chromatid exchanges in phytohaemagglutinin-stimulated human lymphocytes, Chinese hamster Don-6 and Chinese hamster embryonic B-131 cells (Sasaki *et al.*, 1980). In the human fibroblastic cell line HE2144, the chemical induced sister chromatid exchanges but not chromosomal aberrations (Sasaki *et al.*, 1980). In human lymphoblastoid cells, sister chromatid exchanges were induced only when the compound was tested in the presence of polychlorinated biphenyl-induced rat liver 9000 x *g* supernatant (Tohda *et al.*, 1980).

Trp-P-1 induced morphological transformation *in vitro* in primary cultures of Syrian golden hamster embryo cells (Takayama *et al.*, 1977).

(b) Humans

No data were available to the Working Group.

3.3 Case reports and epidemiological studies of carcinogenicity in humans

No data were available to the Working Group.

4. Summary of Data Reported and Evaluation

4.1 Experimental data

Trp-P-1 was tested for carcinogenicity in mice by administration in the diet, by skin application and by bladder implantation, and in rats and hamsters by subcutaneous administration. Hepatic tumours were induced by oral administration in both male and female mice, although the increased incidence was significant only in females. In female rats, there was a significant increase in the incidence of fibrosarcomas at the site of injection; in hamsters there was an increased incidence of subcutaneous sarcomas. Bladder carcinomas were observed in female mice after implantation of paraffin pellets containing Trp-P-1 at this site. The study in mice by skin painting was inadequate for evaluation.

Trp-P-1 is mutagenic to bacteria following metabolic activation. It induced chromosomal anomalies in mammalian cells, including human cells, *in vitro*. It also caused morphological transformation of hamster embryo cells. There is *sufficient evidence* that Trp-P-1 is active in short-term tests.

No data were available to evaluate the teratogenicity of this compound to experimental animals.

4.2 Human data

Trp-P-1 is found in the charred fraction of cooked fish and meat, and the consumption of these foods is a source of exposure for the general population.

No data were available to evaluate the teratogenicity or chromosomal effects of this compound in humans.

No case report or epidemiological study of the carcinogenicity of Trp-P-1 was available to the Working Group.

4.3 Evaluation

There is *sufficient evidence*[1] for the carcinogenicity of Trp-P-1 in experimental animals. No data on humans were available.

---

[1]In the absence of adequate data on humans, it is reasonable, for practical purposes, to regard chemicals for which there is sufficient evidence of carcinogenicity in animals as if they presented a carcinogenic risk to humans.

5. References

Hashida, C., Nagayama, K. & Takemura, N. (1982) Induction of bladder cancer in mice by implanting pellets containing tryptophan pyrolysis products. *Cancer Lett.*, *17*, 101-105

IARC (1981) *Information Bulletin of the Survey of Chemicals Being Tested for Carcinogenicity*, No. 9, Lyon, pp. 78, 82

Ishikawa, T., Takayama, S., Kitagawa, T., Kawachi, T., Kinebuchi, M., Matsukura, N., Uchida, E. & Sugimura, T. (1979a) In vivo *experiments on tryptophan pyrolysis products.* In: Miller, E.C., Miller, J.A., Hirono, I., Sugimura, T. & Takayama, S., eds, *Naturally Occurring Carcinogens-Mutagens and Modulators of Carcinogenesis*, Tokyo/Baltimore, Japan Scientific Societies Press/University Park Press, pp. 159-167

Ishikawa, T., Takayama, S., Kitagawa, T., Kawachi, T. & Sugimura, T. (1979b) Induction of enzyme-altered islands in rat liver by tryptophan pyrolysis products. *J. Cancer Res. clin. Oncol.*, *95*, 221-224

Kasai, H., Nishimura, S., Nagao, M., Takahashi, Y. & Sugimura, T. (1979) Fractionation of a mutagenic principle from broiled fish by high-pressure liquid chromatography. *Cancer Lett.*, *7*, 343-348

Kosuge, T., Tsuji, K., Wakabayashi, K., Okamoto, T., Shudo, K., Hitaka, Y., Itai, A., Sugimura, T., Kawachi, T., Nagao, M., Yahagi, T. & Seino, Y. (1978) Isolation and structure studies of mutagenic principles in amino acid pyrolysates. *Chem. pharm. Bull.*, *26*, 611-619

Matsukura, N., Kawachi, T., Morino, K., Ohgaki, H., Sugimura, T. & Takayama, S. (1981) Carcinogenicity in mice of mutagenic compounds from a tryptophan pyrolysate. *Science*, *213*, 346-347

Nagao, M., Takahashi, Y., Yahagi, T., Sugimura, T., Takeda, K., Shudo, K. & Okamoto, T. (1980) Mutagenicities of γ-carboline derivatives related to potent mutagens found in tryptophan pyrolysates. *Carcinogenesis*, *1*, 451-454

Pezzuto, J.M., Lau, P.P., Luh, Y., Moore, P.D., Wogan, G.N. & Hecht, S.M. (1980) There is a correlation between the DNA affinity and mutagenicity of several 3-amino-1-methyl-5*H*-pyrido-[4,5-*b*]indoles. *Proc. natl Acad. Sci. USA*, *77*, 1427-1431

Pezzuto, J.M., Moore, P.D. & Hecht, S.M. (1981) Metabolic activation of 1-methyl-3-amino-5*H*-pyrido[4,3-*b*]indole and several structurally related mutagens. *Biochemistry*, *20*, 298-305

Sasaki, M., Sugimura, T., Yoshida, M.A. & Kawachi, T. (1980) Chromosome aberrations and sister chromatid exchanges induced by tryptophan pyrolysates, Trp-p-1 and Trp-p-2, in cultured human and Chinese hamster cells. *Proc. Jpn. Acad.*, *56B*, 332-337

Sugimura, T., Nagao, M. & Wakabayashi, K. (1981) *Mutagenic heterocyclic amines in cooked food.* In: Egan, H., Fishbein, L., Castegnaro, M., O'Neill, I.K. & Bartsch, H., eds, *Environmental Carcinogens. Selected Methods of Analysis,* Vol. 4, *Some Aromatic Amines and Azo-Dyes in the General and Industrial Environment (IARC Scientific Publications No. 40),* Lyon, International Agency for Research on Cancer, pp. 251-267

Takayama, S., Katoh, Y., Tanaka, M., Nagao, M., Wakabayashi, K. & Sugimura, T. (1977) *In vitro* transformation of hamster embryo cells with tryptophan pyrolysis products. *Proc. Jpn. Acad., 53B,* 126-129

Tohda, H., Oikawa, A., Kawachi, T. & Sugimura, T. (1980) Induction of sister-chromatid exchanges by mutagens from amino acid and protein pyrolysates. *Mutat. Res., 77,* 65-69

Uyeta, M., Kanada, T., Mazaki, M., Taue, S. & Takahashi, S. (1979) *Assaying mutagenicity of food pyrolysis products using the Ames test.* In: Miller, E.C., Miller, J.A., Hirono, I., Sugimura, T. & Takayama, S., eds, *Naturally Occurring Carcinogens-Mutagens and Modulators of Carcinogenesis,* Tokyo/Baltimore, Japan Scientific Societies Press/University Park Press, pp. 169-176

Yagi, M. (1979) Oxidation of tryptophan-P-1 and P-2 by beef liver catalase-H_2O_2 intermediate: Comparison with horseradish peroxidase. *Cancer Biochem. Biophys., 4,* 105-117

Yamada, M., Tsuda, M., Nagao, M., Mori, M. & Sugimura, T. (1979) Degradation of mutagens from pyrolysates of tryptophan, glutamic acid and globulin by myeloperoxidase. *Biochem. biophys. Res. Commun., 90,* 769-776

Yamaguchi, K., Shudo, K., Okamoto, T., Sugimura, T. & Kosuge, T. (1980) Presence of 3-amino-1,4-dimethyl-5*H*-pyrido[4,3-*b*]indole in broiled beef. *Gann, 71,* 745-746

Yamaizumi, Z., Shiomi, T., Kasai, H., Nishimura, S., Takahashi, Y., Nagao, M. & Sugimura, T. (1980) Detection of potent mutagens, Trp-P-1 and Trp-P-2, in broiled fish. *Cancer Lett., 9,* 75-83

Trp-P-2 (3-AMINO-1-METHYL-5H-PYRIDO[4,3-b]INDOLE) AND ITS ACETATE

A general review on this compound has been published (Sugimura *et al.*, 1981).

1. Chemical and Physical Data

Trp-P-2

1.1 Synonyms and trade names

Chem. Abstr. Services Reg. No.: 62450-07-1

Chem. Abstr. Name: 5H-Pyrido[4,3-b]indol-3-amine, 1-methyl-

IUPAC Systematic Name: 3-Amino-1-methyl-5H-pyrido[4,3-b]indole

Synonyms: 3-Amino-1-methyl-γ-carboline;1-methyl-3-amino-5H-pyrido[4,3-b]indole; TRP-P2; Tryptophan P2

1.2 Structural and molecular formulae and molecular weight

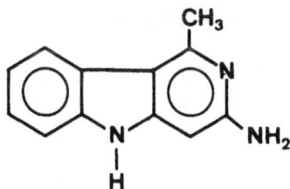

$C_{12}H_{11}N_3$ Mol. wt: 197.2

Trp-P-2 acetate

1.1 Synonyms and trade names

Chem. Abstr. Services Reg. No.: 72254-58-1

Chem. Abstr. Name: 5*H*-Pyrido[4,3-*b*]indol-3-amine, 1-methyl-, monoacetate

IUPAC Systematic Name: 3-Amino-1-methyl-5*H*-pyrido[4,3-*b*]indole acetate

Synonym: TRP-P-2 (acetate)

1.2 Structural and molecular formulae and molecular weight

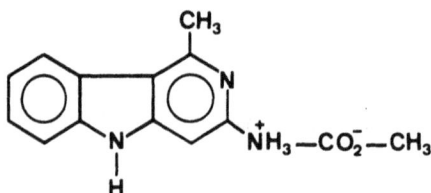

$C_{12}H_{11}N_3.C_2H_4O_2$ Mol. wt: 257.3

1.3 Chemical and physical properties of the acetate salt

From Kosuge *et al.* (1978)

(*a*) *Description*: Brown needles

(*b*) *Melting-point*: 248-250°C (recrystallized from ethyl acetate-methanol)

(*c*) *Spectroscopy data*: λ_{max} nm (methanol): 244, 265, 268, and 290-330. Infra-red, nuclear magnetic resonance, and mass spectral data have been determined.

(*d*) *Solubility*: Soluble in methanol

1.4 Technical products and impurities

No technical product containing Trp-P-2 is available.

2. Production, Use, Occurrence and Analysis

2.1 Production and use

There is no commercial production or use of Trp-P-2.

2.2 Occurrence

Trp-P-2 has been detected in broiled sardines at a level of 13.1 μg/kg (Yamaizumi *et al.*, 1980). It has also been isolated by fractionation of the tar obtained from the pyrolysis of tryptophan (Kosuge *et al.*, 1978; Kasai *et al.*, 1979) and of those of casein (0.75 mg/kg) and of gluten (0.20 mg/kg) (Uyeta *et al.*, 1979).

2.3 Analysis

Trp-P-2 has been determined in broiled fish by gas chromatography-mass spectrometry (Yamaizumi *et al.*, 1980).

3. Biological Data Relevant to the Evaluation of Carcinogenic Risk to Humans

3.1 Carcinogenicity studies in animals

(a) *Oral administration*

Mouse: Groups of 40 male and 40 female CDF$_1$ (BALB/cAnN x DBA/2N, Charles River Japan) mice, seven weeks old, were fed a pellet diet containing 200 mg/kg Trp-P-2 acetate (purity > 99.5%) for 621 days, at which time the experiment was terminated. A group of 40 male and 40 female mice given the basal diet alone served as controls. The numbers of survivors on day 402, when the first hepatic tumour was found, were 25 males and 24 females in both the experimental and control groups. Hepatic tumours were found in 4/25 (16%) treated males and 22/24 (92%) treated females; female mice showed a higher susceptibility to Trp-P-2 carcinogenicity than males. In the control group, a hepatic tumour was found in 1/25 (4%) male mice but in 0/24 females; the increased incidence of hepatic tumours in treated female mice was statistically significant [p < 0.001]. Most hepatic tumours were hepatocellular carcinomas (22 in females, 3 in males); the hepatic tumour found in the control group was a haemangioma (Matsukura et al., 1981).

Rat: Ten male and 10 female inbred ACI rats, five weeks old, were fed a diet containing 100 mg/kg Trp-P-2 acetate (purity > 99%) for 870 days, at which time the experiment was terminated. A control group of 30 male and 30 female rats was fed the normal basal diet. Ten male and 9 female treated and 30 male and 30 female control rats survived for longer than 400 days after the start of feeding. One treated female rat developed a hemangioendothelial sarcoma of the liver and 6 treated females developed neoplastic liver nodules (classified according to Squire et al., 1979) between 666-870 days after the start of feeding. No tumour of the liver was found in treated males or in male or female controls. There was a significant difference in the incidence of liver tumours between treated and control females (p < 0.001) and a significant sex difference in the incidence of liver tumours in treated rats (p < 0.01) (Hosaka et al., 1981).

(b) Skin application

Mouse: The skin of the interscapular region of 20 female ICR mice (Charles River Japan), eight weeks old, was painted with a 0.4% solution of Trp-P-2 in acetone thrice weekly for six months. Twenty animals treated with acetone alone served as controls. Mice were necropsied 12 months after the start of the experiment, but no marked change was observed in either control or experimental groups (Ishikawa et al., 1979). [The Working Group noted the short duration of treatment and observation.]

(c) Subcutaneous administration

Rat: Ten male and 10 female Fischer rats, eight weeks old, received s.c. injections of 1.5 mg Trp-P-2 in 0.1 ml olive oil once a week for 20 weeks; equal numbers of control rats were injected with olive oil alone. All animals were killed 10 months after the first injection. No tumour developed in either the treated or vehicle control group (Ishikawa et al., 1979). [The Working Group noted the short duration of treatment and observation.]

Hamster: Ten male and 10 female, eight-week-old, Syrian golden hamsters received s.c. injections of 1.5 mg Trp-P-2 in 0.1 ml olive oil once a week for 20 weeks. An equal number of animals injected with olive oil alone served as a control group. All surviving animals were killed 10 months after the first injection. No tumour was observed in either treated survivors (3 males and 6 females) or in controls (8 males and 9 females) (Ishikawa et al., 1979). [The Working Group noted the short duration of treatment and observation and the small number of surviving animals.]

(d) Other experimental systems

Bladder implantation: A group of 34 female mice of the ddy strain (18 g bw) received implants of paraffin pellets containing 5% Trp-P-2 into the bladder. Another group of 55 female mice of the same strain were implanted with pellets of paraffin wax alone and served as a control group. The experiment was terminated 40 weeks after pellet implantation. Five out of 22 mice (22.7%) implanted with Trp-P-2 pellets and surviving until termination of the experiment developed bladder carcinomas, whereas only one animal out of 36 surviving controls (2.7%) had a bladder carcinoma (p < 0.025) (Hashida et al., 1982).

3.2 Other relevant biological data

(a) *Experimental systems*

Toxic effects

No LD$_{50}$ value was available to the Working Group. However, it was reported that the acute toxicity of Trp-P-2 was similar to that of Trp-P-1. Trp-P-2 induced a local inflammatory reaction in mice, rats and hamsters when injected subcutaneously (Ishikawa *et al.*, 1979).

Effects on reproduction and prenatal toxicity

No data were available to the Working Group.

Absorption, distribution, excretion and metabolism

No data were available on the absorption, distribution or excretion of Trp-P-2.

The two major microsomal metabolites of Trp-P-2 identified in rat liver *in vitro* are the 3-hydroxyamino and nitroso derivatives. The production of these metabolites by cytochrome P-450-dependent enzymes is increased by pretreatment of rats with either polychlorinated biphenyls or 3-methylcholanthrene (Yamazoe *et al.*, 1980).

Trp-P-2 binds non-covalently to DNA without prior activation by rat liver microsomes (Pezzuto *et al.*, 1980; Shishido *et al.*, 1980). It binds covalently to calf thymus DNA in the presence of hepatic microsomes or a liver 9000 x *g* supernatant fraction from polychlorinated biphenyl-treated rats (Hashimoto *et al.*, 1978; Nemoto *et al.*, 1979; Pezzuto *et al.*, 1980). A base adduct was isolated and identified as (^{8}C-guanyl)-Trp-P-2 (Hashimoto *et al.*, 1979). N-Hydroxy-Trp-P-2, produced by a reconstituted cytochrome P-450 system, bound covalently to calf thymus DNA without the addition of other enzymes or further activation (Mita *et al.*, 1981). Rapid covalent binding to calf thymus DNA has been demonstrated following esterification of N-hydroxy-Trp-P-2 by acetic anhydride (Hashimoto *et al.*, 1980). Seryl-tRNA synthetase acts as an activating enzyme of N-hydroxy-Trp-P-2, as both ATP and L-serine are essential requirements for its covalent binding to DNA (Yamazoe *et al.*, 1981a).

Covalent binding of Trp-P-2 to bovine serum albumin is catalysed by myeloperoxidase in the presence of hydrogen peroxide (Yamada *et al.*, 1980).

Mutagenicity and other short-term tests

Trp-P-2 was a very potent mutagen in *Salmonella typhimurium* strains TA98 and TA100 when tested in the presence of a polychlorinated biphenyl-induced rat liver 9000 x *g* supernatant preparation (Nagao *et al.*, 1980). In all mammalian species examined, N-hydroxylation has been shown to be an obligatory step in the metabolic activation of Trp-P-2 to a mutagen (Yamazoe *et al.*, 1980; Mita *et al.*, 1981; Yamazoe *et al.*, 1981a,b). The presence of a methyl group at position 1 seemed to increase the mutagenic potency of the chemical towards TA98, whereas a methyl group at position 4 decreased the activity. Thus, Trp-P-2 was a stronger mutagen than Trp-P-1. Furthermore, substitution of the methyl group at position 1 by a long alkyl group, a benzyl group or a phenyl group reduced its mutagenic activity (Nagao *et al.*, 1980).

In further experiments with *Salmonella* it was shown that Trp-P-2 is oxidized to a mutagenically inactive form by treatment with oxidizing agents such as beef liver catalase-H_2O_2 and horseradish peroxidase (Yagi, 1979; Yamada *et al.*, 1980).

Trp-P-2 was also mutagenic in a forward mutation assay to 8-azaguanine resistance with *S. typhimurium* TM677 in the presence of a liver microsomal preparation from 3-methylcholanthrene-induced rats (Pezzuto *et al.*, 1981). It was reported in an abstract that Trp-P-2 induced diphtheria toxin-resistant mutations in Chinese hamster lung fibroblasts in the presence of a microsomal activation system (Terada *et al.*, 1982). Trp-P-2, in the absence of exogenous metabolic activation, induced chromosomal aberrations and sister chromatid exchanges in phytohaemagglutinin-stimulated human lymphocytes, Chinese hamster Don-6 and Chinese hamster embryonic B-131 cells but induced neither chromosomal aberrations nor sister chromatid exchanges in the human fibroblast line HE2144 (Sasaki *et al.*, 1980). After metabolic activation with microsomal enzymes, it induced sister chromatid exchanges in a permanent line of human lymphoblastoid cells (Tohda *et al.*, 1980).

Trp-P-2 induced morphological transformation in primary cultures of Syrian golden hamster embryo cells *in vitro* (Takayama *et al.*, 1977); these transformed cells produced tumours when transplanted into the cheek pouches of young hamsters (Takayama *et al.*, 1978).

(b) *Humans*

No data were available to the Working Group.

3.3 Case reports and epidemiological studies of carcinogenicity in humans

No data were available to the Working Group.

4. Summary of Data Reported and Evaluation

4.1 Experimental data

Trp-P-2 was tested for carcinogenicity in mice and rats by administration in the diet, in mice by skin application and bladder implantation and in rats and hamsters by subcutaneous administration. An increased incidence of liver tumours was observed in female mice and female rats following its oral administration. Bladder carcinomas were observed in female mice after implantation of Trp-P-2 in paraffin pellets at this site. The results of the experiments by subcutaneous injection and by skin application were considered inadequate for evaluation.

Trp-P-2 is mutagenic to *Salmonella typhimurium* following metabolic activation. It induced chromosomal anomalies in mammalian cells, including human cells, *in vitro*. It caused neoplastic transformation *in vitro* in Syrian golden hamster cells. There is *sufficient evidence* that Trp-P-2 is active in short-term tests.

No data were available to evaluate the teratogenicity of this compound to experimental animals.

4.2 Human data

Trp-P-2 is found in the charred fraction of cooked fish, and the consumption of this food is a source of exposure for the general population.

No data were available to evaluate the teratogenicity or chromosomal effects of this compound in humans.

No case report or epidemiological study of the carcinogenicity of Trp-P-2 was available to the Working Group.

4.3 Evaluation

There is *sufficient evidence*[1] for the carcinogenicity of Trp-P-2 in experimental animals. No data on humans were available.

5. References

Hashida, C., Nagayama, K. & Takemura, N. (1982) Induction of bladder cancer in mice by implanting pellets containing tryptophan pyrolysis products. *Cancer Lett.*, *17*, 101-105

Hashimoto, Y., Takeda, K., Shudo, K., Okamoto, T., Sugimura, T. & Kosuge, T. (1978) Rat liver microsome-mediated binding to DNA of 3-amino-1-methyl-5*H*-pyrido-[4,3-*b*]indole, a potent mutagen isolated from tryptophan pyrolysate. *Chem.-biol. Interact.*, *23*, 137-140

Hashimoto, Y., Shudo, K. & Okamoto, T. (1979) Structural identification of a modified base in DNA covalently bound with mutagenic 3-amino-1-methyl-5*H*-pyrido[4,3-*b*]indole. *Chem. pharm. Bull.*, *27*, 1058-1060

Hashimoto, Y., Shudo, K. & Okamoto, T. (1980) Activation of a mutagen, 3-amino-1-methyl-5*H*-pyrido[4,3-*b*]indole. Identification of 3-hydroxyamino-1-methyl-5*H*-pyrido[4,3-*b*]indole and its reaction with DNA. *Biochem. biophys. Res. Commun.*, *96*, 355-362

Hosaka, S., Matsushima, T., Hirono, I. & Sugimura, T. (1981) Carcinogenic activity of 3-amino-1-methyl-5*H*-pyrido[4,3-*b*]indole (Trp-P-2), a pyrolysis product of tryptophan. *Cancer Lett.*, *13*, 23-28

Ishikawa, T., Takayama, S., Kitagawa, T., Kawachi, T., Kinebuchi, M., Matsukura, N., Uchida, E. & Sugimura, T. (1979) In vivo *experiments on tryptophan pyrolysis products*. In: Miller, E.C., Miller, J.A., Hirono, I., Sugimura, T. & Takayama, S., eds, *Naturally Occurring Carcinogens-Mutagens and Modulators of Carcinogenesis*, Tokyo/Baltimore, Japan Scientific Societies Press/University Park Press, pp. 159-167

---

[1]In the absence of adequate data on humans, it is reasonable, for practical purposes, to regard chemicals for which there is sufficient evidence of carcinogenicity in animals as if they presented a carcinogenic risk to humans.

Kasai, H., Nishimura, S., Nagao, M., Takahashi, Y. & Sugimura, T. (1979) Fractionation of a mutagenic principle from boiled fish by high-pressure liquid chromatography. *Cancer Lett.*, *7*, 343-348

Kosuge, T., Tsuji, K., Wakabayashi, K., Okamoto, T., Shudo, K., Iitaka, Y., Itai, A., Sugimura, T., Kawachi, T., Nagao, M., Yahagi, T. & Seino, Y. (1978) Isolation and structure studies of mutagenic principles in amino acid pyrolysates. *Chem. pharm. Bull.*, *26*, 611-619

Matsukura, N., Kawachi, T., Morino, K., Ohgaki, H., Sugimura, T. & Takayama, S. (1981) Carcinogenicity in mice of mutagenic compounds from a tryptophan pyrolyzate. *Science, 213*, 346-347

Mita, S., Ishii, K., Yamazoe, Y., Kamataki, T., Kato, R. & Sugimura, T. (1981) Evidence for the involvement of *N*-hydroxylation of 3-amino-1-methyl-5*H*-pyrido[4,3-*b*]indole by cytochrome P-450 in the covalent binding to DNA. *Cancer Res.*, *41*, 3610-3614

Nagao, M., Takahashi, Y., Yahagi, T., Sugimura, T., Takeda, K., Shudo, K. & Okamoto, T. (1980) Mutagenicities of γ-carboline derivatives related to potent mutagens found in tryptophan pyrolysates. *Carcinogenesis, 1*, 451-454

Nemoto, N., Kusumi, S., Takayama, S., Nagao, M. & Sugimura, T. (1979) Metabolic activation of 3-amino-5*H*-pyrido[4,3-*b*]indole, a highly mutagenic principle in tryptophan pyrolysate, by rat liver enzymes. *Chem.-biol. Interact.*, *27*, 191-198

Pezzuto, J.M., Lau, P.P., Luh, Y., Moore, P.D., Wogan, G.N. & Hecht, S.M. (1980) There is a correlation between the DNA affinity and mutagenicity of several 3-amino-1-methyl-5*H*-pyrido[4,3-*b*]indoles. *Proc. natl Acad. Sci. USA*, *77*, 1427-1431

Pezzuto, J.M., Moore, P.D. & Hecht, S.M. (1981) Metabolic activation of 1-methyl-3-amino-5*H*-pyrido[4,3-*b*]indole and several structurally related mutagens. *Biochemistry, 20*, 298-305

Sasaki, M., Sugimura, K., Yoshida, M.A. & Kawachi, T. (1980) Chromosome aberrations and sister chromatid exchanges induced by tryptophan pyrolysates, Trp-p-1 and Trp-p-2 in cultured human and Chinese hamster cells. *Proc. Jpn. Acad.*, *56B*, 332-337

Shishido, K., Tachibana, T. & Ando, T. (1980) Enzymatic studies on binding of mutagenic principles in tryptophan pyrolysate to DNA. *Agric. biol. Chem.*, *44*, 1609-1616

Sugimura, T., Nagao, M. & Wakabayashi, K. (1981) *Mutagenic heterocyclic amines in cooked food.* In: Egan, H., Fishbein, L., Castegnaro, M., O'Neill, I.K. & Bartsch, H., eds, *Environmental Carcinogenis. Selected Methods of Analysis*, Vol. 4, *Some Aromatic Amines and Azo-Dyes in the General and Industrial Environment* (*IARC Scientific Publications No. 40*), Lyon, International Agency for Research on Cancer, pp. 251-267

Takayama, S., Katoh, Y., Tanaka, M., Nagao, M., Wakabayashi, K. & Sugimura, T. (1977) *In vitro* transformation of hamster embryo cells with tryptophan pyrolysis products. *Proc. Jpn. Acad.*, *53B*, 126-129

Takayama, S., Hirakawa, T. & Sugimura, T. (1978) Malignant transformation *in vitro* by tryptophan pyrolysis products. *Proc. Jpn. Acad.*, *54B*, 418-422

Terada, M., Nakayasu, M., Sakamoto, H., Wakabayashi, K., Nagao, M., Rosenkranz, H.S. & Sugimura, T. (1982) *Mutagenic activity of nitropyrenes and heterocyclic aromatic amines on Chinese hamster cells with diphtheria toxin resistance as a marker* (Abstract no. 3P16). In: Sugimura, T., Kondo, S. & Takebe, H., eds, *3rd International Conference on Environmental Mutagens, Tokyo, 1981*, Tokyo, University of Tokyo Press, p. 3P

Tohda, H., Oikawa, A., Kawachi, T. & Sugimura, T. (1980) Induction of sister-chromatid exchanges by mutagens from amino acid and protein pyrolysates. *Mutat. Res.*, *77*, 65-69

Uyeta, M., Kanada, T., Mazaki, M., Taue, S. & Takahashi, S. (1979) *Assaying mutagenicity of food pyrolysis products using the Ames test.* In: Miller, E.C., Miller, J.A., Hirono, I., Sugimura, T. & Takayama, S., eds, *Naturally Occurring Carcinogens-Mutagens and Modulators of Carcinogenesis*, Tokyo/Baltimore, Japan Scientific Societies Press/University Park Press, pp. 169-176

Yagi, M. (1979) Oxidation of tryptophan-P-1 and P-2 by beef liver catalase-H_2O_2 intermediate: comparison with horseradish peroxidase. *Cancer Biochem. Biophys.*, *4*, 105-117

Yamada, M., Mori, M. & Sugimura, T. (1980) Myeloperoxidase-catalyzed binding of 3-amino-1-methyl-5*H*-pyrido[4,3-*b*]indole, a tryptophan pyrolysis product, to protein. *Chem.-biol. Interact.*, *33*, 19-33

Yamaizumi, Z., Shiomi, T., Kasai, H., Nishimura, S., Takahashi, Y., Nagao, M. & Sugimura, T. (1980) Detection of potent mutagens, Trp-P-1 and Trp-p-2, in broiled fish. *Cancer Lett.*, *9*, 75-83

Yamazoe, Y., Ishii, K., Kamataki, T., Kato, R. & Sugimura, T. (1980) Isolation and characterization of active metabolites of tryptophan-pyrolysate mutagen, trp-P-2, formed by rat liver microsomes. *Chem.-biol. Interact.*, *30*, 125-138

Yamazoe, Y., Tada, M., Kamataki, T. & Kato, R. (1981a) Enhancement of binding of *N*-hydroxy-Trp-P-2 to DNA by seryl-tRNA synthetase. *Biochem. biophys. Res. Commun.*, *102*, 432-439

Yamazoe, Y., Kamataki, T. & Kato, R. (1981b) Species difference in *N*-hydroxylation of a tryptophan pyrolysis product in relation to mutagenic activation. *Cancer Res.*, *41*, 4518-4522

T$_2$-TRICHOTHECENE

1. Chemical and Physical Data

1.1 Synonyms and trade names

Chem. Abstr. Services Reg. No.: 21259-20-1

Chem. Abstr. Name: Trichothec-9-ene-3,4,8,15-tetrol, 12,13-epoxy-, 4,15-diacetate 8-(3-methylbutanoate), (3α,4β,8α)-

IUPAC Systematic Name: 12,13-Epoxytrichothec-9-ene-3α,4β,8α,15-tetrol,4,15-diacetate 8-isovalerate or (2*R*,3*R*,4*S*,5*S*,5a*R*,7*S*,9a*R*,10*S*)-2,3,4,5,7,9a-Hexa-hydro-3,4,7-trihydroxy-5,8-dimethyl spiro[2,5-methano-1-benzoxepin-10,2'-oxirane]-5a(6*H*)-methanol, 4,5a-diacetate 7-isovalerate

Synonyms: 8-Isovalerate; fusariotoxine T2; isariotoxin; 8-(3-methylbutyryloxy)-diacetoxyscirpenol; mycotoxin T2; NSC 138780; T-2 mycotoxin; T2 toxin; toxin T2

1.2 Structural and molecular formulae and molecular weight

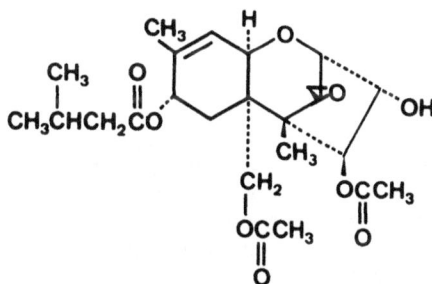

C$_{24}$H$_{34}$O$_9$ Mol. wt: 466.5

1.3 Chemical and physical properties of the pure substance

From Bamburg *et al.* (1968), Yates *et al.* (1968) and Wei *et al.* (1971)

- (*a*) *Description*: White needles (recrystallized from benzene-Skellysolve B)

- (*b*) *Melting-point*: 151-152°C

- (*c*) *Optical rotation*: $[\alpha]_D^{26}$ + 15° (c = 2.58 in 95% ethanol); $[\alpha]_D^{24}$ -50° (c = 0.16 in cyclohexane)

- (*d*) *Spectroscopy data*: Infra-red, nuclear magnetic resonance and mass spectral data have been reported.

- (*e*) *Solubility*: Soluble in acetone, acetonitrile, chloroform, diethyl ether, ethyl acetate and dichloromethane

- (*f*) *Stability*: Stable in the solid state. The ester groups are saponified by alkalis, and the epoxide is opened by strong mineral acids.

1.4 Technical products and impurities

No technical product containing T_2-trichothecene is available.

2. Production, Use, Occurrence and Analysis

2.1 Production and use

(*a*) *Production*

T_2-Trichothecene was first isolated in 1968 (Bamburg *et al.*, 1968) from a culture of the fungus *Fusarium tricinctum*, strain T-2, by ethyl acetate extraction of the whole blended and lyophilized culture. The yield of toxin was 0.5%, based on the dry weight of the lyophilized culture. There is no evidence that T_2-trichothecene is produced commercially, but it can be readily prepared in gram quantities by culturing of *Fusarium tricinctum* on corn (Burmeister, 1971).

(*b*) *Use*

T_2-Trichothecene is not used commercially.

2.2 Occurrence

The mycotoxin T_2-trichothecene has been found in members of the *Fusarium sporotrichioides* (also designated *F. tricinctum*), *F. roseum, F. solani, F. lateritium* and *F. rigidosum* groups, all of which cause moulding of wheat, oats, straw, hay and, particularly, corn. It is also found in *Trichothecium viride* and *T. lignorum* (FAO, 1982). Grain infection probably depends on environmental conditions: it is usually associated with corn that was late to mature or was high in moisture content at harvest. Infection has occurred mostly in the northerly parts of the corn-producing areas of the US (Tuite, 1979) and in the USSR and other countries in eastern Europe, Finland and Japan. Tricothecenes probably occur in other countries which have similar climates (FAO, 1979).

Instances of poisoning by trichothecene toxins from *Fusarium* species date back to 1891, when it was found that 'scabby grain' was toxic to man and animals. Since then, outbreaks of mouldy food-associated diseases have occurred all over the world, some of which have been attributed specifically to *Fusarium* infection. It is not possible to determine whether these outbreaks were caused by T_2-trichothecene toxin alone or if a mixture of different toxins was involved (Saito & Ohtsubo, 1974). The first direct implication of T_2-trichothecene in lethal toxicosis in dairy cattle was made in 1972, when mouldy corn used as feed was found to contain 2×10^5 *Fusarium tricinctum* propagules per gram of corn. Isolation of T_2-trichothecene indicated that it was present at a concentration of 2 mg/kg of dry corn (Hsu *et al.*, 1972).

The natural occurrence of T_2-trichothecene in various parts of the world is shown in Table 1.

Table 1. Natural occurrence of T_2-trichothecene in various parts of the world

Feed	Country	Concentration (mg/kg)	Reference
Corn	USA	2.0	Hsu *et al.* (1972)
Mixed feed	USA	0.076	Mirocha *et al.* (1976)
Barley	Canada	25.0[a]	Puls & Greenway (1976)
Corn	France	0.02	Jemmali *et al.* (1978)
Sweet corn	India	4.0	Ghosal *et al.* (1978)
Safflower	India	5	Ghosal *et al.* (1977)
Sorghum	India	0.5	Rukmini & Bhat (1978)

[a]The identity and quantitation are questionable.

2.3 Analysis

The isolation and analysis of T_2-trichothecene are complicated due, in part, to the large number of compounds with closely related structures (all produced by *Fusarium* species) and to the fact that the T_2-trichothecene molecule contains only a very weak chromophore. Some general methods for its analysis were summarized by Eppley (1979).

Typical methods for the analysis of T_2-trichothecene are summarized in Table 2.

Table 2. Methods for the analysis of T_2-trichothecene

Sample matrix	Sample preparation	Assay procedure[a]	Limit of detection	Reference
Foods	Extract (20% sulphuric acid/4% potassium chloride/acetonitrile); defat (isooctane); transfer to chloroform, clean up (silica gel column)	TLC/FL	500 µg/kg	Takeda *et al.* (1979)
Rice	Extract (acetonitrile/aqueous potassium chloride); partition against hexane and dichloromethane; evaporate; dissolve (methanol); clean up (Sep-Pak C_{18} column)	HPLC/DR	1 µg	Schmidt *et al.* (1981)
Wheat flour and corn meal	Extract (methanol); defat (hexane); purify (Sep-Pak C_{18} column)	ELISA	2.5 pg	Pestka *et al.* (1981)
Milk	Extract (ethyl acetate); evaporate; dissolve (acetonitrile); defat (hexane); evaporate; dissolve (ethyl acetate); purify on TLC plate; derivatize with *N,O*-bis(trimethylsilyl)acetamide	GC/MS	3 µg/kg	Collins & Rosen (1979)
Mixed feeds and other food products	Extract; clean up by extracting with solvents of different pH	TLC/UV	800 µg/kg	Gimeno (1979)
Feedstuffs	Extract (acetonitrile-4% aqueous potassium chloride); defat (isooctane); dilute (water); extract (chloroform); clean up by dialysis	TLC/UV	200 µg/kg	Patterson & Roberts (1979)

Sample matrix	Sample preparation	Assay procedure[a]	Limit of detection	Reference
Cereals grains faeces, urine, tissues	Extract (acetonitrile); clean-up (XAD-2, Flori-sil, Sep-Pak C_{18}); TLC (silica gel); spray (20% sulphuric acid); scrape; denitrate (bis-trimethyl-silyl or trifluoroacetic anhydride)	GC/FID GC/MS	100 μg/kg 1-5 μg/kg	Mirocha (1983)
Serum, urine and milk	Extract (ethyl acetate); wash (water); concen-trate; dissolve (metha-nol); dilute (water); purify (Sep-Pak C_{18} column)	RIA	0.5 μg/kg (serum) 2.5 μg/kg (urine or milk)	Lee & Chu (1981)

[a]Abbreviations: TLC/FL, thin-layer chromatography with fluorescence detection; HPLC/DR, high-performance liquid chromatography with differential refractometry; ELISA, enzyme-linked immunosorbent assay; GC/MS, gas chromatography with mass spectrometry; TLC/UV, thin-layer chromatography with ultra-violet spectrometry; GC/FID, gas chromatography with flame-ionization determination; RIA, radioimmunoassay

3. Biological Data Relevant to the Evaluation of Carcinogenic Risk to Humans

3.1 Carcinogenicity studies in animals

(a) Oral administration

Rat: Approximately 40 Wistar-Porton rats [sex not specified] were given 1-8 doses of 0.2 to 4 mg/kg bw T_2-trichothecene [purity not specified] intragastrically at approximately monthly intervals. Another 30 rats of the same strain received the same treatment but were also given i.p. injections of 200-250 mg/kg bw nicotinamide 10 minutes before and 2 hours after each dosing with T_2-trichothecene. Ten rats were given nicotinamide only, and another 10 rats served as untreated controls. About 65% of the rats treated with T_2-trichothecene alone or with nicotinamide died within a few days after the first or a subsequent T_2-trichothecene treatment. The 25 (22 males) rats surviving for 12 to 27.5 months presented a variety of pathological conditions, including cardiovascular lesions, kidney lesions and tumours at various sites. In 8/16 male rats treated four to eight times, tumours of the exocrine pancreas (1 carcinoma and 7 adenomas) were found; and islet-cell adenomas of the pancreas were found in 5/16 males. Three of four surviving rats treated eight times with both T_2-trichothecene and nicotinamide developed exocrine pancreatic carcinomas. Several other malignant and benign tumours were noted in the stomach, duodenum, brain, pituitary and mammary gland. In the 20 controls, only 4 pituitary adenomas were reported (Schoental *et al.*, 1979). [The Working Group noted the lack of reporting on the particulars of the experimental protocol.]

Trout: Groups of 1000 rainbow trout were given 0.2 or 0.4 mg/kg T_2-trichothecene in ethyl acetate sprayed onto feed for 12 months; control feed was treated with ethyl acetate only. At the end of the experiment, no evidence of neoplasia was found in the livers of the trout [number of trout examined not specified] (Marasas *et al.*, 1969).

(b) Co-carcinogenicity experiments

Mouse: Groups of 20 white mice [strain and sex not specified] received single doses of 10 or 20 µg per mouse of T_2-trichothecene [purity not specified] on the dorsal skin as an initiating agent. Two weeks later, these mice received ten weekly topical applications of croton oil (two drops of a 0.5% solution) as a promotor. The treatment induced no skin papilloma. In a second set of experiments, groups of 20 white mice received 25 µg 7,12-dimethylbenz[a]anthracene (DMBA) as initiator followed by 10 µg T_2-trichothecene after two weeks and then once a week for 10 weeks. Skin papillomas were observed in 2/20 mice (Marasas *et al.*, 1969). [The Working Group noted the incomplete reporting of the experiment, in that no information was available on strain or sex of mice or on their survival, the lack of solvent controls, and the lack of data on tumours in positive controls.]

Groups of eight CD-1 female mice, six weeks old, received single doses of 50 µg DMBA as initiator on the shaved back, followed four days later by topical skin application of 10 µg weekly or 25 µg every three weeks of T_2-trichothecene for 22 weeks. Positive (DMBA and croton oil), T_2-trichothecene-treated and solvent controls were also available. The administration of DMBA followed by 25 µg T_2-tichothecene resulted in the development of skin papillomas in 1/8 mice. Of the positive controls (DMBA and croton oil), 8/8 mice had papillomas. No such tumour was observed in the solvent controls, nor in T_2-trichothecene-treated mice (Lindenfelser *et al.*, 1974).

3.2 Other relevant biological data

The toxicology and pharmacology of T_2-trichothecene have been reviewed (Saito & Ohtsubo, 1974; Ueno, 1977).

(a) Experimental systems

Toxic effects

The oral LD_{50} of T_2-trichothecene in rats and swine is about 4 mg/kg bw (Kosuri et *al.*, 1971; Smalley, 1973). The i.p. LD_{50} in mice is 5.2 mg/kg bw (Ueno, 1977). The oral LD_{50} in guinea-pigs is 3 mg bw (DeNicola *et al.*, 1978), and the i.v. LD_{50} in swine is 1.2 mg/kg bw (Weaver *et al.*, 1978).

T_2-Trichothecene causes inflammatory reactions when applied to the skin of rats and rabbits; the rabbit was more sensitive than the rat (Hayes & Schiefer, 1979). T_2-Trichothecene also caused an irreversible depigmentation of dark C57Bl mouse skin (Schoental *et al.*, 1978).

Guinea-pigs treated orally with 0.5 mg/kg bw for 21 days and then 0.75 mg/kg bw for 21 days remained clinically normal and had no gross or microscopic lesion; however, moderate leucopenia and absolute lymphopenia were observed. Oral administration of a single dose of 2.5 or 5 mg/kg bw T_2-trichothecene caused irritation of the gut with subsequent necrosis, ulceration and hyperaemia of the gastric mucosa (DeNicola et al., 1978).

Pyknotic nuclei and karyorrhexis appeared in the epithelial cells of the gastrointestinal mucosa and in crypt cells of the jejunum and ileum of swine receiving 0.1-3 mg/kg bw T_2-trichothecene (Weaver et al., 1978).

Anaemia, lymphophenia and thymic atrophy were produced in mice given diets containing 20 mg/kg T_2-trichothecene for six weeks (Hayes et al., 1980). In rats fed diets containing 25 mg/kg, no pathological change was seen, but in rhesus monkeys given 0.5 or 1 mg/kg bw T_2-trichothecene orally for 15 days, severe leucocytopenia was observed in males (Rukmini et al., 1980).

Focal fatty changes and cytoplasmic degeneration were observed in the livers of rats given diets containing of 5-15 mg/kg T_2-trichothecene for three weeks (Marasas et al., 1969).

T_2-Trichothecene inhibits DNA and protein synthesis in a variety of cell types obtained from guinea-pigs and rabbits (Ueno et al, 1973; Ueno, 1977), and in cultured human fibroblasts, in which the LD_{50} was estimated to be 0.7 µg/ml (Oldham et al., 1980).

T_2-Trichothecene binds in vitro to active SH groups of creatine phosphokinase, lactate dehydrogenase and alcohol dehydrogenase, inhibiting their catalytic activity (Ueno, 1977).

Effects on reproduction and prenatal toxicity

The effects of prenatal exposure to T_2-trichothecene and other mycotoxins have been reviewed (Hayes & Hood, 1976; Hayes, 1978).

Pregnant mice were injected intraperitoneally with 0.5, 1.0 or 1.5 mg/kg bw T_2-trichothecene on one of days 7-11 of gestation. With the two higher doses there was significant maternal mortality and decreased prenatal survival. In eight litters evaluated from the group receiving 1.0 mg/kg on day 10, foetal weight was decreased and 38% of the foetuses had gross malformations, including missing tails, limb malformations, exencephaly, open eyes and retarded jaws (Stanford et al., 1975).

Doses of 0.5 mg/kg bw T_2-trichothecene given intraperitoneally to pregnant CD-1 mice induced tail and limb anomalies in 12.5% of the offspring when given on day 10 of gestation (Hood et al., 1976, 1978).

The feeding or i.p. injection of T_2-trichothecene to pregnant rats at doses of 0.1, 0.2 or 0.4 mg/kg bw daily on day 14 to 20 of gestation produced a decrease in thymus weight in newborn rats that lasted about a week (Bertin et al., 1978).

Absorption, distribution, excretion and metabolism

T_2-Trichothecene is readily absorbed through the skin and the gut in pigs and rats (Smalley, 1973).

The radioactivity of orally administered ^{3}H-T_2-trichothecene (1 mg/kg bw) to mice and rats was recovered in faeces (55%) and urine (15%) within 72 hours. It was distributed in the liver, kidneys and other organs, without specific accumulation. Analysis of the radioactivity recovered in the faeces of rats revealed that 2.7% of the dose was excreted as unchanged T_2-trichothecene and 7.5% as 4-O-deacetylated T_2-trichothecene (HT$_2$-trichothecene) (Matsumoto et al., 1978), which has approximately half the toxicity of T_2-trichothecene (Ueno, 1977); the remaining faecal excretion products were not identified. In the urine, HT$_2$-trichothecene, representing 1.4% of the total dose and 8-hydroxydiacetoxyscirpenol (1.8%) were identified; three unidentified metabolites of T_2-trichothecene were also isolated (Matsumoto et al., 1978).

The epoxide moeity of T_2-trichothecene seems to be essential for its toxicological activity; the liver detoxifies T_2-trichothecene, probably through epoxide hydrolase (Patterson, 1973).

In vitro, rat liver homogenate metabolizes T_2-trichothecene to HT$_2$-trichothecene, T_2-trichothecene tetraol, 4-deacetylneosolaniol (TMR-1) and neosolaniol (TMR-2). The same metabolites were obtained from HT$_2$-trichothecene, indicating that T_2-trichothecene was preferentially hydrolysed at the C-4 position to give HT$_2$-trichothecene (Yoshizawa et al., 1980).

Mutagenicity and other short-term tests

The genetic effects of mycotoxins, including T_2-trichothecene, have been reviewed (Stark, 1980).

T_2-Trichothecene was negative in a Bacillus subtilis rec assay measuring DNA damage when tested at 20 and 100 μg/plate (Ueno & Kubota, 1976). It was not mutagenic to Salmonella typhimurium TA1535, TA1537, TA1538, TA98 or TA100, either with or without exogenous metabolic activation with doses of up to 500 μg/plate T_2-trichothecene (Ueno, 1977; Kuczuk et al., 1978; Wehner et al., 1978). No increase in genetic changes at the ade 2 locus of the D3 strain of Saccharomyces cerevisiae was observed after treatment with 50 or 100 μg/plate T_2-trichothecene with or without exogenous metabolic activation (Kuczuk et al., 1978).

In a test for sex-linked recessive lethals in Drosophila melanogaster, no effect was found after feeding diets containing 100-1000 mg/kg T_2-trichothecene to adults for 2-3 days. After feeding 30-60 mg/kg to larvae, a slight increase in the incidence of recessive lethals was noted (p = 0.04). A significant increase in chromosomal loss and nondisjunction of sex chromosomes was observed (Sorsa et al., 1980). These findings on chromosomal disjunction are supported by observations of c-mitotic effects in root-tip cells of Allium species (Linnainmaa et al., 1979). The high affinity of T_2-trichothecene and other trichothecenes to SH compounds (Ueno, 1977) provides a molecular basis for an interaction with the spindle fibre mechanism.

T_2-Trichothecene was reported to induce unscheduled DNA synthesis in human fibroblasts (at doses of 0.005-0.5 μg/ml), but the observed effect was not dose-dependent (Oldham et al., 1980). No increase in unscheduled DNA synthesis was observed in human fibroblasts after treatment with 0.006-20 μg/ml T_2-trichothecene. The 4-O-deacylated metabolite of T_2-trichothecene, HT$_2$-trichothecene, however, induced unscheduled DNA synthesis in human fibroblasts in the presence of a rat liver 9000 x g supernatant fraction (Agrelo & Schoental, 1980).

A slight increase in the incidence of chromatid aberrations was induced in Chinese hamster bone-marrow cells after i.p. injection of 2.7-3.7 mg/kg bw T_2-trichothecene. No increase in the number of micronuclei was noted in bone-marrow erythrocytes after i.p. injection of 3 mg/kg bw (Norppa et al., 1980).

(b) Humans

Toxic effects

Accidental contact of laboratory workers with crude extracts containing T_2-trichothecene (approximately 100 mg/l) caused severe irritation, loss of sensitivity and desquamation of the skin of the hands. A solution of crude toxin caused dermatitis of the hands and face of laboratory workers (Saito & Ohtsubo, 1974).

Outbreaks of human disease attributed to poisoning by Fusarium metabolites, including T_2-trichothecene and closely related trichothecenes, have been characterized by widespread haemorrhage, necrotic ulcers in the gut and disturbances of the haematopoietic system (Rodricks & Eppley, 1974; Saito & Ohtsubo, 1974).

Effects on reproduction and prenatal toxicity

No data were available to the Working Group.

Absorption, distribution, excretion and metabolism

Human liver enzymes deacetylate T_2-trichothecene to HT_2-trichothecene in vitro (Ellison & Kotsonis, 1974).

Mutagenicity and chromosomal effects

No data were available to the Working Group.

3.3 Case reports and epidemiological studies of carcinogenicity in humans

No data were available to the Working Group..

4. Summary of Data Reported and Evaluation

4.1 Experimental data

T_2-Trichothecene was tested for carcinogenicity in rats by intragastric administration, in trout by administration in the diet and in mice by skin painting studies to investigate initiating and promoting activity. These studies were inadequate for evaluation.

T_2-Trichothecene was not mutagenic to bacteria or yeast. It induced chromosomal loss, non-disjunction of sex chromosomes and a slight increase in recessive lethal mutations in *Drosophila melanogaster*. Its 4-*O*-deacylated metabolite induced unscheduled DNA synthesis in human fibroblasts *in vitro*. Chromatid aberrations but not micronuclei were induced in hamsters exposed *in vivo*. There is *limited evidence* that T_2-trichothecene is active in short-term tests.

T_2-Trichothecene is embryolethal and teratogenic to mice, inducing tail and limb anomalies and exencephaly.

4.2 Human data

T_2-Trichothecene is a naturally occurring mycotoxin which was first isolated in 1968. There is exposure to this toxin from the consumption of cereals contaminated with T_2-trichothecene.

No data were available to assess the teratogenicity or chromosomal effects of this compound in humans.

No case report or epidemiological study of the carcinogenicity of T_2-trichothecene was available to the Working Group.

4.3 Evaluation

No evaluation of the carcinogenicity of T_2-trichothecene to experimental animals could be made. In the absence of epidemiological data, no evaluation of the carcinogenicity of T_2-trichothecene to humans could be made.

5. References

Agrelo, C.E. & Schoental, R. (1980) Synthesis of DNA in human fibroblasts treated with T-2 toxin and HT-2 toxin (the trichothecene metabolites of *Fusarium* species) and the effects of hydroxyurea. *Toxicol. Lett.*, 5, 155-160

Bamburg, J.R., Riggs, N.V. & Strong, F.M. (1968) The structures of toxins from two strains of *Fusarium tricinctum*. *Tetrahedron*, 24, 3329-3336

Bertin, G., Chakor, K., Lafont, P. & Frayssinet, C. (1978) Transmission to the progeny of contamination of maternal diet by mycotoxins (Fr.). *Collect. Med. leg. Toxicol. med.*, 107, 95-100

Burmeister, H.R. (1971) T-2 toxin production by *Fusarium tricinctum* on solid substrate. *Appl. Microbiol.*, 21, 739-742

Collins, G.J. & Rosen, J.D. (1979) Gas-liquid chromatographic/mass spectrometric screening method for T-2 toxin in milk. *J. Assoc. off. anal. Chem.*, *62*, 1274-1280

DeNicola, D.B., Rebar, A.H. & Carlton, W.W. (1978) T-2 toxin mycotoxicosis in the guinea-pig. *Food Cosmet. Toxicol.*, *16*, 601-609

Ellison, R.A. & Kotsonis, F.N. (1974) *In vitro* metabolism of T-2 toxin. *Appl. Microbiol.*, *27*, 423-424

Eppley, R. M. (1979) Trichothecenes and their analysis. *J. Am. Oil. Chem. Soc.*, *56*, 824-829

FAO (1979) *Perspective on Mycotoxins* (*FAO Food and Nutrition Paper No. 13*), Rome, p. 31

FAO (1982) *Mycotoxin Surveillance. A Guideline* (*FAO Food Control Series No. 4*), Rome, pp. 20, 23

Ghosal, S., Chakrabarti, D.K. & Chaudhary, K.C.B. (1977) The occurrence of 12,13-epoxytrichothecenes in seeds of safflower infected with *Fusarium oxysporum* F. sp. carthami. *Experientia*, *33*, 574-575

Ghosal, S., Biswas, K., Srivastava, R.S., Chakrabarti, D.K. & Chaudhary, K.C.B. (1978) Toxic substances produced by *Fusarium*. V: Occurrence of zearalenone, diacetoxys-cirpenol and T-2 toxin in moldy corn infected with *Fusarium moniliforme* shield. *J. pharm. Sci.*, *67*, 1768-1769

Gimeno, A. (1979) Thin layer chromatographic determination of aflatoxins, ochratoxins, sterigmatocystin, zearalenone, citrinin, T-2 toxin, diacetoxyscirpenol, penicillic acid, patulin, and penitrem A. *J. Assoc. off. anal. Chem.*, *62*, 579-585

Hayes, A.W. (1978) *Mycotoxin teratogenicity.* In: Rosenberg, P., ed., *Toxins: Animal, Plant and Microbial*, New York, Pergamon Press, pp. 739-758

Hayes, A.W. & Hood, R.D. (1976) Effect of prenatal exposure to mycotoxins. *Proc. Eur. Soc. Toxicol.*, *17*, 209-219

Hayes, M.A. & Schiefer, H.B. (1979) Quantitative and morphological aspects of cutaneous irritation by trichothecene mycotoxins. *Food Cosmet. Toxicol.*, *17*, 611-621

Hayes, M.A., Bellamy, J.E.C. & Schiefer, H.B. (1980) Subacute toxicity of dietary T-2 toxin in mice: morphological and hematological effects. *Can. J. comp. Med.*, *44*, 203-218

Hood, R.D., Kuczuk, M.H. & Szczech, G.M. (1976) Prenatal effects in mice of mycotoxins in combination: ochratoxin A and T-2 toxin (Abstract). *Teratology*, *13*, 25A

Hood, R.D., Kuczuk, M.H. & Szczech, G.M. (1978) Effects in mice of simultaneous prenatal exposure to ochratoxin A and T-2 toxin. *Teratology*, *17*, 25-30

Hsu, I.-C., Smalley, E.B., Strong, F.M. & Ribelin, W.E. (1972) Identification of T-2 toxin in moldy corn associated with a lethal toxicosis in dairy cattle. *Appl. Microbiol.*, *24*, 684-690

Jemmali, M., Ueno, Y., Ishii, K., Frayssinet, C. & Etienne, M. (1978) Natural occurrence of trichothecenes (nivalenol, deoxynivalenol, T_2) and zearalenone in corn. *Experientia, 34*, 1333-1334

Kosuri, N.R., Smalley, E.B. & Nichols, R.E. (1971) Toxicologic studies of *Fusarium tricinctum* (corda) Snyder et Hansen from moldy corn. *Am. J. vet. Res., 32*, 1843-1850

Kuczuk, M.H., Benson, P.M., Heath, H. & Hayes, A.W. (1978) Evaluation of the mutagenic potential of mycotoxins using *Salmonella typhimurium* and *Saccharomyces cerevisiae. Mutat. Res., 53*, 11-20

Lee, S. & Chu, F.S. (1981) Radioimmunoassay of T-2 toxin in biological fluids. *J. Assoc. off. anal. Chem., 64*, 684-688

Lindenfelser, L.A., Lillehoj, E.B. & Burmeister, H.R. (1974) Aflatoxin and trichothecene toxins: Skin tumor induction and synergistic acute toxicity in white mice. *J. natl Cancer Inst., 52*, 113-116

Linnainmaa, K., Sorsa, M. & Ilus, T. (1979) Epoxytrichothecene mycotoxins as c-mitotic agents in *Allium. Hereditas, 90*, 151-156

Marasas, W.F.O., Bamburg, J.R., Smalley, E.B., Strong, F.M., Ragland, W.L. & Degurse, P.E. (1969) Toxic effects on trout, rats, and mice of T-2 toxin produced by the fungus *Fusarium tricinctum* (Cd.) Snyd. et Hans. *Toxicol. appl. Pharmacol., 15*, 471-482

Matsumoto, H., Ito, T. & Ueno, Y. (1978) Toxicological approaches to the metabolites of *Fusaria*. XII. Fate and distribution of T-2 toxin in mice. *Jpn. J. exp. Med., 48*, 393-399

Mirocha, C.J. (1983) *Analysis of T-2 toxin and other trichothecenes in cereal grains*. In: Egan, H., Stoloff, L., Castegnaro, M., Scott, P., O'Neill, I.K. & Bartsch, H., eds., *Environmental Carcinogens. Selected Methods of Analysis*, Vol. 5, *Some Mycotoxins (IARC Scientific Publications No. 44)*, Lyon, International Agency for Research on Cancer, pp. 373-383

Mirocha, C.J., Pathre, S.V., Schauerhamer, B. & Christensen, C.M. (1976) Natural occurrence of *Fusarium* toxins in feedstuff. *Appl. environ. Microbiol., 32*, 533-556

Norppa, H., Penttilä, M., Sorsa, M., Hintikka, E.-L. & Ilus, T. (1980) Mycotoxin T-2 of *Fusarium tricinctum* and chromosome changes in Chinese hamster bone marrow. *Hereditas, 93*, 329-332

Oldham, J.W., Allred, L.E., Milo, G.E., Kindig, O. & Capen, C.C. (1980) The toxicological evaluation of the mycotoxins T-2 and T-2 tetraol using normal human fibroblasts *in vitro. Toxicol. appl. Pharmacol., 52*, 159-168

Patterson, D.S.P. (1973) Mycotoxins: Metabolism and liver injury. *Biochim. Soc. Trans., 1*, 917-922

Patterson, D.S.P. & Roberts, B.A. (1979) Mycotoxins in animal feedstuffs: Sensitive thin layer chromatographic detection of aflatoxin, ochratoxin A, sterigmatocystin, zearalenone, and T-2 toxin. *J. Assoc. off. anal. Chem., 62*, 1265-1267

Pestka, J.J., Lee, S.C., Lau, H.P. & Chu, F.S. (1981) Enzyme-linked immunosorbent assay for T-2 toxin. *J. Am. Oil Chem. Soc.*, *58*, 940A-944A

Puls, R. & Greenway, J.A. (1976) Fusariotoxicosis from barley in British Columbia. II. Analysis and toxicity of suspected barley. *Can. J. comp. Med.*, *40*, 16-19

Rodricks, J.V. & Eppley, R.M. (1974) *Stachybotrys and stachybotryotoxicosis*. In: Purchase, I.F.H., ed., *Mycotoxins*, Amsterdam, Elsevier, pp. 181-197

Rukmini, C. & Bhat, R.V. (1978) Occurrence of T-2 toxin in *Fusarium*-infested sorghum from India. *J. agric. Food Chem.*, *26*, 647-649

Rukmini, C., Prasad, J.S. & Kao, K. (1980) Effects of feeding T-2 toxin to rats and monkeys. *Food Cosmet. Toxicol.*, *18*, 267-269

Saito, M. & Ohtsubo, K. (1974) *Trichothecene toxins of* Fusarium *species*. In: Purchase, I.F.H., ed., *Mycotoxins*, Amsterdam, Elsevier, pp. 263-281

Schmidt, R., Ziegenhagen, E. & Dose, K. (1981) High-performance liquid chromatography of trichothecenes. I. Detection of T-2 toxin and HT-2 toxin. *J. Chromatogr.*, *212*, 370-373

Schoental, R., Joffe, Z.A. & Yagen, B. (1978) Irreversible depigmentation of dark mouse hair by T-2 toxin (a metabolite of *Fusarium sporotrichioides*) and by calcium pantothenate. *Experientia*, *34*, 763-764

Schoental, R., Joffe, A.Z. & Yagen, B. (1979) Cardiovascular lesions and various tumors found in rats given T-2 toxin, a trichothecene metabolite of *Fusarium*. *Cancer Res.*, *39*, 2179-2189

Smalley, E.B. (1973) T-2 toxin. *J. Am. vet. med. Assoc.*, *163*, 1278-1281

Sorsa, M., Linnainmaa, K. , Penttilä, M. & Ilus, T. (1980) Evaluation of the mutagenicity of epoxytrichothecene mycotoxins in *Drosophila melanogaster*. *Hereditas*, *92*, 163-165

Stanford, G.K., Hood, R.D. & Hayes, A.W. (1975) Effect of prenatal administration of T-2 toxin to mice. *Res. Commun. chem. Pathol. Pharmacol.*, *10*, 743-746

Stark, A.-A. (1980) Mutagenicity and carcinogenicity of mycotoxins: DNA binding as a possible mode of action. *Ann. Rev. Microbiol.*, *34*, 235-262

Takeda, Y., Isohata, E., Amano, R. & Uchiyama, M. (1979) Simultaneous extraction and fractionation and thin layer chromatographic determination of 14 mycotoxins in grains . *J. Assoc. off. anal. Chem.*, *62*, 573-578

Tuite, J. (1979) *Field and storage conditions for the production of mycotoxins and geographic distribution of some mycotoxin problems in the United States*. In: *Interactions of Mycotoxins in Animal Production*, Washington DC, National Academy of Sciences, pp. 19-39

Ueno, Y. (1977) Mode of action of trichothecenes. *Pure appl. Chem.*, *49*, 1737-1745

Ueno, Y. & Kubota, K. (1976) DNA-attacking ability of carcinogenic mycotoxins in recombination-deficient mutant cells of *Bacillus subtilis*. *Cancer Res.*, *36*, 445-451

Ueno, Y., Nakajima, M., Sakai, K., Ishii, K., Sato, N. & Shimada, N. (1973) Comparative toxicology of trichothec mycotoxins: inhibition of protein synthesis in animal cells. *J. Biochem.*, *74*, 285-296

Weaver, G.A., Kurtz, H.J., Bates, F.Y., Chi, M.S., Mirocha, C.J., Behrens, J.C. & Robison, T.S. (1978) Acute and chronic toxicity of T-2 mycotoxin in swine. *Vet. Rec.*, *9*, 531-535

Wehner, F.C., Marasas, W.F.O. & Thiel, P.G. (1978) Lack of mutagenicity to *Salmonella typhimurium* of some *Fusarium* mycotoxins. *Appl. environ. Microbiol.*, *35*, 659-662

Wei, R.-D., Strong, F.M., Smalley, E.B. & Schnoes, H.K. (1971) Chemical interconversion of T-2 and HT-2 toxins and related compounds. *Biochem. biophys. Res. Commun.*, *45*, 396-401

Yates, S.G., Tookey, H.L., Ellis, J.J. & Burkhardt, H.J. (1968) Mycotoxins produced by *Fusarium nivale* isolated from tall fescue (*Festuca arundinacea* Schreb.). *Phytochemistry*, *7*, 139-146

Yoshizawa, T., Swanson, S.P. & Mirocha, C.J. (1980) *In vitro* metabolism of T-2 toxin in rats. *Appl. environ. Microbiol.*, *40*, 901-906

ZEARALENONE

1. Chemical and Physical Data

1.1 Synonyms and trade names

Chem. Abstr. Services Reg. No.: 17924-92-4

Chem. Abstr. Name: 1*H*-2-Benzoxacyclotetradecin-1,7(8*H*)-dione, 3,4,5,6,9,10-hexa-hydro-14,16-dihydroxy-3-methyl-, [*S*-(*E*)]-

IUPAC Systematic Name: (-)-(3*S*,11*E*)-3,4,5,6,9,10-Hexahydro-14,16-dihydroxy-3-methyl-1*H*-2-benzoxacyclotetradecin-1,7(8*H*)-dione

Synonyms: Compound F-2; F2; fermentation estrogenic substance; FES; (*S*)-(-)-3,4,5,6,9, 10-hexahydro-14, 16-dihydroxy-3-methyl-1*H*-2-benzoxacyclotetradecin-1,7 (8*H*)-dione; 6-(10-hydroxy-6-oxo-*trans*-1-undecenyl)-β-resorcylic acid lactone; mycotoxin F2; toxin F2; (-)-zearalenone; (*S*)-zearalenone; *trans*-zearalenone; (10*S*)-zearalenone

1.2 Structural and molecular formulae and molecular weight

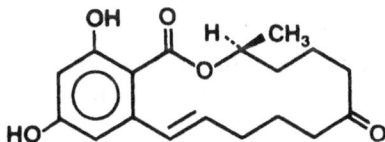

$C_{18}H_{22}O_5$ Mol. wt: 318.4

1.3 Chemical and physical properties of the pure substance

From Urry *et al.* (1966) and Windholz (1976), unless otherwise specified

    (*a*) *Description*: White crystals

    (*b*) *Melting-point*: 164-165°C

    (*c*) *Optical rotation*: $[\alpha]^{25}_{546}$ -170.5° (c = 1.0 in methanol)

    (*d*) *Spectroscopy data*: λ_{max} 236 nm, A^1_1 = 933; 274 nm, A^1_1 = 437; 316 nm, A^1_1 = 189; mass spectrometry data have been reported (NIH/EPA Chemical Information System, 1982).

    (*e*) *Solubility*: Solubilities at 25°C in % by wt are: water, 0.002; *n*-hexane, 0.05; benzene, 1.13; acetonitrile, 8.6; dichloromethane, 17.5; methanol, 18; ethanol, 24; and acetone, 58 (Hidy *et al.*, 1977).

    (*f*) *Stability*: Stable in the solid state; stable to hydrolysis

1.4 Technical products and impurities

No technical product containing zearalenone is available.

2. Production, Use, Occurrence and Analysis

2.1 Production and use

    (*a*) *Production*

Zearalenone was first isolated in 1962 (Stob *et al.*, 1962) from the mycelia of the fungus *Gibberella zeae* (*Fusarium graminearum*). The structure determination was carried out by classical chemistry as well as by spectrometric studies in 1966 (Urry *et al.*, 1966), and the total synthesis and determination of the absolute configuration were accomplished in 1968 (Taub *et al.*, 1967, 1968).

Zearalenone is produced commercially by large-scale biosynthesis, using submerged fermentation of glucose (Hidy *et al.*, 1977).

In the US, only one company produces zearalenone, as an intermediate in the manufacture of other chemicals. Whether it is isolated during this process is not known. Zearalenone is not believed to be produced commercially in western Europe or Japan.

(b) *Use*

Zearalenone appears to be used exclusively as an intermediate for the manufacture of zearalanol, a mixture of the diastereoisomers of the alcohol derivative produced by catalytic reduction with a nickel catalyst of both the keto group and the double bond adjacent to the aromatic ring. Zeranol, one of these isomers, was reported to have been evaluated in the US and some other countries for use in human medicine for the treatment of the postmenopausal syndrome (Hidy *et al.*, 1977); however, no evidence was found that it is presently being used in this way.

Zeranol (Ralgro[R]) is approved for use in the US as a subcutaneous ear implantation in beef cattle, feedlot lambs, and suckling beef calves (US Food & Drug Administration, 1980).

2.2 Occurrence

Zearalenone is a natural product produced primarily by members of the *Fusaria* group (*Fusarium culmorum, F. equiseti , F. gibbosum, F. lateritium, F. moniliforme, F. tricinctum, F. Avenaceum, F. roseum, F. roseum Graminearum* (*Gibberella zeae*), *F. roseum Culmorum, F. roseum Equiseti, F. roseum Gibbasum* (Pathre & Mirocha, 1976; FAO, 1982). It has been detected in a variety of agricultural commodities, such as hay feed, corn, pig feed, sorghum, dairy rations and barley, at levels in the range of 0.01-2900 mg/kg. Zearalenone-containing commodities have caused mycotoxicosis in farm animals in Finland, France, the UK, the US and Yugoslavia (Shotwell, 1977). The outbreaks are closely connected with growing conditions and have been severe in the years when unusually wet weather has delayed planting and harvest (FAO, 1979). A comprehensive report of a United Nations-sponsored meeting in 1977 gives detailed information on the reported occurrence of zearalenone in agricultural products throughout the world (FAO, 1979). [For several examples, see Table 1.]

Table 1. Natural occurrence of zearalenone in feeds in various parts of the world

Feed	Country (years)	Number of positive samples/Number of samples studied	Concentration (mg/kg)	References
Maize	USA (1968-1969)	6/576	0.45-0.8	Shotwell *et al.* (1970, 1971)
Maize	USA (1972)	38/223	0.1-5.0	Eppley *et al.* (1974)
Maize	USA (1974)	23/372	<0.1-10.4	Stoloff *et al.* (1976)
Maize	USA	-	0.43-7.62	Shotwell *et al.* (1976)
Maize	USA	-	0.9-7.8	Bennett *et al.* (1976)

Feed	Country (years)	Number of positive samples/Number of samples studied	Concentration (mg/kg)	References
Maize	France (1974)	62/75	up to 170	FAO (1979)
Maize	Yugoslavia (1972)	23/54	0.7-37.5	FAO (1979)
Maize	Hungary (1968)	-	70-80	FAO (1979)
Wheat	Hungary	3	5-10	FAO (1979)
Feed	USA (1968-1970)	28/65	0.1-2909	Mirocha & Christensen (1974)
Feed	Finland	-	25	FAO (1979)
Hay	USA	-	14	Mirocha et al. (1968)
Fermented feed	Swaziland	6/55	0.8-5.3	FAO (1979)

In a study of cereal products in Italy in 1975-1977, three out of 52 samples were found to contain zearalenone at levels of 0.4-2.0 mg/kg. The toxin was found in very few samples of freshly harvested maize. In 66 samples of wheat kernels collected in 1976 (when there were unusually heavy rains during ripening), no toxin was found (Bottalico, 1979).

Zearalenone was found in 1974 in samples of beer in Zambia at levels of 0-2.47 mg/l and in 17/140 samples in Lesotho at levels of 0.3-2 mg/kg (FAO (1979).

2.3 Analysis

General methods for the isolation and analysis of zearalenone have been summarized (Hidy et al., 1977; Shotwell, 1977; FAO, 1982). Typical methods for the analysis of zearalenone published more recently are summarized in Table 2.

Table 2. Methods for the analysis of zearalenone

Sample matrix	Sample preparation	Assay procedure[a]	Limit of detection	Reference
Cereals, grains and foodstuffs	Extract (aqueous methanol); purify in two steps (Amberlite XAD-4 and Florisil columns)	TLC or GC/FID	10 μg/kg	Kamimura et al. (1981)

Sample matrix	Sample preparation	Assay procedure[a]	Limit of detection	Reference
Foods and mixed feeds	Extract (acetic acid/diethyl ether); evaporate dissolve (chloroform); purify by several extractions at different pHs	HPLC/FL	2 μg/kg	Schweighardt et al. (1980)
	Extract and clean up by extracting with solvents of different pHs	TLC/UV	410-430 μg/kg	Gimeno (1980)
Maize and barley	Extract (ethyl acetate); evaporate; dissolve (chloroform); partition (aqueous sodium hydroxide); concentrate	TLC/FL GC/MS UV GC/FL MID	0.1 μg not given 0.1 μg/ml <50 μg/kg 10 ng	Mirocha et al. (1974)
Maize	Extract (chloroform/water); clean up (liquid-liquid chromatography)	HPLC/FL	10 μg/kg	Ware & Thorpe (1978)
	Add zearalenone internal standard; extract (ethyl acetate); purify (TLC); derivatize (N,O-bis(trimethylsilyl)triflu oroacetamide, trimethylchlorosilane and methoxyamine hydrochloride)	GC/FID	100 μg/kg	Thouvenot & Morfin (1979)
	Extract (aqueous methanol); partition (hexane/dichloromethane); evaporate; dissolve (benzene/acetonitrile); evaporate; dissolve (ethanol); purify (Sep-Pak C_{18} column)	HPLC/LF	5 μg/kg	Diebold et al. (1979)
Blood serum	Elute (column chromatography); base-acid extract (dichloromethane); add epicoprostanol internal standard; evaporate; derivatize (N-methyl-N-trimethylsilyltrif luoroacetamide)	GC/FID	100 μg/l	Trenholm et al. (1980)

[a]Abbreviations: TLC, thin-layer chromatography; GC/FID, gas chromatography with flame-ionization detection; HPLC/FL, high-performance liquid chromatography with fluorescence detection; TLC/UV, thin-layer chromatography with ultra-violet spectrometry; TLC/FL, thin-layer chromatography with fluorescence detection; GC/MS, gas chromatography with mass spectrometry; UV, ultra-violet spectrometry; GC/FL, gas chromatography with fluorescence detection; MID; multiple ion detection; HPLC/LF, high-performance liquid chromatography with laser fluorimetry

3. Biological Data Relevant to the Evaluation of Carcinogenic Risk to Humans

3.1 Carcinogenicity studies in animals

Oral administration

Mouse: Groups of 50 $B6C3F_1$ mice of each sex, seven weeks old, were fed diets containing 0, 50 or 100 mg/kg (maximum tolerated dose) zearalenone for 103 weeks. (Examination of the compound by thin-layer chromatography indicated the presence of a trace impurity in all three batches used; a minor impurity was detected by high-pressure liquid chromatography in one batch.) All survivors were killed 105-108 weeks after the start of treatment. No significant reduction in body weight gain was apparent in treated mice, and no significant difference in survival was observed between groups: 42/50 (84%) controls, 40/50 (80%) low-dose and 44/50 (88%) high-dose males lived to termination of the study; and 37/50 (74%) controls, 37/50 (74%) low-dose and 32/50 (64%) high-dose females were still alive at that time. Hepatocellular adenomas were found in 3/50 (6%) and 7/49 (14%) males given the low and high doses, respectively (compared with 4/50 (8%) in the controls), and in 2/49 (4%) and 7/49 (14%) females given the low and high doses, respectively (compared with 0/50 in the controls). The incidence in the high-dose female group was statistically significantly different (p $\leqslant$ 0.006) in individual comparisons with the control group. The incidence of hepatocellular adenomas in untreated historical control female $B6C3F_1$ mice at the institute where the study took place was 14/498 (2.8%). Pituitary adenomas occurred in both male and female mice in a statistically significant positive trend (p $\leqslant$ 0.022 for males and p $\leqslant$ 0.001 for females); they occurred in 4/45 (9%) and 6/44 (14%) males given the low and high doses (compared with 0/40 in the controls) and in 2/43 (5%) and 13/42 (31%) females given the low and high doses, respectively (compared with 3/46 (7%) in the respective controls). The increased incidences of pituitary adenomas were statistically significant in high-dose males (p $\leqslant$ 0.032) and in high-dose females (p $\leqslant$ 0.003). The incidences of pituitary adenomas and carcinomas in untreated historical control female and male $B6C3F_1$ mice at the institute where the study was undertaken were 21/428 (4.9%) and 0/399, respectively (National Toxicology Program, 1982).

Rat: Groups of 50 Fischer 344 rats of each sex, five weeks old, were fed diets containing 0, 25 or 50 mg/kg (maximum tolerated dose) zearalenone for 103 weeks. (Examination of the compound by thin-layer chromatography indicated the presence of a trace impurity in all three batches used; a minor impurity was detected by high-pressure liquid chromatography in one batch). All survivors were killed at 104-106 weeks. Mean body weight gains of treated rats were lower than those of controls; depression in mean body weight was dose related. Survival rates of dosed and control rats were comparable: of the male rats, 39/50 (78%) of the controls, 38/50 (76%) of the low-dose and 37/50 (74%) of the high-dose group were still alive at termination of the study; of the female rats, 40/50 (80%) of the controls, 38/50 (76%) of the low-dose, and 41/50 (82%) of the high-dose group were alive at the end of the study. No compound-related increase in tumour incidence was observed (National Toxicology Program, 1982).

3.2 Other relevant biological data

(a) *Experimental systems*

Toxic effects

The major effects of zearalenone are oestrogen-like. It caused atrophy of the seminal vesicles and testes and fibromuscular hyperplasia of the prostate in 90-100% of male rats fed diets containing 1000 or 3000 mg/kg for 13 weeks (National Toxicology Program, 1982).

Zearalenone interacts with oestrogen receptors in human breast cancer cells grown *in vitro* (Martin *et al.*, 1978).

Osteopetrosis occurred in a dose-related incidence in all groups of female rats administered diets containing 30-3000 mg/kg zearalenone for 13 weeks. Incidences of 90-100% were found in females administered 100 mg/kg or more, and in males given 1000 or 3000 mg/kg. The same dose-related effect was seen in male and female mice given 100-3000 mg/kg of the compound in the diet (National Toxicology Program, 1982).

Effects on reproduction and prenatal toxicity

Groups of 10 Wistar rats received 1, 5 or 10 mg/kg bw per day zearalenone by oral intubation on days 6-15 of gestation. The mean foetal weight was significantly reduced in the high-dose group, and there was a higher than normal incidence of minor skeletal anomalies in foetuses (Ruddick *et al.*, 1976).

Groups of 100 male and female rats received 0.1, 1.0 or 10.0 mg/kg bw dietary levels of zearalenone daily. Fertility was greatly impaired in high-dose females, with only 26 pregnancies from 50 matings; and the number of resorptions and stillborns was greatly increased, with 56% of the high-dose dams showing complete litter resorption. Foetal examination indicated no teratogenic response at any level (Bailey *et al.*, 1976).

In pigs fed 100 mg/kg zearalenone in the diet throughout pregnancy, complete infertility occurred. At lower concentrations (25 or 50 mg/kg), small litters and low birth weights were observed (Chang *et al.*, 1979). After intramuscular injections of 5 mg zearalenone throughout the last month of pregnancy, 3/20 piglets were stillborn and 13/20 were affected with a splay-leg condition (Miller *et al.*, 1973).

Absorption, distribution, excretion and metabolism

Comparative metabolic studies have indicated that zearalenone is well absorbed after oral administration in the rat, rabbit and pig (Mirocha *et al.*, 1981). The primary metabolites of zearalenone are the reduction products, α- and β-zearalenol, and the glucurono conjugates of both the parent compound and the metabolites (Ueno & Ayaki, 1976; Kiessling & Pettersson, 1978; Ueno & Tashiro, 1981). The reduction is catalysed by a 3α-hydroxy-steroid dehydrogenase (Olsen *et al.*, 1981). There are large species variations with regard to the extent of formation and excretion of the reduced metabolites (Mirocha *et al.*, 1981).

Zearalenone promotes cell proliferation and RNA and protein synthesis in the uterus of ovariectomized mice and rats (Ueno *et al.*, 1974; Ueno & Yagasaki, 1975). Both zearalenone and its metabolites, α- and β-zearalenol, bind to uterine cytoplasmic receptors and elicit the translocation of the cytosol-receptor complex into the nucleus. Zearalenone also binds to the mammary gland oestrogen receptor (National Toxicology Program, 1982).

Mutagenicity and other short-term tests

The genetic effects of mycotoxins, including zearalenone, have been reviewed (Stark, 1980).

In two studies of DNA damaging effects with the *rec* assay in *Bacillus subtilis*, zearalenone gave positive results (Ueno & Kubota, 1976; Boutibonnes & Loquet, 1979).

Zearalenone is not mutagenic to *Salmonella typhimurium* TA1535, TA1537, TA1538, TA98 or TA100, with or without rat liver 9000 x *g* supernatant preparations (Wehner *et al.*, 1978; Kuczuk *et al.*, 1978; Boutibonnes & Loquet, 1979; Bartholomew & Ryan, 1980; Ingerowski *et al.*, 1981). The zearalenone derivatives, zeranol and zearalanone, also gave negative results in these *Salmonella* strains (Ingerowski *et al.*, 1981). β-Zearalenol, a metabolite of zearalenone, was also negative in *S. typhimurium* TA98 and TA100 (Ueno *et al.*, 1978). The bacteriotoxic effect of zearalenone and its derivatives, however, makes the suitability of *Salmonella* test system questionable, as pointed out by Ingerowski *et al.* (1981).

No increase in genetic changes at the *ade2* locus of *Saccharomyces cerevisiae* was observed after treatment with 50 or 100 μg/plate zearalenone, with or without microsomal activation (Kuczuk *et al.*, 1978).

(b) Humans

Toxic effects

No data were available to the Working Group.

Effects on reproduction and prenatal toxicity

No data were available to the Working Group.

Absorption, distribution, excretion and metabolism

An adult man was given a single oral dose of 100 mg zearalenone and his urine collected during the following 24 hours; glucuronide conjugates of zearalenone, α- and β-zearalenol were detected (Mirocha *et al.*, 1981).

Mutagenicity and chromosomal effects

No data were available to the Working Group.

3.3 Case reports and epidemiological studies of carcinogenicity in humans

In a descriptive study, Marasas *et al.* (1979) examined the amounts of deoxynivalenol and zearalenone in 200 samples of mouldy corn from randomly selected areas in both the high-risk and low-risk oesophageal cancer regions of the Republic of Transkei in southern Africa where corn is the main dietary staple. The level of contamination of corn kernels with each of these two *Fusarium* mycotoxins was apparently higher in the pooled samples from the high-risk than the low-risk region. [However, the actual number of kernels infected specifically with *Fusarium* included in the tabulated data is not specified. Statistical evaluation of the data was not possible.]

4. Summary of Data Reported and Evaluation

4.1 Experimental data

Zearalenone was tested for carcinogenicity in mice and rats by administration in the diet. Increased incidences of hepatocellular adenomas in female mice and of pituitary adenomas in mice of both sexes were observed. There was no evidence of a carcinogenic effect in rats.

Zearalenone was positive in a bacterial repair test but was not mutagenic in bacteria or yeast. The data were *inadequate* to evaluate the activity of zearalenone in short-term tests.

Zearalenone induces multiple reproductive deficiencies, such as infertility and small litters, in rats and pigs. The data were inadequate to assess its teratogenicity to experimental animals.

4.2 Human data

Zearalenone is a mycotoxin found on a variety of agricultural commodities, and there is widespread human exposure.

No data were available to assess the teratogenicity or chromosomal effects of this compounds in humans.

The one available epidemiological study was considered inadequate to evaluate the carcinogenicity of zearalenone to humans.

4.3 Evaluation

There is *limited evidence*[1] for the carcinogenicity of zearalenone in experimental animals. In the absence of adequate epidemiological data, no evaluation of the carcinogenicity of zearalenone to humans could be made.

---

[1]See preamble, p. 18.

5. References

Bailey, D.E., Cox, G.E., Morgareidge, K. & Taylor, J. (1976) Acute and subacute toxicity of zearalenone in the rat (Abstract no. 126). *Toxicol. appl. Pharmacol., 37,* 144

Bartholomew, R.M. & Ryan, D.S. (1980) Lack of mutagenicity of some phytoestrogens in the *Salmonella*/mammalian microsome assay. *Mutat. Res., 78,* 317-321

Bennett, G.A., Peplinski, A.J., Brekke, O.L & Jackson, L.K. (1976) Zearalenone: distribution in dry-milled fractions of contaminated corn. *Cereal Chem., 53,* 299-307

Bottalico, A. (1979) On the occurrence of zearalenone in Italy. *Mycopathologia, 67,* 119-121

Boutibonnes, P. & Loquet, C. (1979) Antibacterial activity, DNA-attacking ability and mutagenic ability of the mycotoxin zearalenone. *Int. Res. Commun. System med. Sci., 7,* 204

Chang, K., Kurtz, H.J. & Mirocha, C.J. (1979) Effects of the mycotoxin zearalenone on swine reproduction. *Am. J. vet. Res., 40,* 1260-1267

Diebold, G.J., Karny, N. & Zare, R.N. (1979) Determination of zearalenone in corn by laser fluorimetry. *Anal. Chem., 51,* 67-69

Eppley, R.M., Stoloff, L., Trucksess, M.W. & Chung, C.W. (1974) Survey of corn for *Fusarium* toxins. *J. Assoc. off. anal. Chem., 57,* 632-635

FAO (1979) *Perspectives on Mycotoxins (FAO Food and Nutrition Paper 13),* Rome, pp. 15-120

FAO (1982) *Mycotoxin Surveillance. A Guideline (FAO Food Control Series No. 4),* Rome, pp. 20-21, 23

Gimeno, A. (1980) Improved method for thin layer chromatographic analysis of mycotoxins. *J. Assoc. off. anal. Chem., 63,* 182-186

Hidy, P.H., Baldwin, R.S., Greasham, R.L., Keith, C.L. & McMullen, J.R. (1977) *Zearalenone and some derivatives: production and biological activities.* In: Perlman, D., ed., *Advances in Applied Microbiology,* Vol. 22, New York, Academic Press, pp. 59-82

Ingerowski, G.H., Scheutwinkel-Reich, M. & Stan, H.-J. (1981) Mutagenicity studies on veterinary anabolic drugs with *Salmonella*/microsome test. *Mutat. Res., 91,* 93-98

Kamimura, H., Nishijima, M., Yasuda, K., Saito, K., Ibe, A., Nagayama, T., Ushiyama, H. & Naoi, Y. (1981) Simultaneous detection of several *Fusarium* mycotoxins in cereals, grains, and foodstuffs. *J. Assoc. off. anal. Chem., 64,* 1067-1073

Kiessling, K.-H. & Pettersson, H. (1978) Metabolism of zearalenone in rat liver. *Acta pharmacol. toxicol., 43,* 285-290

Kuczuk, M.H., Benson, P.M., Heath, H. & Hayes, A.W. (1978) Evaluation of the mutagenic potential of mycotoxins using *Salmonella typhimurium* and *Saccharomyces cerevisiae. Mutat. Res., 53,* 11-20

Marasas, W.F.O., van Rensburg, S.J. & Mirocha, C.J. (1979) Incidence of *Fusarium* species and the mycotoxins, deoxynivalenol and zearalenone, in corn produced in esophageal cancer areas in Transkei. *J. agric. Food Chem.*, *27*, 1108-1112

Martin, P.M., Horwitz, K.B., Ryan, D.S. & McGuire, W.L. (1978) Phytoestrogen interaction with estrogen receptors in human breast cancer cells. *Endocrinology*, *103*, 1860-1867

Miller, J.K., Hacking, A., Harrison, J. & Gross, V.J. (1973) Stillbirths, neonatal mortality and small litters in pigs associated with the ingestion of *Fusarium* toxin by pregnant sows. *Vet. Rec.*, *93*, 555-559

Mirocha, C.J. & Christensen, C.M. (1974) *Oestrogenic mycotoxins synthesized by* Fusarium. In: Purchase, I.F.H., ed., *Mycotoxins*, Amsterdam, Elsevier, pp. 129-148

Mirocha, C.J., Harrison, J., Nichols, A.A. & McClintock, M. (1968) Detection of a fungal estrogen (F-2) in hay associated with infertility in dairy cattle. *Appl. Microbiol.*, *16*, 797-798 [*Chem. Abstr.*, *69*, 16629x]

Mirocha, C.J., Schauerhamer, B. & Pathre, S.V. (1974) Isolation, detection, and quantitation of zearalenone in maize and barley. *J. Assoc. off. anal. Chem.*, *57*, 1104-1110

Mirocha, C.J., Pathre, S.V. & Robison, T.S. (1981) Comparative metabolism of zearalenone and transmission into bovine milk. *Food Cosmet. Toxicol.*, *19*, 25-30

National Toxicology Program (1982) *Carcinogenesis Bioassay of Zearalenone* (*NTP 81-54, DHHS Publ. No. (NIH) 81-1791*), Washington DC

NIH/EPA Chemical Information System (1982) *Mass Spectral Search System*, Washington DC, CIS Project, Information Services Corporation

Olsen, M., Petterson, H. & Kiessling, K.H. (1981) Reduction of zearalenone to zearalenol in female rat liver by 3a-hydroxysteroid dehydrogenase. *Acta Pharmacol. Toxicol.*, *48*, 157-161

Pathre, S.V. & Mirocha, C.J. (1976) *Zearalenone and related compounds*. In: Rodricks, J.V., ed., *Mycotoxins and Other Fungal Related Food Problems* (*Adv. Chem. Ser. No. 149*), Washington DC, Americal Chemical Society, pp. 178-225

Ruddick, J.A., Scott, P.M. & Harwig, J. (1976) Teratological evaluation of zearalenone administered orally to the rat. *Bull. environ. Contam. Toxicol.*, *15*, 678-681

Schweighardt, H., Böhm, J., Abdelhamid, A.M., Leibetseder, J., Schuh, M. & Glawischnig, E. (1980) Analysis of the fusariotoxins zearalenone and vomitoxin (deoxynivalenol) in human foods and animal feeds by high-performance liquid chromatography (HPLC). *Chromatographia*, *13*, 447-450

Shotwell, O.L. (1977) *Assay methods for zearalenone and its natural occurrence*. In: Rodricks, J.V., Hesseltine, C.W. & Mehlman, M.A., eds, *Mycotoxins in Human and Animal Health*, Park Forest South, IL, Pathotox Publishers, pp. 403-413

Shotwell, O.L., Hesseltine, C.W., Goulden, M.L. & Vandegraft, E.E. (1970) Survey of corn for aflatoxin, zearalenone and ochratoxin. *Cereal Chem.*, *47*, 700-707

Shotwell, O.L., Hesseltine, C.W., Vandegraft, E.E. & Goulden, M.L. (1971) Survey of corn from different regions for aflatoxin, ochratoxin and zearalenone. *Cereal Sci. Today*, *16*, 266-273

Shotwell, O.L., Goulden, M.L. & Bennett, G.A. (1976) Determination of zearalenone in corn: collaborative study. *J. Assoc. off. anal. Chem.*, *59*, 666-670

Stark, A.-A. (1980) Mutagenicity and carcinogenicity of mycotoxins: DNA binding as a possible mode of action. *Ann. Rev. Microbiol.*, *34*, 235-262

Stob, M., Baldwin, R.S., Tuite, J., Andrews, F.N. & Gillette, K.G. (1962) Isolation of an anabolic, uterotrophic compound from corn infected with *Gibberella zeae*. *Nature*, *196*, 1318

Stoloff, L., Henry, S. & Francis, O.J., Jr (1976) Survey for aflatoxins and zearalenone in 1973 crop corn stored on farms and in country elevators. *J. Assoc. off. anal. Chem.*, *59*, 118-121

Taub, D., Girotra, N.N., Hoffsommer, R.D., Kuo, C.H., Slates, H.L., Weber, S. & Wendler, N.L. (1967) Total synthesis of the macrolide, zearalenone. *Chem. Commun.*, 225-226

Taub, D., Girotra, N.N., Hoffsommer, R.D., Kuo, C.H., Slates, H.L., Weber, S. & Wendler, N.L. (1968) Total synthesis of the macrolide, zearalenone. *Tetrahedron*, *24*, 2443-2461

Thouvenot, D.R. & Morfin, R.F. (1979) Quantitation of zearalenone by gas-liquid chromatography on capillary glass columns. *J. Chromatogr.*, *170*, 165-173

Trenholm, H.L., Warner, R. & Farnworth, E.R. (1980) Gas chromatographic detection of the mycotoxin zearalenone in blood serum. *J. Assoc. off. anal. Chem.*, *63*, 604-611

Ueno, Y. & Ayaki, S. (1976) Metabolism of zearalenone, an uterotrophic mycotoxin, in rats (Abstract no. 116). *Jpn. J. Pharmacol., Suppl.*, *26*, 91P

Ueno, Y. & Kubota, K. (1976) DNA-attacking ability of carcinogenic mycotoxins in recombination-deficient mutant cells of *Bacillus subtilis*. *Cancer Res.*, *36*, 445-451

Ueno, Y. & Tashiro, F. (1981) α-Zearalenol, a major hepatic metabolite in rats of zearalenone, an estrogenic mycotoxin of *Fusarium* species. *J. Biochem.*, *89*, 563-571

Ueno, Y. & Yagasaki, S. (1975) Toxicological approaches to the metabolites of *Fuseria*. X. Accelerating effect of zearalenone on RNA and protein syntheses in the uterus of ovariectomized mice. *Jpn. J. exp. Med.*, *45*, 199-205

Ueno, Y., Shimada, N., Yagasaki, S. & Enomoto, M. (1974) Toxicological approaches to the metabolites of *Fusaria*. VII. Effects of zearalenone on the uteri of mice and rats. *Chem. pharm. Bull.*, *22*, 2830-2835

Ueno, Y., Kubota, K., Ito, T. & Nakamura, Y. (1978) Mutagenicity of carcinogenic mycotoxins in *Salmonella typhimurium*. *Cancer Res.*, *38*, 536-542

Urry, W.H., Wehrmeister, H.L., Hodge, E.B. & Hidy, P.H. (1966) The structure of zearalenone. *Tetrahedron Lett.*, *27*, 3109-3114

US Food & Drug Administration (1980) Foods and drugs. *US Code Fed. Regul., Title 21*, part 522, pp. 192, 239

Ware, G.M. & Thorpe, C.W. (1978) Determination of zearalenone in corn by high pressure liquid chromatography and fluorescence detection. *J. Assoc. off. anal. Chem., 61*, 1058-1062

Wehner, F.C., Marasas, W.F.O. & Thiel, P.G. (1978) Lack of mutagenicity to *Salmonella typhimurium* of some *Fusarium* mycotoxins. *Appl. environ. Microbiol., 35*, 659-662

Windholz, M., ed. (1976) *The Merck Index*, 9th ed., Rahway, NJ, Merck & Co., Inc., p. 1306

SUPPLEMENTARY CORRIGENDA TO VOLUMES 1-30

Corrigenda covering Volumes 1-6 appeared in Volume 7; others appeared in Volumes 8, 10-13, 15-28

Volume 8

p. 311   line 7   *delete*

Volume 19

p. 119   3.2 (a)   *replace* LD_{50} *by* LC_{50}
         Acute toxicity
         line 1

Volume 21

p. 404   4.1   *replace* subcutaneous
         line 2   *by* intramuscular

Volume 27

p. 230   3.1 *Mouse*   *replace* 12/13 *by* 12/31
         line 12

Supplement 3

p. 63   line 35   *delete* Diaminobenzidine *see*
                                         p-Dimethylaminoazobenzene
                                         8 125

Supplement 4

p. 262   last line   *replace* vinyl chloride
                                         by vinylidene chloride

CUMULATIVE INDEX TO IARC MONOGRAPHS
ON THE EVALUATION OF THE CARCINOGENIC RISK
OF CHEMICALS TO HUMANS

Numbers in italics indicate volume, and other numbers indicate page. References to corrigenda are given in parentheses. Compounds marked with and asterisk(*) were considered by the working groups, but monographs were not prepared becaused adequate data on carcinogenicity were not available.

2-Amino-5-(5-nitro-2-furyl)-1,3,4-thiadiazole	*7*, 143
4-Amino-2-nitrophenol	*16*, 43
2-Amino-4-nitrophenol*	
2-Amino-5-nitrophenol*	
2-Amino-5-nitrothiazole	*31*, 71
6-Aminopenicillanic acid*	
Amitrole	*7*, 31
	Suppl. 4, 38
Amobarbital sodium*	
Anaesthetics, volatile	*11*, 285
	Suppl. 4, 41
Aniline	*4*, 27 (corr. *7*, 320)
	27, 39
	Suppl. 4, 49
Aniline hydrochloride	*27*, 40
ortho-Anisidine and its hydrochloride	*27*, 63
para-Anisidine and its hydrochloride	*27*, 65
Anthranilic acid	*16*, 265
Apholate	*9*, 31
Aramite	*5*, 39
Arsenic and arsenic compounds	*1*, 41
	2, 48
	23, 39
	Suppl. 4, 50

Arsanilic acid
Arsenic pentoxide
Arsenic sulphide
Arsenic trioxide
Arsine
Calcium arsenate
Dimethylarsinic acid
Lead arsenate
Methanearsonic acid, disodium salt
Methanearsonic acid, monosodium salt
Potassium arsenate
Potassium arsenite
Sodium arsenate
Sodium arsenite
Sodium cacodylate

Asbestos	*2*, 17 (corr. *7*, 319)
	14 (corr. *15*, 341)
	(corr. *17*, 351)
	Suppl. 4, 52

Actinolite
Amosite
Anthophyllite
Chrysotile
Crocidolite
Tremolite
Asiaticoside*

Auramine	*1*, 69 (corr. *7*, 319)
	Suppl. 4, 53

Carpentry and joinery	*25*, 139
	Suppl. 4, 139
Carrageenans (native)	*10*, 181 (corr. *11*, 295)
	31, 79
Catechol	*15*, 155
Chloramben*	
Chlorambucil	*9*, 125
	26, 115
	Suppl. 4, 77
Chloramphenicol	*10*, 85
	Suppl. 4, 79
Chlordane	*20*, 45 (corr. *25*, 391)
	Suppl. 4, 80
Chlordecone (Kepone)	*20*, 67
Chlordimeform	*30*, 61
Chlorinated dibenzodioxins	*15*, 41
	Suppl. 4, 211, 238
Chlormadinone acetate	*6*, 149
	21, 365
	Suppl. 4, 192
Chlorobenzilate	*5*, 75
	30, 73
1-(2-Chloroethyl)-3-cyclohexyl-1-nitrosourea (CCNU)	*26*, 137
	Suppl. 4, 83
Chloroform	*1*, 61
	20, 401
	Suppl. 4, 87
Chloromethyl methyl ether	*4*, 239
	Suppl. 4, 64
4-Chloro-*ortho*-phenylenediamine	*27*, 81
4-Chloro-*meta*-phenylenediamine	*27*, 82
Chloroprene	*19*, 131
	Suppl. 4, 89
Chloropropham	*12*, 55
Chloroquine	*13*, 47
Chlorothalonil	*30*, 319
para-Chloro-*ortho*-toluidine and its hydrochloride	*16*, 277
5-Chloro-*ortho*-toluidine*	
Chlorotrianisene	*21*, 139
Chlorpromazine*	
Cholesterol	*10*, 99
	31, 95
Chromium and chromium compounds	*2*, 100
	23, 205
	Suppl. 4, 91

  Barium chromate
  Basic chromic sulphate
  Calcium chromate
  Chromic acetate
  Chromic chloride
  Chromic oxide
  Chromic phosphate

Dienoestrol	*21*, 161
	Suppl. 4, 183
Diepoxybutane	*11*, 115 (corr. *12*, 271)
Di-(2-ethylhexyl) adipate	*29*, 257
Di-(2-ethylhexyl) phthalate	*29*, 269
1,2-Diethylhydrazine	*4*, 153
Diethylstilboestrol	*6*, 55
	21, 173 (corr. *23*, 417)
	Suppl. 4, 184
Diethylstilboestrol dipropionate	*21*, 175
Diethyl sulphate	*4*, 277
	Suppl. 4, 115
Diglycidyl resorcinol ether	*11*, 125
Dihydrosafrole	*1*, 170
	10, 233
Dihydroxybenzenes	*15*, 155
Dihydroxymethylfuratrizine	*24*, 77
Dimethisterone	*6*, 167
	21, 377
	Suppl. 4, 193
Dimethoate*	
Dimethoxane	*15*, 177
3,3'-Dimethoxybenzidine (*ortho*-Dianisidine)	*4*, 41
	Suppl. 4, 116
para-Dimethylaminoazobenzene	*8*, 125 (corr. *31*, 295)
para-Dimethylaminobenzenediazo sodium sulphonate	*8*, 147
trans-2[(Dimethylamino)methylimino]-5-[2-(5-nitro-2-furyl)vinyl]-1,3,4-oxadiazole	*7*, 147 (corr. *30*, 407)
3,3'-Dimethylbenzidine (*ortho*-Tolidine)	*1*, 87
Dimethylcarbamoyl chloride	*12*, 77
	Suppl. 4, 118
1,1-Dimethylhydrazine	*4*, 137
1,2-Dimethylhydrazine	*4*, 145 (corr. *7*, 320)
Dimethyl sulphate	*4*, 271
	Suppl. 4, 119
Dimethylterephthalate*	
Dinitrosopentamethylenetetramine	*11*, 241
1,4-Dioxane	*11*, 247
	Suppl. 4, 121
2,4'-Diphenyldiamine	*16*, 313
Diphenylthiohydantoin*	
Direct Black 38	*29*, 295
	Suppl. 4, 59
Direct Blue 6	*29*, 311
	Suppl. 4, 59
Direct Brown 95	*29*, 321
	Suppl. 4, 59
Disulfiram	*12*, 85
Dithranol	*13*, 75
Dulcin	*12*, 97

O
Ochratoxin A   *10*, 191
                                                      31, 191
Oestradiol-17β   *6*, 99
                                                      21, 279
                                                      Suppl. 4, 190
Oestradiol 3-benzoate   *21*, 281
Oestradiol dipropionate   *21*, 283
Oestradiol mustard   *9*, 217
Oestradiol-17β-valerate   *21*, 284
Oestriol   *6*, 117
                                                      21, 327
Oestrone   *6*, 123
                                                      21, 343 (corr. *25*, 391)
                                                      Suppl. 4, 191
Oestrone benzoate   *21*, 345
                                                      Suppl. 4, 191
Oil Orange SS   *8*, 165
Orange I   *8*, 173
Orange G   *8*, 181
Oxazepam   *13*, 58
Oxymetholone   *13*, 131
                                                      Suppl. 4, 203
Oxyphenbutazone   *13*, 185

P
Panfuran S (Dihydroxymethylfuratrizine)   *24*, 77
Parasorbic acid   *10*, 199 (corr. *12*, 271)
Parathion   *30*, 153
Patulin   *10*, 205
Penicillic acid   *10*, 211
Pentachlorophenol   *20*, 303
                                                      Suppl. 4, 88, 205
Pentobarbital sodium*
Petasitenine   *31*, 207
Phenacetin   *13*, 141
                                                      24, 135
                                                      Suppl. 4, 47
Phenazopyridine (2,6-Diamino-3-phenylazopyridine) and *8*, 117
    its hydrochloride   *24*, 163 (corr. *29*, 399)
                                                      Suppl. 4, 207
Phenelzine and its sulphate   *24*, 175
                                                      Suppl. 4, 207
Phenicarbazide   *12*, 177
Phenobarbital and its sodium salt   *13*, 157
                                                      Suppl. 4, 208
Phenoxybenzamine and its hydrochloride   *9*, 223
                                                      24, 185
Phenylbutazone   *13*, 183
                                                      Suppl. 4, 212

Propylene oxide	*11*, 191
Propylthiouracil	*7*, 67
	Suppl. 4, 222
The pulp and paper industry	*25*, 157
	Suppl. 4, 144
Pyrazinamide*	
Pyrimethamine	*13*, 233
Pyrrolizidine alkaloids	*10*, 333

Q

Quercetin	*31*, 213
Quinoestradol*	
Quinoestrol*	
para-Quinone	*15*, 255
Quintozene (Pentachloronitrobenzene)	*5*, 211

R

Reserpine	*10*, 217
	24, 211 (corr. *26*, 387)
	(corr. *30*, 407)
	Suppl. 4, 222
Resorcinol	*15*, 155
Retrorsine	*10*, 303
Rhodamine B	*16*, 221
Rhodamine 6G	*16*, 233
Riddelliine	*10*, 313
Rifampicin	*24*, 243
Rotenone*	
The rubber industry	*28* (corr. *30*, 407)
	Suppl. 4, 144

S

Saccharated iron oxide	*2*, 161
Saccharin	*22*, 111 (corr. *25*, 391)
	Suppl. 4, 224
Safrole	*1*, 169
	10, 231
Scarlet red	*8*, 217
Selenium and selenium compounds	*9*, 245 (corr. *12*, 271)
	(corr. *30*, 407)
Semicarbazide hydrochloride	*12*, 209 (corr. *16*, 387)
Seneciphylline	*10*, 319
Senkirkine	*10*, 327
	31, 231
Simazine*	
Sodium cyclamate	*22*, 56 (corr. *25*, 391)
	Suppl. 4, 97
Sodium diethyldithiocarbamate	*12*, 217
Sodium equilin sulphate	*21*, 148

Sodium oestrone sulphate   *21*, 147
Sodium saccharin   *22*, 113 (corr. *25*, 391)
                                                   Suppl. 4, 224
Soot, tars and minerals oils   *3*, 22
                                                   Suppl. 4, 227
Spironolactone   *24*, 259
                                                   Suppl. 4, 229
Sterigmatocystin   *1*, 175
                                                   10, 245
Streptozotocin   *4*, 221
                                                   17, 337
Styrene   *19*, 231
                                                   Suppl. 4, 229
Styrene-acrylonitrile copolymers   *19*, 97
Styrene-butadiene copolymers   *19*, 252
Styrene oxide   *11*, 201
                                                   19, 275
                                                   Suppl. 4, 229
Succinic anhydride   *15*, 265
Sudan I   *8*, 225
Sudan II   *8*, 233
Sudan III   *8*, 241
Sudan brown RR   *8*, 249
Sudan red 7B   *8*, 253
Sulfafurazole (Sulphisoxazole)   *24*, 275
                                                   Suppl. 4, 233
Sulfallate   *30*, 283
Sulfamethoxazole   *24*, 285
                                                   Suppl. 4, 234
Sulphamethazine*
Sunset yellow FCF   *8*, 257
Symphytine   *31*, 239

T
2,4,5-T and esters   *15*, 273
                                                   Suppl. 4, 211, 235
Tannic acid   *10*, 253 (corr. *16*, 387)
Tannins   *10*, 254
Terephthalic acid*
Terpene polychlorinates (Strobane^R)   *5*, 219
Testosterone   *6*, 209
                                                   21, 519
Testosterone oenanthate   *21*, 521
Testosterone propionate   *21*, 522
2,2',5,5'-Tetrachlorobenzidine   *27*, 141
Tetrachlorodibenzo-*para*-dioxin (TCDD)   *15*, 41
                                                   Suppl. 4, 211, 238
1,1,2,2-Tetrachloroethane   *20*, 477
Tetrachloroethylene   *20*, 491
                                                   Suppl. 4, 243
Tetrachlorvinphos   *30*, 197

www.ingramcontent.com/pod-product-compliance
Lightning Source LLC
Chambersburg PA
CBHW081804200326
41597CB00023B/4139